ETHICS IN
HEALTH SERVICES
MANAGEMENT

ETHICS IN HEALTH SERVICES MANAGEMENT

FIFTH EDITION

by

KURT DARR, J.D., SC.D., FACHE
THE GEORGE WASHINGTON UNIVERSITY
WASHINGTON, D.C.

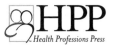

Baltimore • London • Sydney

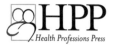

Health Professions Press, Inc.
Post Office Box 10624
Baltimore, Maryland 21285-0624

www.healthpropress.com

Cover design by Erin Geoghegan.
Typeset by Blue Heron Typesetting.

Manufactured in the United States of America by Versa Press, East Peoria, Illinois.

Certain case studies in this book are based on well-known news accounts and use real names and details as reported in the media. Others are based on real stories, but names and identifying details have been changed to protect identities. Still other case studies are composite or fictional accounts that do not represent the lives or experiences of specific individuals, and no implications should be inferred.

Library of Congress Cataloging-in-Publication Data

Darr, Kurt.
   Ethics in health services management / by Kurt Darr. — 5th ed.
     p. ; cm.
   Includes bibliographical references and index.
   ISBN 978-1-932529-68-5 (pbk.)
   1. Health services administration—Moral and ethical aspects.
2. Medical ethics. I. Title.
   [DNLM: 1. Health Services Administration—ethics—Case Reports.
2. Ethics, Medical—Case Reports. W 84.1]
   RA394.D35 2011
   174'.2—dc23   2011017931

British Library Cataloguing in Publication data are available from the British Library.

CONTENTS

To Anne

ABOUT THE AUTHOR

Kurt Darr, J.D., Sc.D., FACHE, is Professor of Hospital Administration in the Department of Health Services Management and Leadership at The George Washington University. He holds the Doctor of Science from The Johns Hopkins University and a Master of Hospital Administration and the Juris Doctor from the University of Minnesota.

Professor Darr completed his administrative residency at Rochester (Minnesota) Methodist Hospital and subsequently worked as an administrative associate at Mayo Clinic. After being commissioned in the U.S. Navy, he served in administrative and educational assignments at St. Albans Naval Hospital and Bethesda Naval Hospital. He completed post-doctoral fellowships with the Department of Health and Human Services, the World Health Organization, and the Accrediting Commission on Education for Health Services Administration.

Dr. Darr is a fellow of the American College of Healthcare Executives and a member of the District of Columbia and Minnesota Bars. He is a mediator for the Superior Court of the District of Columbia. He is a commissioner on the Accreditation Council of the Commission on Accreditation of Healthcare Management Education.

Professor Darr educates in the areas of health services ethics, management theory, hospital organization and management, quality improvement, and application of the Deming method in health services delivery. In addition, he is a consultant and educator to hospital ethics committees. Professor Darr has authored, co-authored, and edited books used in health services management education programs and numerous articles on various health services topics.

PREFACE

The fifth edition of *Ethics in Health Services Management* continues the intention of the first four. It seeks to help students of health services management and nascent and experienced managers of health services organizations hone their skills in applied managerial and biomedical ethics. Suggesting a methodology to identify and solve ethical problems and positing tools to guide ethical decision making should make the reader a more effective problem solver. *Brevity* and *organization* continue as watchwords.

Numerous cases and vignettes are included. This edition adds seven new cases, including attention to public health. Sources for the cases and vignettes include the author's personal experience, information from colleagues, and reports in the media and professional literature. Some are fully analyzed for the reader's scrutiny and critique. Others invite the reader's dissection and provide an opportunity to identify the ethical issues and consider their solution. All offer lessons in normative and applied ethics.

Rarely are ready answers available in either managerial or ethical problem solving. As in medicine, the "cookbook" approach is inadequate; it fails to account for nuances of fact, setting, and personalities in each situation. Were ready answers available, the challenge of ethical problems and the satisfaction of solving them would be absent from a manager's professional life.

Virtue ethics is given greater attention in this edition. The principles of respect for persons, beneficence, nonmalfeasance, and justice continue as the focus for managers, their duties, and their relationships with patients, staff, and profession. The virtues supplement the principles and offer managers specific attributes and qualities that should be intrinsic to the virtuous manager.

One's personal ethic is key. Plato said that the unexamined life is not worth living; his pupil, Aristotle, a bit snidely perhaps, added that the unplanned life is not worth examining. These aphorisms are useful guides to us as managers. We cannot be effective as managers (or, likely, as human beings) without having a lodestar by which to navigate our personal and professional lives. The moral certainty of a well-developed personal ethic is an essential element of personal and professional success. It is hoped that the fifth edition will benefit those examining or reconsidering their personal ethic.

This reorganized, updated, and enhanced fifth edition has 14 chapters in five sections. Section I sets the framework for identifying and solving ethical problems. It includes discussion of the moral philosophies and derivative principles, as supplemented by the virtues, and a methodology for solving ethical problems. Section II identifies the importance of the organizational philosophy—its values, as complemented by the personal ethic of managers and supported by professional codes. In addition, organizational responses to ethical issues are identified. The importance of culture is emphasized. Section III considers administrative ethical issues. Included are conflicts of interest and the organization's ethical obligations to patients, staff, and community, as led by managers whose moral agency makes them the organization's conscience. The ethical dimensions of human immunodeficiency virus/acquired immunodeficiency syndrome (HIV/AIDS) are found in Chapters 7 and 8 and have been supplemented by consideration of hepatitis B and hepatitis C.

Section IV addresses major biomedical ethical issues, including consent, dying and death, and patient autonomy as expressed through the paradigm of physician-assisted suicide. Their effects on managerial decision making and the health services organization are emphasized. Section V considers ethical issues relating to marketing and managed care, resource allocation, and the social responsibility of health services organizations. Simultaneously, these areas are new, emerging, and continuing. Resource allocation and social responsibility reflect the greater organizational and societal concern directed toward them. Appendixes include valuable resource material; a detailed index makes the book user friendly and enhances its value as a reference and use in the classroom.

The genesis of this book lies 30 years in the past. Each edition was written in an environment that presented seemingly insurmountable challenges to those who manage what are among the most important and complex organizations in American society. As managers must do more with less, compete aggressively but fairly, meet an increasingly oppressive regulatory and payment environment, and provide a broader range of services, it is hoped that this fifth edition will provide a measure of help in their work. If so, I will have accomplished the goal that was first set three decades ago.

ACKNOWLEDGMENTS

This book was conceived as a vehicle to assist health services managers to identify and solve the numerous and complex ethical issues they confront. This goal came to fruition with publication of the first edition in 1987. Publication of the second edition only four years later was a response to the rapid pace of change in health services management. Subsequent editions have built on the strengths of their predecessors. Each has been complemented with new ethical concerns, cases, and insights.

Writing and publishing five editions of a book require help from many individuals and organizations. Those instrumental in preparing the first four editions have my continuing thanks. My late friend and colleague, Robert G. Shouldice, was helpful in preparing the managed care section in the first two editions. I hope that he is at peace. Robert Burke, Chair of the Department of Health Services Management and Leadership, and Lynn Goldman, Dean of the School of Public Health and Health Services, both at The George Washington University, were supportive as they have striven to create an environment that stresses research and writing. A special thanks is owed Donald Lehman, formerly Executive Vice President for Academic Affairs, and Steven Knapp, President of The George Washington University, for approving the sabbatical that enabled me to prepare the manuscript for the fifth edition.

Research and other assistance for the fifth edition were provided by Carey Anne Lafferty, who worked industriously and cheerfully, often under daunting time constraints. She has earned my sincere appreciation and has my best wishes for every future success.

At Health Professions Press, Mary Magnus, Director of Publications and patient taskmistress, was consistently encouraging and helpful. She has my gratitude. Cecilia González, Production Manager, effectively managed the editorial process. I thank her for her help.

INTRODUCTION

Two themes underlie *Ethics in Health Services Management*: the autonomy, primacy, and protection of the patient* and the health services manager as moral agent and leader of the health services organization.

This book is intended to assist health services managers develop a personal ethic and gain an understanding of administrative and biomedical ethical issues, and it suggests a methodology for solving the problems that these issues raise. The emphasis is on normative ethics (*what should be done*). Some attention is paid to descriptive ethics (*what is actually done*) and metaethics (*study of ethical systems*) because they assist in understanding normative ethics. The theories of ethical relativism and ethical nihilism are not considered. Ethical relativism holds that there are no absolutes and that all answers to ethical questions are morally correct, depending on circumstances and culture. Nihilists consider no choice correct. Neither theory helps managers meet the needs of patients, staff, and organizations nor aids them in resolving ethical problems. Furthermore, ethical relativism and nihilism do not help the manager formulate and reconsider a personal ethic.

For the health services manager, a personal ethic is a moral framework for relationships with patients, staff members, organization, and community. In these relationships, the manager morally affects and is morally affected by what is done or not done. This places special emphasis on misfeasance, malfeasance, and nonfeasance. Management's decisions are not value-free; in a moral sense, they affect the organization's environment and are touched by them.

---

*To ease reading, *patient* is used to describe anyone served by a health services organization.

The patient relies on the health services organization and its staff to perform services unique in society. Managers' responsibilities to patients take precedence over their fiduciary duty to their organizations. Protecting the patient is more than providing safe surroundings and competent staff. It is more than licensure, accreditation, and compliance. It is more than a surplus at the end of the fiscal year. The manager is the organization's conscience. This responsibility is exemplified by the organization's willingness, prompted and led by management, to recognize the inherent human dignity of the patient and do so through effective programs that make it a reality. It means using effective consent forms and procedures and ascertaining that all who have contact with patients are qualified and work for the patients' good. It means not considering patients as adversaries and not deserting them should something go wrong in the care process. An organization that has done its best can face the consequences of an error honestly, mitigate the injury, and find a fair solution. The loop is closed when management determines the cause of the problem, prevents or minimizes the probability of its recurrence, and strives to improve quality continuously. At times, justice requires a decision process that prospectively includes the criteria of cost–benefit analysis and utilitarianism (*the greatest good for the greatest number*). Even here, the organization recognizes the dignity and worth of people as yet unserved or only partially served.

How does the health services organization develop and implement a "just" policy? How does it strive to treat patients as equals and work to serve their interests? Implementation of a just policy begins with the organizational philosophy,* which should explicitly state the nature of the relationship between patient and organization. This philosophy should reflect the view that the patient is autonomous and is entitled to be treated with respect and dignity. In a sense, there is a contract—an implicit but verifiable understanding between patient and provider, grounded in mutual trust and confidence. It recognizes that whenever possible, patients retain control of their lives.

Once enunciated, the organization's philosophy must be reflected in all derivative mission and vision statements, policies, procedures, and rules, but especially in relationships with patients and community. If not operationalized, the organization and its managers will be judged as cynical about themselves and those they serve. This cynicism is easily recognized by staff and, in turn, will be reflected in staff's relationship with patients.

Organizational philosophy is used as a generic concept to include values, core values, shared values, ministry, healing ministry, philosophy, or similar terms used to convey the philosophical framework in which services are delivered.

Staff may not succumb to the negative implications of this inconsistency, but it will be an underlying, festering incongruity, nonetheless.

A major participant in developing and maintaining the appropriate relationship with patients is the physician,* necessarily a primary actor. Physicians must respect decisions made by a patient or an appropriate proxy. The roles of physician and organization are complementary, but the organization remains morally (ethically) accountable for the physician's activities performed in the organization.

CONCERN ABOUT ETHICS

Ethics is a word used frequently in healthcare. Questions are asked daily about making the ethically right choice. Seemingly straightforward and value-free management decisions have ethical implications for patients, staff, organization, community, and society. Many decisions that cause ethical dilemmas are the result of the continuing revolution in biology and technology. Fiscal constraints, competition, and new means of delivering services exacerbate existing ethical problems and raise new ones. Beyond these causes is an enhanced level of awareness resulting from the research and writing of ethicists and the work of government commissions on experimentation and bioethics.

Ethical *dilemmas* occur when decision makers are drawn in two directions by competing courses of action that are based on differing moral frameworks, varying or inconsistent elements of the organizational philosophy, conflicting duties or moral principles, or an ill-defined sense of right and wrong. For example, staff members may be asked to follow rules they consider inappropriate or unjust, or two moral principles may conflict with each other. A nurse's duty to preserve life clashes with the patient's wishes not to be kept alive artificially. Another source of ethical dilemmas is the existence of two compelling, ethically defensible positions on an issue, such as the possible conception of a genetically defective infant. Required genetic screening and counseling for people at risk conflict with individual autonomy for those who wish not to know. Conclusions vary when decision makers put different weight on various principles, such as personal liberty or privacy competing with societal interests and economic considerations. Politics, laws, and regulations also affect ethical decisions.

---

*To ease reading, *physician* includes medical doctors and other practitioners of the medical and healing arts licensed to independently treat patients (e.g., dentists, nurse midwives, clinical psychologists, podiatrists, chiropractors). Such persons are often known as *licensed independent practitioners (LIPs)*.

Reasonable persons could differ as to the ethically "right" result on some issues. With few exceptions, one answer emerges as morally superior. Ethical problems are often characterized as *dilemmas* because that emphasizes the difficulty of finding the morally best solution. Solving ethical problems may be demanding, but few are properly labeled dilemmas.

Are laws and regulations the problem or the solution? Some perceive that ethical problems arise because laws or regulations fail to guide actions. Others perceive that laws force organizations and managers to act in ways that contravene their moral frameworks. Depending on the issue and facts, both views have merit. Even when there are external rules, decision makers in organizations must decide when the rules apply, how they are interpreted, and whether to obey them. In fact, by designating and clarifying rules, there is less middle ground, the ethical problems are starker, and solving them may be more difficult. Some people may ignore the rules and apply a personal ethic. Others will apply rules dogmatically, choosing not to think about the underlying philosophy or resulting ethical issues. Conversely, some ethical problems occur because no external rules assist decision makers. For others, there is no consensus as to what the rules should be. A further complication is that some ethical problems have developed more quickly than the ability of the health services field or society to solve them.

ETHICS DEFINED

Defining ethics is difficult because it can have several meanings. For philosophers, ethics is the formal study of morality. Sociologists see ethics as the mores, customs, and behavior of a culture. For physicians, ethics means meeting the expectations of profession and society and interacting with patients in certain ways. Health services managers should consider ethics a special charge and a responsibility to patients, staff, and organization, to themselves and profession, and, ultimately but less directly, to society. Managers are confronted with the normative question "What ought I to do?"

Distinctions often blur, but ethical problems may be divided into biomedical and administrative. Biomedical ethical problems involve individual patients or groups of patients in their relationships with one another or with providers and organizations. Depending on the issue, the manager is involved less directly in biomedical ethical problems. Beyond biomedical ethical problems, some of which become dilemmas that receive great media attention, is the need to identify and solve management problems with ethical dimensions. Administrative ethical problems involve manager and profession, organization, patients, and society. Administrative ethical issues less frequently involve competing, ethically defensible choices. Solving these problems is usually a matter of recognition and resolve—doing what is morally right.

SOURCES OF LAW

The relationship between law and ethics (morality) is dynamic. Thus, it is useful to begin a book about ethics by briefly reviewing development of law. Organized societies have a code or system of rules that distinguishes acceptable behavior from unacceptable behavior and prescribes penalties for transgressors. *Law* may be defined as a system of principles and rules of human conduct recognized or prescribed by an authority. This definition includes criminal and civil law. In contrast, ethics is the study of standards of moral judgment and conduct. For individuals this is the personal ethic. For a profession it is the guiding system or code of ethics.

The moral underpinnings in criminal law are especially clear in reflecting society's sense of right and wrong, or its ethics (morality). In a democratic society criminal law derives from and reflects the views of justice and fairness held by the majority. This is less true in civil law, which governs relations among individuals and includes torts and contracts. The common law tradition of the United States means that a great deal of law is based on the precedents established by court decisions. Civil law emphasizes predictability, stability, and property rights.

If laws in a democracy reflect the moral values of the majority, substantial minorities may hold contrary views. They may consider a law or government action so unjust that they risk the penalties of breaking it. A historical example is the 18th Amendment to the U.S. Constitution. Adopted in 1919, it prohibited the manufacture, sale, or transportation of intoxicating liquors. Violation was widespread until the amendment's repeal in 1933. Contemporary examples are draft resistance during the Vietnam War, common disregard of roadway speed limits, and widespread use of marijuana.

Some cultures regarded the law as a gift from the gods. Plato's *Republic* postulated the ideal state as one based on rational order and ruled by philosopher-kings. Plato considered written law a regrettable oversimplification that could not take into account the differences and conditions in parties and situations involved in legal disputes. He believed that it was best to have a philosopher apply an unwritten law. His own experience proved this theory impossible, and he accepted a written law administered without regard to the circumstances of the individuals involved.[1] This concept of a rule of law, not of men, became established in Anglo-American legal tradition. Because absurd results can occur when civil law is applied without considering the situations of the parties, the concept of unwritten law preferred by Plato was continued, but in a limited manner. Parallel court systems in law and in equity developed at common law; civil actions could be brought in either. Some states have courts of equity that hear cases in which fairness is the primary concern; most, however, have merged law and equity into one court system.

Because of the link between societal views of right and wrong and the law, morality is reflected in all types of law, whether formal or nonformal. A leading jurisprudent, Edgar Bodenheimer,[2] identified formal sources of law as constitutions, statutes, executive orders, administrative regulations, ordinances, charters and bylaws of autonomous or semiautonomous bodies, treaties, and judicial precedents. Nonformal sources of law have not received an authoritative, or at least articulated, formulation and embodiment in a formalized legal document. Sources of nonformal law include standards of justice, principles of reason and consideration of the nature of things (*natura rerum*), equity for individuals, public policies, moral convictions, social trends, and customary law.

Bodenheimer's inclusion of the charters and bylaws of autonomous and semiautonomous bodies in the list of formal sources of law has significance for health services management. Such documents include the articles of incorporation and bylaws of the organization. General references to the organizational philosophy and mission may be included in both, but are usually expanded in other documents. These are key. Medical staff bylaws and rules and regulations are formal sources of law for the organization. They should reflect the organizational philosophy and mission and must be consistent with them.

In addition to their importance in reflecting the philosophy and mission, the corporate charter and its bylaws are an organization's basic laws. Persons affected by the organization—staff members, physicians, patients—look to them for guidance as derivative policies, procedures, and rules. Formal sources of law such as the medical staff bylaws detail the rights and obligations of physicians. Should a legal controversy develop, courts and other reviewing bodies are guided by these documents.

Bodenheimer's definition of formal law is broad enough to include professional codes of ethics. A code can be effectively implemented only when interpreted and enforced. Such activities guide a code's application and related decision making, give it dynamism and life, and ensure the important qualities of consistency and predictability.

RELATIONSHIP BETWEEN ETHICS AND LAW

The relationship between law and ethics might seem to be one-to-one: anything lawful is ethical and vice versa. This is not necessarily true. Most important is that the law states the minimum standard of morality established by society to guide interactions among individuals, and between them and government. Law concentrates on prohibitions—the "thou shalt nots." It contains few positive duties.

For professions, ethics is much more than obeying the law. Professions expect members to comply with the law, but they add to this standard and include positive duties to patients, society, and one another. The result is that a professional code of ethics may require an action that the law does not. For the professional, then, performing (or not performing) a particular activity may be legal but unethical.

Positive duties are not exclusive to professions. Individuals may hold themselves to a standard obligating them to aid others or work on their behalf. In many respects this positive duty means practicing the Golden Rule: "Do unto others as you would have them do unto you." This duty is far more demanding than merely refraining from interfering with someone or enacting a law that protects one person from another.

As noted previously, it is paradoxical that law both prevents and causes ethical problems. Choices must be made regardless of whether there is a public law. Absent public law, managers rely on the formal law of the organization, such as statements of the organizational philosophy (its ethic/values) and mission. Also important in guiding decision making is the informal law present in the manager's personal ethic. Public law may not be determinative in solving a problem. Even when it is clear, ethical problems may remain. An example is the U.S. Supreme Court decision that a woman has an unfettered constitutional right to an abortion during the first trimester of pregnancy. The controversy over the morality (ethics) of abortion continues.

Statutes, court decisions, and codes of ethics are formal sources of law, but the latter affect only members of an identified group, usually one of voluntary association. Belonging to an association may not be completely voluntary because colleagues have expectations and demands, employers may consider memberships important in judging qualifications, and better-informed consumers ask questions and express views about an individual's professional memberships. At root, however, participating in professional groups is voluntary.

Licensure is ubiquitous for clinical personnel. Of health services managers, only nursing facility managers must be licensed. Including ethical standards in licensing statutes gives them the force of law. This does not relieve the professional association of the need to regulate members' behavior by adopting more stringent guidelines. Groups whose codes are not reflected in statutes or regulations bear a heavier burden. Their codes are only private statements of acceptable behavior; the groups themselves must do the monitoring. The obligation to protect and serve society is the hallmark of a profession and greatly heightens its need to monitor members.

In disciplinary proceedings pursuant to a licensing statute, the actions of public regulatory bodies are distinct from those of private groups. Expulsion from the professional group usually occurs only after a separate, private hearing and review process. If a license is necessary for membership in a professional group, its loss means automatic expulsion.

The relationship between law and ethics is shown in Figure 1, a model developed by Henderson. It shows a succession of events leading to corporate decisions being scrutinized by the public and a determination that they are legal and/or ethical. This judgment is necessarily after the fact, despite management's efforts to predict consequences of a decision. The model suggests that for many corporate actions it cannot be known with certainty whether those who finally judge the decision will consider it legal (as determined by law enforcement officials) or ethical (as determined by the profession or the general public). This adds a high degree of uncertainty to decision making inside and outside health services. It is usually easier to predict that an action will be seen as legal than to predict whether it will be perceived to be ethical.

Figure 2 is a matrix developed by Henderson. It shows the combinations of legal, illegal, ethical, and unethical. In Quadrant I, managers act legally and ethically.

Quadrant II includes decisions that are ethical but illegal. The American College of Healthcare Executives' Code of Ethics requires affiliates to comply with all laws and regulations. This suggests the virtual impossibility that health services managers can justify as ethical an illegal act. There are exceptions, however. For example, it is morally justifiable to break the law to prevent greater harm or injury. Someone who engages

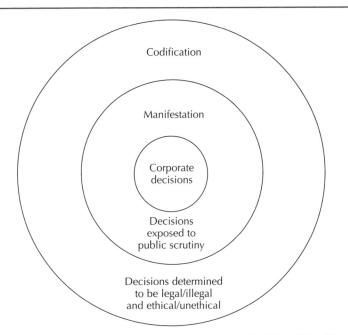

Figure 1. The relationship between law and ethics. (Reprinted from "The Ethical Side of Enterprise" by V.E. Henderson, *MIT Sloan Management Review, 23,* 1982, pp. 37–43, by permission of the publisher. Copyright © 1982 by Massachusetts Institute of Technology. All rights reserved.)

in civil disobedience or breaks other laws must be prepared to suffer the penalties imposed.

Quadrant III includes decisions that are unethical but legal. It incorporates the concept that ethical standards, especially those of a profession, hold the member to a higher standard than does the law. Examples include failing to take reasonable steps to protect the patient from incompetent medical care and preventing manager self-aggrandizement at the expense of patients.

Quadrant IV includes activities that are illegal and unethical. Embezzlement falls into this quadrant, as does ignoring local fire safety requirements or filing false Medicare or Medicaid reports.

It is important to stress the dynamic between law and ethics: each affects and is affected by the other. Professional codes and conduct reflect society's perceptions of a profession as well as that profession's self-image. To the extent that law codifies society's need to protect itself and regulate conduct, licensure laws further clarify what is expected of a profession. Morality reflected in the law evolves but often lags behind private morality

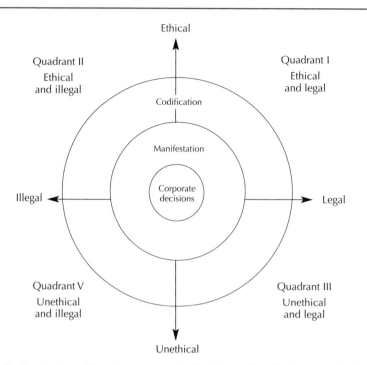

Figure 2.   A matrix of possible outcomes concerning the ethics and legality of corporate decisions. (Reprinted from "The Ethical Side of Enterprise" by V.E. Henderson, *MIT Sloan Management Review,* 23, 1982, pp. 37–43, by permission of the publisher. Copyright © 1982 by Massachusetts Institute of Technology. All rights reserved.)

and ethics. In this regard, the law leads some subsets of society but follows others.

CONCLUSION

Gandhi said, "Noncooperation with evil is as much a duty as cooperation with good." Edmund Burke said, "The only thing necessary for the triumph of evil is for good men to do nothing." Both philosophies are germane to health services, especially to its managers. Understanding and meeting their ethical obligations are essential.

Contemporary demands on health services organizations and managers may seem inconsistent with the often-idealized statements found in codes of ethics. Managers must recognize their responsibility, however, and strive to transform the ideal into reality. Managers must see themselves as others see them: moral agents with a critical role in the organization and its efforts to serve, protect, and further the interests of patient and community.

There is ample evidence of ethical and legal problems in the world of business. Despite occurring less often and having less impact on the economy and society, there have been enough ethical and legal misadventures in the health services management field to know that it faces important challenges. A number of these misadventures are described in the book. There is much of concern beyond the moral lapses and illegality, however. What about a manager's relationships with persons served by the organization or its staff? Managing health services organizations will always be among the most demanding work in society. No one said it would be easy; few in the field expect kudos for their work. But we raise the pride of profession and self and meet our responsibilities when we act as moral agents whose primary duty is to protect patients' interests and further their care. This is the continuing challenge of health services management.

NOTES

1. A useful discussion of Plato's political philosophy is found in Jeremy Waldron. (1995). What Plato would allow. In Ian Shapiro & Judith Wagner DeCew (Eds.), *Theory and practice: Nomos XXXVII* (pp. 138–178). New York: New York University Press.
2. Edgar Bodenheimer. (1974). *Jurisprudence: The philosophy and method of the law* (p. 6). Cambridge, MA: Harvard University Press.

Identifying and Solving Ethical Problems

Chapters 1 and 2 contain information basic to identifying, understanding, analyzing, and solving administrative and biomedical ethical problems. A generic background and methodology are developed and applied to the actual case of an impaired infant, Baby Boy Doe. The nature of ethical problems evolves and new types appear, but the framework and process described here have continued usefulness for managers.

Chapter 1 identifies and discusses moral philosophies and derivative principles—a background essential to analyzing and solving administrative and biomedical ethical problems. Understanding the philosophies and derivative principles, supplemented by virtue ethics, is key to managers who are developing and reconsidering a vibrant and robust personal ethic.

The theory and use of a generic problem-solving method are part of management education. The methodology detailed in Chapter 2 builds on that generic skill and enables managers to more readily identify, analyze, and resolve ethical problems. Managers should read the discussion of the moral philosophies and derivative principles, as supplemented by virtue ethics, in the context of their own problem-solving education and experience, as well as their personal ethic.

Solving administrative ethics cannot be exclusive to managers, nor can solving biomedical ethical problems be exclusive to clinicians. Meeting an organization's ethical imperative is vital and inextricably linked to successfully meeting its mission and objectives. Managers who act only as technocrats ignore their role as moral agents. Moral agency requires each of us to be morally accountable for nonfeasance, misfeasance, and malfeasance. Managers must participate fully in solving all types of ethical problems. This task is too important to be left to others.

CHAPTER 1

CONSIDERING MORAL PHILOSOPHIES AND PRINCIPLES

W hat sources guide us in ethical decision making? How do they help us identify and act on the morally correct choice? Philosophers, theologians, and others grapple with such questions. The clearest tradition of ethics in Western medicine dates from the ancient Greeks. Throughout the 20th century and into the 21st century, managers and nurses have formally sought to clarify, establish, and, sometimes, enforce ethical standards. Their codes and activities incorporate philosophies about the ethical relationships of providers to one another, to patients, and to society. For managers, the appropriate relationship with the organizations that employ them is an added dimension of their codes.

A natural starting point for discussing ethics and understanding how to resolve ethical problems is to review the moral philosophies that have had a major influence on Western European thought and values. Among the most prominent of these philosophies are utilitarian teleology; Kantian deontology; natural law as formulated by St. Thomas Aquinas; and the work of the 20th-century American philosopher John Rawls. The latter part of the 20th century saw renewed interest in casuistry and virtue ethics. Its emphasis on the individual makes virtue ethics especially helpful in guiding action for managers. In addition, the ethics of care is considered briefly.

Principles derived from these moral philosophies provide the framework or moral (ethical) underpinnings for delivery of health services by organizations. These principles will assist managers (and health services caregivers) in honing a personal ethic. The derivative operative principles are respect for persons, beneficence, nonmaleficence, and justice. Virtue ethics stands on its own as a moral philosophy; also, it helps supplement the principles when they lack rigor in analyzing or solving ethical problems.

The following case about Baby Boy Doe is true. State and federal law would prevent it today. Its simplicity and starkness make it a useful paradigm against which to apply the moral philosophies and derivative principles discussed in this chapter.

Baby Boy Doe

In 1970, a male infant born at a major East Coast medical center was diagnosed with mental retardation and duodenal atresia (the absence of a connection between the stomach and intestine). Surgeons determined that although the baby was very small, the atresia was operable, with a high probability of success. The surgery would not alter the baby's mental retardation, but would permit him to take nourishment by mouth.

The baby's parents decided to forego the surgery—something they had the legal right to do—and over the course of the following 2 weeks, the infant was left to die from dehydration and starvation. No basic determination of the extent of mental impairment had been made, nor could it have been, at the time the infant died. Neither hospital personnel nor state family and social services sought to aid him.

This case sends a shudder through most people. Feelings or emotions, however, are insufficient. If managers are to be effective in addressing and solving—or, preferably, preventing—such problems, they must identify and understand the issues involved, know the roles of staff and organization, and apply guidelines for ethical decision making. Following a discussion of moral philosophies and ethical principles, the case of Baby Boy Doe is analyzed.

MORAL PHILOSOPHIES

Utilitarianism

Utilitarians are consequentialists: They evaluate an action in terms of its effect rather than the action's intrinsic attributes. Synonymous with utilitarians are teleologists (from the Greek *telos*, meaning end or goal). Utilitarianism has historical connections to hedonism (Epicureanism), which measured morality by the amount of pleasure obtained from an act or a rule as to how to act—greater pleasure was equated with greater morality. This theory was refined by two 19th-century English philosophers, Jeremy Bentham and John Stuart Mill. Mill's elaboration of utilitarianism was the most complete. Unlike Bentham, Mill sought to distinguish pleasures (the good) on qualitative grounds. Questions about the superiority of certain pleasures, such as listening to a piano concerto, were to be answered by consulting a person of sensitivity and broad experience, even though requiring such judgments diminished the objectivity of utilitarianism. Mill stressed individual freedom. In *On Liberty*, he noted that freedom is requisite to producing happiness and that this makes it unacceptable for the rights of any group or individual to be infringed in significant ways.

In determining the morally correct choice, utilitarians ignore the means of achieving an end and judge the results of an action by comparing the good produced by a particular action to the good produced by alternatives or the amount of evil avoided. Modified utility theory is the basis for the cost–benefit analysis commonly used by economists and managers. "The greatest good for the greatest number" and "the end justifies the means" are statements attributable to utilitarians. However, these statements are only crude gauges of utilitarianism, inappropriately applied without qualification.

Utilitarianism is divided into *act utility* and *rule utility*. Both measure consequences, and the action that brings into being the most good (understood in a nonmoral sense) is deemed the morally correct choice.

Act utilitarians judge each action independently, without reference to preestablished guidelines (rules). They measure the amount of good, or (nonmoral) value brought into being, and the amount of evil, or (nonmoral) disvalue avoided by acting on a particular choice. Each person affected is counted equally, which seems to assign a strong sense of objectivity to this moral philosophy. Because it is episodic and capricious, act utilitarianism is incompatible with developing and deriving the ethical principles needed for a personal ethic, organizations' philosophies, and codes of ethics. Therefore, it receives no further attention.

Rule utilitarians are also concerned only with consequences, but they have prospectively considered various actions and the amount of good or evil brought into being by each. These assessments are used to develop rules (guidelines) for action, because it has been determined that, overall, certain rules produce the most good and result in the least evil or "ungood." Therefore, these rules determine the morally correct choice. The rules are followed for all similar situations, even if they sometimes do not produce the best results. The rule directs selection of the morally correct choice. Rule utilitarianism assists in developing moral principles for health services management. Following Mill, however, it must be stressed that the underlying context and requirement is that liberty be maximized for all.

Deontology

Deontologists adhere to a formalist moral philosophy (in Greek, *deon* means duty). The foremost proponent of deontology was Immanuel Kant, an 18th-century German philosopher. Kant's basic precept was that relations with others must be based on duty. An action is moral if it arises solely from "good will," not from other motives. According to Kant, good will is that which is good without qualification. Unlike utilitarians, deontologists view the end as unimportant, because, in Kant's view, persons have duties to one another as moral agents, duties that take precedence over the consequences of actions. Kantians hold that certain absolute duties are always in force. Among the most important is respect, or the Golden Rule ("Do unto others as you would have them do unto you"). Kant argued that all persons have this duty; respect toward others must always be paid.

Actions that are to be taken under the auspices of this duty must first be tested in a special way, a test Kant termed the *categorical imperative*. The categorical imperative requires that actions under consideration be universalized. In other words, if a principle of action is thought to be appropriate, a determination is made as to whether it can be consistently applied to all persons in all places at all times. There are no exceptions, nor can allowances be made for special circumstances. If the action under consideration meets the test of universality, it is accepted as a duty. The action fails the test if it is contradictory to the overriding principle that all persons must be treated as moral equals and, therefore, are entitled to respect. Truth telling is a prominent example of a duty that meets the categorical imperative. Because the categorical imperative tests the results (ends) of actions, Kantian deontology must be considered teleological (ends-based).

For the Kantian deontologist, it is logically inconsistent to argue that terminally ill persons should be euthanized, because this amounts to the self-contradictory conclusion that life can be improved by ending it. Similarly, caregivers should not lie to patients to improve the efficiency of healthcare delivery; such a policy fails the test of the categorical imperative because it treats patients as means to an end—efficiency—rather than as moral equals. The Golden Rule is the best summary of Kant's philosophy. Having met the test of the categorical imperative, Kantian deontology does not consider results or consequences. This does not mean that managers must ignore consequences, but that the consequences of an action are neither included nor weighed in ethical decision making using Kantian deontology.

Natural Law

Mill defined morally right actions by the happiness or nonmoral value produced. Kant rejected all ethical theories based on desire or inclination. Unlike Mill and Kant, natural law theorists contend that ethics must be based on concern for human good. They also contend that good cannot be defined simply in terms of subjective inclinations. Rather, there is a good for human beings that is objectively desirable, although not reducible to desire.[1] Natural law holds that divine law has inscribed certain potentialities in all things, which constitute the good of those things. In this sense, the theory is teleological because it is concerned with ends. Natural law is based on Aristotelian thought as interpreted and synthesized with Christian dogma by St. Thomas Aquinas (1225–1274).[2]

The potentiality of human beings is based on a uniquely human trait, the ability to reason. Natural law bases ethics on the premise that human beings will do what is rational, and that this rationality will cause them to tend to do good and avoid evil. Natural law presumes a natural order in relationships and a predisposition by rational individuals to do or to refrain from doing certain things. Our capability for rational thought enables us to discover what we should do. In that effort, we are guided by a partial notion of God's divine plan that is linked to our capacity for rational thought. Because natural law guides what rational human beings do, it serves as a basis for positive law, some of which is reflected in statutes. Our natural inclination directs us to preserve our lives and to do such rational things as avoid danger, act in self-defense, and seek medical attention when needed. Our ability to reason shows that other human beings are like us and therefore entitled to the same respect and dignity we seek. A summary statement of the basic precepts of natural law is "do good and avoid evil." Using natural law, theologians have developed moral guidelines about medical services, which are described in Chapters 10 and 11.

Rawls's Theory

The contemporary American moral philosopher John Rawls died in 2002. Rawls espoused a hybrid theory of ethics that has applications in health services allocation and delivery. His theories were expounded in his seminal work, *A Theory of Justice*, originally published in 1971. They are redistributive in nature, and the philosophical construct that he used results, with some exceptions, in egalitarianism in health services.

Rawls's theory uses an elaborate philosophical construct in which persons are in the "original position," behind a veil of ignorance. Such persons are rational and self-interested but know nothing of their individual talents, intelligence, social and economic situations, and the like. Rawls argues that persons in the original position behind a veil of ignorance will identify certain principles of justice. First, all persons should have equal rights to the most extensive basic liberty compatible with similar liberty for others (the *liberty principle*). Second, social and economic inequalities should be arranged so that they are both reasonably expected to be to everyone's advantage and attached to positions and offices open to all (the *difference principle*).[3] According to Rawls's theory, the liberty principle governing political rights is more important and precedes the difference principle, which governs primary goods (distributive rights), including health services.

Rawls argued that hypothetical rational and self-interested persons in the original position will reject utilitarianism and select the concepts of right and justice as precedent to the good. Rawls concluded that rational self-interest dictates that one will act to protect the least well-off because (from the perspective of the veil of ignorance) anyone could be in that group. He termed this *maximizing the minimum position (maximin)*.

When applied to primary goods, one of which is health services, Rawlsian moral theory requires egalitarianism. *Egalitarianism* is defined to mean that rational, self-interested persons may limit the health services available to people in certain categories, such as particular diseases or age groups, or limit services provided in certain situations. It is also rational and self-interested for persons in the original position not to make every good or service available to everyone at all times.

Rawls's theory permits disproportionate distribution of primary goods to some groups, but only if doing so benefits the least advantaged. This is part of the difference principle and justifies elite social and economic status for persons such as physicians and health services managers if their efforts ultimately benefit the least advantaged members of society.

Casuistry and the Ethics of Care

Casuistry   Many historical definitions of casuistry are not flattering. They include a moral philosophy that uses sophistry and encourages rationalizations for desired ethical results, uses evasive reasoning, and is quibbling. Despite these unflattering definitions and a centuries-long hiatus, advocates of casuistry see it as a pragmatic approach to understanding and solving problems of modern biomedical ethics. *Casuistry* can be defined as a kind of case-based reasoning in historical context. A claimed strength is that it avoids excessive reliance on principles and rules, which, it is argued, provide only partial answers and often fall short of comprehensive guidance for decision makers.

A significant effort to rehabilitate casuistry was undertaken by Jonsen and Toulmin,[4] who argued that

> Casuistry redresses the excessive emphasis placed on universal rules and invariant principles by moral philosophers. . . . Instead we shall take seriously certain features of moral discourse that recent moral philosophers have too little appreciated: the concrete circumstances of actual cases, and the specific maxims that people invoke in facing actual moral dilemmas. If we start by considering similarities and differences between particular types of cases on a practical level, we open up an alternative approach to ethical theory that is wholly consistent with our moral practice.

At its foundation casuistry is similar to the law, in which court cases and the precedents they establish guide decision makers. Beauchamp and Walters[5] stated that

> In case law, the normative judgments of a majority of judges become authoritative, and . . . are the primary normative judgments for later judges who assess other cases. Cases in ethics are similar: Normative judgments emerge through majoritarian consensus in society and in institutions because careful attention has been paid to the details of particular problem cases. That consensus then becomes authoritative and is extended to relevantly similar cases.

In fact, this process occurs in organizations when ethics committees, for example, develop a body of experience with ethical issues of various types—their reasoning uses paradigms and analogies.

Clinical medicine is case focused. Increasingly, cases are being used in management education. This development has made it natural to employ a case approach in health services. Traditionally, ethics problem solving in health services has applied moral principles to cases—from the general to the specific, or deductive reasoning. Classical casuists, however, used a kind of inductive reasoning—from the specific to the general. They began by stating a paradigm case with a strong maxim (e.g., "thou shalt not kill") set in its most obvious relevance to circumstances (e.g., a vicious attack on a defenseless person). Subsequent cases added circumstances that made the relevance of the maxim more difficult to understand (e.g., if defense is possible, is it moral?). Classical casuists progressed from being deontologists to teleologists and back again, as suited the case, and adhered to no explicit moral theory.[6] Jonsen[7] argued that modern casuists can profitably copy the classical casuists' reliance on paradigm cases, reference to broad consensus, and acceptance of probable certitude (defined as assent to a proposition but acknowledging that its opposite might be true). Casuistry has achieved a prominent place in applied administrative and biomedical ethics. Increasing numbers of cases and a body of experience will lead to consensus and greater certainty in identifying morally right decisions.

Ethics of Care   Medicine is based on caring, the importance of which is reflected historically and in contemporary biomedical ethics. *Care* focuses on relationships; in clinical practice, this means relationships between caregivers and patients. Effective management also depends on relationships between managers and staff, and through them to patients. As the ethics of care evolves, it may become more applicable to management; at this point, however, it applies almost exclusively to clinical relationships.

The interest in the ethics of care beginning in the 1980s has been attributed to the feminist movement.[8] Its proponents argue that various interpersonal relationships and the obligations and virtues they involve "lack three central features of relations between moral agents as understood by Kantians and contractarians, e.g., Rawls—it is intimate, it is unchosen, and is between unequals."[9] Thus, the ethics of care emphasizes the attachment of relationships rather than the detachment of rules and duties.

A clear link to virtue ethics exists in that the ethics of care focuses on character traits such as compassion and fidelity that are valued in close personal relationships. It has been suggested that the basis for the ethics of care is found in the paradigmatic relationship between mother and child. It is claimed that this paradigm sets it apart from the predominantly male experience, which often uses the economic exchange between buyer and seller as the paradigmatic human relationship, and which, it is argued, characterizes moral theory, generally.[10]

A leading exponent of the ethics of care, Carol Gilligan,[11] argued that unlike traditional moral theories, the ethics of care is grounded in the assumption that

> Self and other are interdependent, an assumption reflected in a view of action as responsive and, therefore, as arising in relationships rather than the view of action as emanating from within the self and, therefore, "self-governed." Seen as responsive, the self is by definition connected to others, responding to perceptions, interpreting events, and governed by the organizing tendencies of human interaction and human language. Within this framework, detachment, whether from self or from others, is morally problematic, since it breeds moral blindness or indifference—a failure to discern or respond to need. The question

of what responses constitute care and what responses lead to hurt draws attention to the fact that one's own terms may differ from those of others. Justice in this context becomes understood as respect for people in their own terms.

Similar to virtue ethics and the renewed interest in casuistry, the ethics of care is a reaction to the rules and systems building of traditional theories. Its proponents argue that the ethics of care more closely reflects the real experiences in clinical medicine and of caregivers, who are expected to respond with, for example, warmth, compassion, sympathy, and friendliness, none of which fits well into a system of rules and duties. "Ethical problems are considered in a contextual framework of familial relationships and intrapersonal relationships combined with a focus on goodness and a reflective understanding of care."[12]

Virtue Ethics

Western thought about the importance of virtue can be traced to Plato, but more particularly to Aristotle.[13] Like natural law, virtue ethics is based on theological ethics but does not focus primarily on obligations or duties. "Virtue" is that "state of a thing that constitutes its peculiar excellence and enables it to perform its function well." It is "in man, the activity of reason and of rationally ordered habits."[14] Virtue ethics prescribes no rules of conduct. "Instead, the virtue ethical approach can be understood as an invitation to search for standards, as opposed to strict rules, that ought to guide the conduct of our individual lives."[15] As with casuistry, virtue ethics is receiving increased attention. MacIntyre's *After Virtue* and Foot's *Virtues and Vices*[16] reaffirmed the importance of virtue ethics as a moral philosophy with 20th-century relevance.

Some of this attention resulted from a perception that traditional rule- or principle-based moral philosophies deal inadequately with the realities of ethical decision making. That is to say, rules (as derived from moral principles) take us only so far in solving ethical problems; when there are competing ethical rules or situations to which no rules apply, something more than a coin toss is needed. This is where virtue ethicists claim to have a superior moral philosophy. Rule utilitarians and Kantian moral philosophies provide principles to guide actions, thus allowing someone to decide how to act in a given situation. By contrast, virtue ethics focuses on what makes a good person rather than on what makes a good action.[17] "Virtuous persons come to recognize both things that should be avoided and those that should be embraced."[18] Action comes from within and is not guided by external rules and expectations.

Contemporary authors Pellegrino and Thomasma[19] argue that virtue ethics has three levels. The first two are 1) observing the laws of the land and 2) observing moral rights and fulfilling moral duties that go beyond the law. The third and highest level is the practice of virtue.

> Virtue implies a character trait, an internal disposition habitually to seek moral perfection, to live one's life in accord with a moral law, and to attain a balance between noble intention and just action. . . .
> In almost any view the virtuous person is someone we can trust to act habitually in a good way—courageously, honestly, justly, wisely, and temperately.[20]

Thus, virtuous managers (or physicians) are disposed to the right and good that is intrinsic to the practice of their profession, and they will work for the good of the patient. As Pellegrino noted, "Virtue ethics expands the notions of benevolence, beneficence, conscientiousness, compassion, and fidelity well beyond what strict duty might require."[21]

Some virtue ethicists argue that, as with any skill or expertise, practice and constant striving to achieve virtuous traits (good works) improves one's ability to be virtuous. Other virtue ethicists argue that accepting in one's heart the forgiveness and reconciliation offered by God (faith) "would lead to a new disposition toward God (trust) and the neighbor (love), much as a physician or patient might be judged to be a different (and better) person following changed dispositions toward those persons with whom . . . (they) are involved."[22]

As noted, the virtues are character traits, a disposition well entrenched in the possessor. The fully virtuous do what they should without any struggle against contrary desires.[23] Most of us are less than fully virtuous, however. We are continent—we need to control a desire or temptation to do otherwise than be virtuous. Another way to describe a virtue is that it is a tendency to control a certain class of feeling and to act rightly in a certain kind of situation.[24]

Plato identified only four cardinal virtues: wisdom, courage, self-control, and justice.[25] Aristotle expanded these four virtues in ways that need not concern us. Beauchamp and Childress identified five "focal virtues" that are appropriate for health professionals: compassion, discernment, trustworthiness, integrity, and conscientiousness.[26] Virtues appropriate for health services managers include those selected by Plato and by Beauchamp and Childress, and several more that can be added, including honesty, punctuality, temperance, friendliness, cooperativeness, fortitude, caring, truthfulness, courteousness, thrift, veracity, candor, and loyalty. The goal of the virtuous manager is to achieve a mean between a virtue's excess and its absence. For example, courage is a virtue, but its excess is rashness; its absence is cowardice. Another example is friendliness. In excess, it is obsequiousness; its absence is sullenness. Neither extreme is acceptable in the virtuous manager.[27] A way to understand the virtues is to identify the vices or character flaws managers should avoid. These include being irresponsible, feckless, lazy, inconsiderate, uncooperative, harsh, intolerant, dishonest, selfish, mercenary, indiscreet, tactless, arrogant, unsympathetic, cold, incautious, unenterprising, pusillanimous, feeble, presumptuous, rude, hypocritical, self-indulgent, materialistic, grasping, shortsighted, vindictive, calculating, ungrateful, grudging, brutal, profligate, disloyal, and so on.[28]

All people should live virtuous lives, but those in the caring professions have a special obligation to do so, which is to say that virtuous managers and physicians are not solely virtuous persons practicing a profession. They are expected to work for the patient's good even at the expense of personal sacrifice and legitimate self-interest.[29] Virtuous physicians place the good of their patients above their own and seek that good, unless pursuing it imposes injustice on them or their families or violates their conscience.[30] Thus, virtuous physicians place themselves at risk of contracting a deadly infectious disease to comfort and treat their patients, and they provide large amounts of uncompensated treatment even though doing so diminishes their economic circumstances. Similarly, virtuous managers place the good of the patient (through the organization) above their own. This means that they speak out to protect the patient from harm because of incompetent care, even though doing so risks their continued employment, and they work the hours necessary to ensure that needed services are provided, despite a lack of commensurate remuneration. Meeting the responsibility to protect the patient requires virtues such as courage, perseverance, fortitude, and compassion.

Virtues may come into conflict. For example, the virtue of compassion conflicts with the virtue of honesty when a patient asks a caregiver, "Am I going to die?" Moreover, the virtue of loyalty to the employing organization conflicts with the virtue of fair treatment of staff. Such conflicts cause an ethical dilemma. They may be resolved by asking questions such as

> Which of the alternative courses of action is more distant from the virtue that is relevant to it? Which of these virtues is more central with the role relationship that the agent(s) plays in the lives of the others with whom (they) are involved? Which of these roles is more significant in the life of the moral patient, the person to be affected by the agent's behavior?[31]

Answers to these questions enable the decision maker to choose a course of action that does no violence to their effort to be virtuous.

The concept of virtue and a moral philosophy based on it goes well beyond Western philosophical thought. Hindu ethics as discussed in the Hindu scripture the Bhagavad Gita identify duty, but duty coexists with virtue.[32] Confucianism exhibits attention to the virtues, but the virtues are present only in the context of filial piety—a pattern of interpersonal connectedness. This connectedness diminishes the extent to which individuals can be analyzed as autonomous entities. Thus, being virtuous for Confucius is to have traits that render trait-based explanations of behavior inadequate on their own.[33]

Summary

The moral philosophies described in this section span a wide spectrum. Health services managers are likely to be eclectic in selecting those that become part of the organization's philosophy and those that will influence the content of their personal ethic, as well as its reconsideration and evolution. Most important is that managers recognize that a basic understanding of moral philosophies is vital.

LINKING THEORY AND ACTION

Ethical theories are drawn from abstractions that are often stated broadly. Principles developed from these theories establish a relationship and suggest a course of action. Rules can be derived from the principles; the specific judgments and actions to be applied are the result. Figure 3 was developed by Beauchamp and Childress to demonstrate the relationship between ethical theories (moral philosophies) and actions implementing decisions.

Ethical theories do not necessarily conflict. Diverse philosophies may reach the same conclusion, albeit through different reasoning, by various constructs, or by focusing on divergent criteria (e.g., the rule utilitarian's use of ends versus the Kantian's use of duty). The principles discussed here, supplemented by various of the virtues, are considered crucial and should be reflected in the organization's philosophy and the personal ethic of health services managers.

Linking ethical theories and derivative principles permits the development of usable guidelines. To aid in that process, this discussion identifies four principles that provide a context for managing in health services environments: 1) respect for persons, 2) beneficence, 3) nonmaleficence, and 4) justice. Utility is sometimes treated as a distinct principle, but that

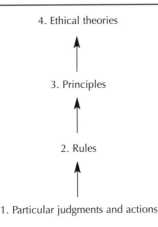

4. Ethical theories

3. Principles

2. Rules

1. Particular judgments and actions

Figure 3.   Hierarchy of relationships. (From Beauchamp, T.L., & Childress, J.F. [1983]. *Principles of biomedical ethics* [2nd ed., p. 5]. New York: Oxford University Press. Reprinted by permission.)

construct is somewhat artificial and potentially confusing. Here, utility is included as an adjunct to the principle of beneficence.

Respect for Persons

The theories discussed in this chapter support the conclusion that respect for persons is an important ethical principle. This principle has four elements. The first, autonomy, requires that one act toward others in ways that allow them to be self-governing—to choose and pursue courses of action. To do so, a person must be rational and uncoerced. Sometimes patients are or become nonautonomous (e.g., some persons with physical or cognitive disabilities). They are owed respect nonetheless, even though special means are required. Recognizing the patient's autonomy is the reason that consent for treatment is obtained, and it is a general basis for the way an organization views and interacts with patients and staff.

Autonomy is in dynamic tension with paternalism, the concept that one person knows what is best for another. Paternalism is an established tradition in health services. The earliest evidence of it is found in the Hippocratic oath, which is reproduced in Appendix B. It directs physicians to act in what they believe to be the patient's best interests. Stressing autonomy does not eliminate paternalism, but paternalism should be used in limited circumstances (e.g., when patients cannot communicate and there is no one to speak for them).

The second element of respect for persons is truth telling, which requires managers to be honest in all activities. Depending on how absolute a position is taken, this element prohibits fibs or white lies, even if they are told because it is correctly believed that knowing the truth would harm someone. The morality of insisting that patients be told the truth may also be problematic, depending on the circumstances. Some patients would suffer mental and physical harm if told the truth about their illnesses. In doing so, physicians would not meet their obligation of primum non nocere or "first, do no harm." The modern expression of this concept is nonmaleficence, which is discussed later in the chapter.

Confidentiality is the third element of the principle of respect for persons. It requires managers as well as clinicians to keep what they learn about patients confidential. Morally justified exceptions to confidentiality are made, for example, when the law requires that certain diseases and conditions be reported to government. For managers, the obligation of confidentiality extends beyond patients. It applies to information about staff, organization, and community that becomes known to them in the course of their work.

The fourth element of respect for persons is fidelity: doing one's duty or keeping one's word. Sometimes, this is called "promise keeping." We treat persons with respect when we do what we are expected to do or what we have promised to do. Fidelity enables managers to meet the principle of respect for persons. Here, too, if exceptions are made, they cannot be made lightly. Breaking a promise must be justified on moral grounds; it must never be done merely for convenience or self-interest.

Beneficence

Like respect for persons, the principle of beneficence is supported by most of the moral philosophies described previously, although utilitarians would require it to meet the consequences test they apply. Beneficence is rooted in Hippocratic tradition and in the history of the caring professions. Beneficence may be defined as acting with charity and kindness. Applied as a principle in health services, beneficence has a similar but broader definition. It suggests a positive duty, as distinct from the principle of nonmaleficence, which requires refraining from actions that aggravate a problem or cause other negative results. Beneficence and nonmaleficence may be viewed as opposite ends of a continuum.

Beauchamp and Childress[34] divide beneficence into two categories: 1) providing benefits and 2) balancing benefits and harms (utility). Conferring benefits is firmly established in medical tradition, and failure to provide them when one is in a position to do so violates the moral agency of both clinician and manager. Balancing benefits against harms provides a philosophical basis for cost–benefit analysis, as well as other considerations of risks balanced against benefits. In this sense, it is similar to the principle of utility espoused by the utilitarians. However, here, utility is only one of several considerations and has more limited application.

The positive duty suggested by the principle of beneficence requires organizations and managers to do all they can to aid patients. A lesser duty exists to aid those who are potential rather than actual patients. This distinction and its importance vary with the philosophy and mission of the organization and whether it serves a defined population, as would a health maintenance organization. Thus, under a principle of beneficence, the hospital operating an emergency department has no duty to scour the neighborhoods for individuals needing its assistance. However, when they become patients, this relationship changes.

The second aspect of beneficence is balancing the benefits and harms that could result from certain actions. This is a natural consequence of a positive duty to act in the patient's best interests. Beyond providing benefits in a positive fashion, one cannot act with kindness and charity when risks outweigh benefits. Regardless of its interpretation, utility cannot be used to justify overriding the interests of individual patients and sacrificing them to the greater good.

Nonmaleficence

The third principle applicable to managing health services organizations is nonmaleficence. Like beneficence, it is supported by most of the ethical theories discussed previously (it must meet the consequences test to claim utilitarianism as a basis). Nonmaleficence means primum non nocere. This dictum to physicians is equally applicable to health services managers. Beauchamp and Childress[35] noted that although nonmaleficence gives rise to specific moral rules, neither the principle nor the derivative rules can be absolute because it is often appropriate (with the patient's consent) to cause some risk, discomfort, or even harm in order to avoid greater harm or to prevent a worse situation from occurring. Beauchamp and Childress included the natural law concepts of extraordinary and ordinary care and double effect in the principle of nonmaleficence. (Extraordinary and ordinary care are considered later in this chapter under the subheading "Application of the Principles and Virtues.") Nonmaleficence also leads managers and clinicians to avoid risks, unless potential results justify them.

Justice

The fourth principle, justice, is especially important for administrative (and clinical) decision making in resource allocation, but it applies to areas of management such as human resources policies as well. What is just, and how does one know when justice has been achieved? Although all moral philosophies recognize the importance of achieving justice, they define it differently. Rawls defined justice as fairness. Implicit in that definition is that persons get what is due them. But how are fairness and "just deserts" defined? Aristotle's concept of justice, which is reflected in natural law, is that equals are treated equally, unequals unequally. This concept of fairness is used commonly in policy analysis. Equal treatment of equals is reflected in liberty rights (e.g., universal freedom of speech). Unequal treatment of unequal individuals is used to justify progressive income taxation and redistribution of wealth: It is argued that those who earn more should pay higher taxes. This concept is expressed in health services delivery by expending greater resources on individuals who are sicker and thus in need of more services.

These concepts of justice are helpful, but they do not solve the problems of definition and opinion, which are always troublesome. Macro- and microallocation of resources have received extensive consideration in the literature, but there is little agreement as to operational definitions. Each organization must determine how its resources will be allocated. An essential measure of whether organizations and their clinicians and managers are acting justly is that they consistently apply clear criteria in decision making.

Summary

Philosophers call respect for persons, beneficence, nonmaleficence, and justice prima facie (at first view, self-evident) principles, or prima facie duties. None is more important; none has greater weight. Health services managers are expected to meet all four. A principle can be violated only with clear moral justification, and then negative results must be minimized. Virtue ethics holds a special place in the work of managers, and the virtues are applied to supplement and complement the prima facie duties.

MORAL PHILOSOPHY AND THE PERSONAL ETHIC

This examination of moral philosophies and derivative principles provides a framework for developing a personal ethic and subsequently analyzing ethical problems. Like philosophers, managers are unlikely to agree with all elements of a moral philosophy and make it their own. Most managers are eclectic as they develop and reconsider their personal ethic. In general, however, the principles and virtues described here are essential to establishing and maintaining appropriate relationships among patients, managers, and organizations, and they should be part of the ethic of health services managers and the value system of the organizations they manage. It should be stressed that the four derivative principles may appropriately carry different weights, depending on the ethical issue being considered. The principle of justice requires, however, that there be a consistent ordering and weighing when the same types of ethical problems are considered.

Application of the Principles and Virtues

How do the principles and virtues identified and discussed in the preceding section and their underlying moral philosophies assist in solving ethical problems in cases such as Baby Boy Doe? (see p. 16). The principle of respect for persons implies certain duties and relationships, including autonomy. Nonautonomous persons, however, must have decisions made for them by a surrogate. The parents of Baby Boy Doe, a nonautonomous person, had to make decisions on behalf of their son. Surrogates cannot exercise unlimited authority, especially when it is uncertain that a decision is in the patient's best interests. If the infant's and parents' interests differ, caregivers (including managers) are duty bound under the principles of beneficence and nonmaleficence to try to persuade parents to take another course of action. Such efforts by caregivers and managers should have been attempted for Baby Boy Doe.

Extending the principles of beneficence and nonmaleficence, it is acceptable for the organization to seek legal intervention and obtain permission to treat an infant against the parents' wishes. The moral compulsion to do so is especially great when the parents are not acting in the child's best interests, but this moral duty should be exercised only as a last resort. Courts intervene under the theory of *parens patriae* (parent of the nation) to permit a hospital or social welfare agency to stand *in loco parentis* (in the role or in place of a parent). Courts take this step reluctantly because of the common law tradition that gives parents control over reproductive and family matters, including decisions about children. As noted, although it is an element of beneficence, utility is not an overriding concept that permits trampling on the rights of the person, as happened to Baby Boy Doe.

Intervention has limits. Absent an emergency, treating the infant against the parents' wishes without a court order is unethical because it breaks the law. If persons caring for the infant cannot continue because of their personal ethic, they should be permitted to withdraw. Or they may engage in whistle-blowing or other actions to bring attention to the situation. In doing so, however, they must accept the consequences of their actions. The option to remove oneself from an ethically intolerable situation should be reflected in the organization's philosophy and policies.

In applying the principle of nonmaleficence, one must consider whether the ethically superior choice would have been to shorten Baby Boy Doe's life through active euthanasia. This consideration raises the question of the moral difference between killing and letting die. Some argue that the identical results make them morally indistinguishable. The analysis cannot end there, however; to do so ignores critical aspects of medical decision making.

When caregivers apply the principle of nonmaleficence, they refrain from doing harm, which includes minimizing pain and suffering. Asking caregivers dedicated to preserving life to end it will cause significant role conflict. Furthermore, physicians and nurses in such roles are on a slippery slope that may lead to more exceptions and increasing use of positive acts to shorten lives that are deemed to be not worth living.

The concept of extraordinary care is a part of the principle of nonmaleficence that developed from natural law. *Ordinary care* is treatment that is provided without excessive expense, pain, or inconvenience and that offers reasonable hope of benefit. Care is *extraordinary* if it is available only in conjunction with excessive expense, pain, or other inconvenience or if it does not offer any reasonable hope of benefit.[36] With no reasonable hope of benefit, *any* expense, pain, or inconvenience is excessive. Beauchamp and Childress[37] concluded that the "ordinary-extraordinary distinction thus collapses into the balance between benefits and burdens, where the latter category includes immediate detriment, inconvenience, risk of harm, and other costs." For Baby Boy Doe, there was hope of benefit, even though correcting the atresia would not reverse his mental retardation. Surgery would have given Baby Boy Doe a normal life for someone with his cognitive abilities. That benefit justifies the use of treatment involving significant expense, pain, and/or inconvenience.

Justice is the final principle to be applied, a principle that was previously noted to have rather divergent definitions. Rawls defined justice as fairness. Applied to the case of Baby Boy Doe, one could conclude that the result was just. Fairness is arguably compatible with an enlightened self-interest expressed by persons in the original position behind a veil of ignorance—the Rawlsian philosophical construct. Rational persons could decide that no life is preferable to one of significantly diminished quality, even though this arguably limits the liberty principle, which Rawls considered ultimately important.

For a Kantian or an adherent to natural law, the outcome in the Baby Boy Doe case is abhorrent because the infant was used as a means rather than as an end—the parents' apparent unwillingness to accept and raise a less-than-perfect child. Conversely, rule utilitarians would find the result acceptable. Other definitions of justice produce different conclusions. For example, if justice is defined as getting one's just deserts, it is clear that Baby Boy Doe fared badly. Applying an even cruder standard—that individuals equally situated should be treated equally—it is clear that if an adult had been in a similar situation, the necessary treatment would have been rendered. For Baby Boy Doe, the results of applying the principle of justice are uncertain.

The final regulations about infant care published by the U.S. Department of Health and Human Services (DHHS) in April 1985 focus on beneficence and nonmaleficence. In implementing the Child Abuse Amendments of 1984 ([PL 98-457], amending the Child Abuse Prevention and Treatment Act of 1974 [PL 93-247]), DHHS placed no weight on the parents' traditional right to judge what should be done for infants with cognitive and/or physical impairments and life-threatening conditions. The potential problem caused by parents who may not fully understand the implications of the diagnosis (of both the impairments and the life-threatening conditions) and the effects of their decision is obviated by the regulations because medical criteria applied by a knowledgeable, reasonable physician are used. Quality of life criteria cannot be considered. The preliminary regulations to implement the law made specific reference to a case similar to that of Baby Boy Doe and stated that appropriate medical treatment had to be rendered. The final regulations contain no examples, however. Nevertheless, it is likely that DHHS will view narrowly any decisions to forego treatment of infants with impairments and life-threatening conditions. Specifics of the regulations are discussed in Chapter 10.

As with most governmental efforts to regulate ethical decision making, these regulations are likely to be modified in the future. From an ethical standpoint, it is more important to bear in mind the moral considerations that should underlie public policy than to be preoccupied with the semantics of a particular enactment.

Implications for Management

What are the implications of cases like that of Baby Boy Doe for health services managers? Such events place a heavy burden on caregivers. Whatever the decision, these cases split the staff. The resulting controversy diminishes morale. In addition, criticism may be leveled against management, governance, and medical staff by individuals who question the morality of the decision and the organization's role in it. In extreme cases, legal action may ensue.

It is crucial that the health services organization implement a view (a philosophy) about matters such as these that is reflected in its policies and procedures. This means the organization has explicitly formulated a course of action that it will take when confronted with such problems. Having a philosophy in place permits a deliberate response rather than one that is reactive, inadequately considered, or governed by (rather than governing) events. At the very least, the organization must consider these issues prospectively and within the constraints of its organizational philosophy.

Paradoxically, prior to the 1984 Child Abuse Amendments, the health services organization could legally do to Baby Boy Doe what the parents could not. Had the parents taken the infant home and allowed him to starve and dehydrate until he died, it is likely that they would have been charged with child neglect or some degree of homicide or manslaughter. However, the organization did not face the same liability. In fact, had it surgically repaired the atresia without parental consent it would have committed battery on the infant, for which it could have been sued for civil damages and for which the staff might have been charged criminally. Criminal charges are unlikely, but the hospital is legally obligated to obtain consent from the parents or legal guardian for a minor when no emergency exists.

CONCLUSION

This chapter helps the manager develop a personal ethic and stimulates the organization to formulate a philosophy. Few managers will disagree as to the importance of the principles of respect for persons, beneficence, nonmaleficence, justice, and various other complementary virtues. However, not all managers will embrace unequivocally the principles and underlying moral philosophies discussed here. It is even more unlikely that they will agree about their weighing or priority. Chapter 2 suggests a methodology that managers can use in solving ethical problems.

NOTES

1. Robert Hunt & John Arras, Eds. (1983). *Issues in modern medicine* (2nd ed., p. 27). Palo Alto, CA: Mayfield Publishing.
2. Edgar Bodenheimer. (1974). *Jurisprudence: The philosophy and method of the law* (Rev. ed., pp. 23–24). Cambridge, MA: Harvard University Press.
3. John Rawls. (1971). *A theory of justice* (p. 60). Cambridge, MA: Belknap Press.

4. Albert R. Jonsen & Stephen Toulmin. (1988). *The abuse of casuistry: A history of moral reasoning* (p. 13). Berkeley, CA: University of California Press.

5. Tom L. Beauchamp & LeRoy Walters, Eds. (1994). *Contemporary issues in bioethics* (4th ed., p. 21). Belmont, CA: Wadsworth Publishing.

6. Albert R. Jonsen. (1986). Casuistry and clinical ethics. *Theoretical Medicine, 7,* p. 70.

7. *Ibid.*, p. 71.

8. Beauchamp & Walters, p. 19.

9. Annette C. Baier. (1987). Hume, the women's moral theorist? In Eva Feder Kittay & Diana T. Meyers (Eds.), *Women and moral theory* (p. 44). Totowa, NJ: Rowman & Littlefield.

10. Virginia Held. (1987). Feminism and moral theory. In Eva Feder Kittay & Diana T. Meyers (Eds.), *Women and moral theory* (p. 111). Totowa, NJ: Rowman & Littlefield.

11. Carol Gilligan. (1987). Moral orientation and moral development. In Eva Feder Kittay & Diana T. Meyers (Eds.), *Women and moral theory* (p. 24). Totowa, NJ: Rowman & Littlefield.

12. James J. Finnerty, JoAnn V. Pinkerton, Jonathan Moreno, & James E. Ferguson. (2000, August). Ethical theory and principles: Do they have any relevance to problems arising in everyday practice? *American Journal of Obstetrics and Gynecology 183*(2), pp. 301–308.

13. Rosalind Hursthouse. (2003, July 18). Virtue ethics. *Stanford encyclopedia of philosophy.* Retrieved December 18, 2003, from http://plato.stanford.edu/entries/ethics-virtue.

14. Glenn R. Morrow. (2011). Virtue. *Dictionary of philosophy.* Retrieved January 7, 2001, from http://www.ditext.com/runes//v.html.

15. Marcel Becker. (2004). Virtue ethics, applied ethics, and rationality twenty-three years after *After Virtue. South African Journal of Philosophy* 23(3), p. 267.

16. Alasdair MacIntyre. (1984). *After virtue.* Notre Dame, IN: University of Notre Dame Press; Philippa Foot. (2003). *Virtues and vices.* New York: Oxford University Press.

17. Virtue ethics contrasted with deontology and consequentialism. (2003, November 17). *Wikipedia: The free encyclopedia.* Retrieved November 30, 2003, from http://en.wikipedia.org/wiki/Virtue_ethics.

18. Ann Marie Begley. (2005, November). Practising virtue: A challenge to the view that a virtue centred approach to ethics lacks practical content. *Nursing Ethics* 12, p. 630.

19. Edmund D. Pellegrino & David C. Thomasma. (1988). *For the patient's good: The restoration of beneficence in health care* (p. 121). New York: Oxford University Press.

20. *Ibid.*, p. 116.

21. Edmund D. Pellegrino. (1994). The virtuous physician and the ethics of medicine. In Tom L. Beauchamp & LeRoy Walters (Eds.), *Contemporary issues in bioethics* (4th ed., p. 55). Belmont, CA: Wadsworth Publishing.

22. Frederick S. Carney. (1978). Theological ethics. In Warren T. Reich (Ed.), *Encyclopedia of bioethics: Vol. 1* (pp. 435–436). New York: The Free Press.

23. Hursthouse.

24. William David Ross. (1995). *Aristotle* (6th ed., p. 209). New York: Routledge.
25. *Ibid.*
26. Tom L. Beauchamp & James F. Childress. (2001). *Principles of biomedical ethics* (5th ed., pp. 32–37). New York: Oxford University Press.
27. *Ibid.*, p. 210.
28. Hursthouse.
29. Pellegrino & Thomasma, p. 121.
30. Pellegrino, p. 53.
31. J.L.A. Garcia. (2008). Anscombe's three theses revisited: Rethinking the foundations of medical ethics. *Christian Bioethics* 14(2), p. 132.
32. Bina Gupta. (2006). *Bhagavad Gita as duty and virtue ethics: Some reflections. Journal of Religious Ethics* 34(3), pp. 373–395.
33. Jesse Prinz. (2009). The normativity challenge: Cultural psychology provides the real threat to virtue ethics. *Journal of Ethics* 13(2/3), p. 135.
34. Tom L. Beauchamp & James F. Childress. (1989). *Principles of biomedical ethics* (3rd ed., p. 195). New York: Oxford University Press.
35. *Ibid.*, p. 122.
36. Gerald Kelly. (1951, December 12). The duty to preserve life. *Theological Studies*, p. 550.
37. Beauchamp & Childress, p. 153.

CHAPTER 2

RESOLVING
ETHICAL ISSUES

Managers are problem solvers. It is the reason they are hired—organizations without problems need no managers. Some problems burst on the scene. Something is clearly amiss when a wildcat strike occurs among the nursing staff or when a newspaper editorial attacks the organization. Other problems are hard to uncover and often provide no clear evidence or warning. They must be identified and treated early; undetected, they will grow and may threaten the organization's survival. The aphorism "a stitch in time saves nine" is never truer. Solving them is similar to detection and early treatment of disease.

Successful managers possess highly developed conceptual and problem identification skills. Preventing (if possible) or identifying and solving ethical problems with the least disruption to the organization are as critical as solving management problems affecting personnel or finances. Ethical problems have implications for traditional management areas, and traditional management problems have ethical dimensions. It is important to note in using this comparison that the techniques and skills employed in solving ethical problems have many similarities to those needed to solve management problems. Problem solving is a generic process applicable to both.

IDENTIFYING ETHICAL PROBLEMS

Often, managers believe that they are inadequately prepared to recognize ethical problems and even less able to solve them. This view understates the typical manager's credentials and abilities. Identifying ethical issues that could become problems is primarily a matter of mind-set, attitude, sensitivity, and application of common sense when reviewing or analyzing a situation. Identifying an ethical problem and its dimensions is often less difficult than developing and implementing morally acceptable alternative solutions. Developing and implementing solutions will likely require assistance from elsewhere in the organization or even from outside it.

Managers who see their function only as solving problems of staffing, directing, budgeting, controlling, organizing, coordinating, integrating, and planning are more in need of increased awareness of ethical issues than postgraduate education in philosophy. Methodologies similar to those used to solve traditional management problems can be used to solve ethical problems, whether they are administrative or biomedical. (This generic process is examined later in the chapter.) However, traditional management issues often overshadow and may even overwhelm the ethical dimensions that invariably accompany them. In addition, the ethical dimensions of managerial problems can be subtle, which complicates initially identifying and then solving them.

Managers use authority delegated by the governing body to represent the organization. As discussed in Chapter 3, the organization's philosophy provides a general context for the manager's activities and decision making. The presence of an organizational philosophy, however, does not eliminate the manager's need for a personal ethic. A personal ethic provides a framework—a grounding—for decisions and permits greater refinement of principles, rules, and particular judgments (as well as actions or nonactions) than is likely using only the organization's statement of philosophy. It bears repeating that each human being is a moral agent whose actions, nonactions, and misactions have moral consequences. Morally unacceptable conduct cannot be excused because someone was "following orders" or policy, regardless of their source. Orders from lawfully constituted authorities, such as courts, pose a special problem. Moral agents who consider such orders unjust or immoral may engage in civil disobedience, but in doing so, they must be prepared to bear societally imposed sanctions. The ethical (moral) implications of acts must be considered independently.

Occasionally, there is conflict between the organization's ethic, as expressed in its philosophy, and the manager's personal ethic. The organization is a bureaucracy and the manager must carefully consider the implications of acquiescing to its values. This follows from the concept of moral agency. Often, it seems easier to "go along to get along" than to risk one's position by speaking out. Professional dissent or whistle-blowing are rare, despite evidence that sharp or dishonest practices, criminal behavior, or activities that pose a danger to the public are not uncommon in organizations, even those in the health services field. Managers must recognize both the distinction between and the integration of an organizational and a personal ethic. They must not perform their daily tasks with little thought to the ethical context or implications of what they do, fail to do, or do badly.

In terms of the problem-solving methodology described below, the organization's philosophy and the individual's personal ethic are vital. They provide the framework and context in which the manager functions, and they enhance sensitization to and identification and solution of ethical problems so that managers can approach these problems as they would those of traditional management.

Another technique that may be useful in identifying ethical problems is the ethics audit. Conducted much like a financial audit, an ethics audit uses a set of criteria to compare actual with desired performance. Small increases in some measures should alert managers to actual or potential ethical problems: patient complaints, incident reports, and legal actions; employee grievances, resignations, terminations, and wrongful discharge complaints; medical staff complaints and resignations; problems with suppliers and other vendors; and adverse publicity. The ethics audit has three steps. First, analyze key documents (e.g., mission, vision, and values statements) and their operationalization in policies and procedures, with special attention paid to issues such as uncompensated care, confidentiality, consent, conflicts of interest, and sexual harassment. Second, survey representative board members, managers, physicians, employees, volunteers, and community residents and organizations to determine whether actual performance matches that desired. Third, address deficiencies through education or other appropriate strategies.[1] Compliance or noncompliance with laws and regulations raises other ethical (and legal) issues.

Administrative Ethical Issues

Leadership is essential in management. It includes setting goals, establishing direction, and guiding the organization. These tasks are more ethics-sensitive than are many routine managerial activities. Day-to-day activities (i.e., transactional leadership) seem less tied to values, but even these are based on earlier decisions rooted in ethical principles, whether or not those principles are identified and expressly stated. However management functions are interpreted, human beings cannot escape their role as moral agents. Managers set a tone and establish a context for the organization and staff. They can neither avoid scrutiny of their personal ethic nor ignore its congruence with the organization's philosophy.

Managers hold positions of trust, which may not be used for personal advantage or personal aggrandizement. These are essential elements of a personal ethic if one seeks to be an effective leader. Managers must not act in any ways that raise the slightest hint of wrongdoing. Actions (and nonactions and misactions) should be judged by applying the ethical principles and virtues discussed in Chapter 1. Another effective way to clarify the pragmatic effect of an action is to step back, as though one were an outsider, and view what is being done or contemplated. One should ask, "How would the public and my colleagues see this decision?" This "as seen through the eyes of others," or "in the light of public scrutiny," standard for judging managerial decisions is helpful. A cynic's standard is not useful—meeting it is impossible because cynics see problems when it is unreasonable to do so. Skepticism is a useful criterion for managers to apply as they seek to understand how their actions might be interpreted. A standard of discovery is unacceptable because the concept of "if you don't get caught, it's okay" negates the need for ethics and substitutes deviousness and deceit.

In a way quite different from a personal ethic or an organization's philosophy, the law is a baseline of what is considered ethical. The Introduction noted that laws provide useful comparisons; however, they guide us only partially because the law is a minimum standard of conduct, and no manager is effective by meeting minimum requirements. The manager qua leader must set an example that substantially surpasses what is expected of others. Professional codes also guide conduct and provide frames of reference. These codes have a more demanding level of performance than the law; however, they should be seen only as partially incorporating expectations of ethical performance.

Is it persuasive to argue that where one stands on administrative ethics depends on where one sits? Does the concept of "rank hath its privileges" apply to managing health services? Many senior managers act as though it does. One readily finds situations in which subordinates are reprimanded for behavior unpunished at the upper echelons. Here, it is "do as I say, not as I do" or "what is sauce for the goose is not sauce for the gander." Few will fail to distinguish words from actions. This double standard sends staff a clear message of cynicism and inconsistency and greatly diminishes the manager's ability to lead; respect is lost.

Managers can become sensitive to administrative ethical issues in several ways. They should be voracious readers of the popular press and professional literature because what happens elsewhere could become a problem for them. Codes of ethics are valuable guides to understanding the concerns of the profession and the parameters of acceptable action. Asking whether the Golden Rule is being met also helps identify ethical problems. Not to be forgotten is intuition and hunch, which form that sixth sense that something is wrong. Both can be nurtured to alert managers to the presence of ethical problems.

Identifying ethical problems means focusing on the principles of respect for persons, beneficence, nonmaleficence, and justice, as complemented by the virtues. One must ask if the actions contemplated violate them and then determine whether the violation is justified by special circumstances. A questioning mind permits managers to consider the situation further or seek assistance, as appropriate. Identifying administrative ethical problems requires attention to detail and constant vigilance.

Biomedical Ethical Issues

All contemplated and actual interactions with patients present potential sources of ethical problems, which range from paternalism to consent and from truth telling to decisions at the end of life. Managers may feel uncomfortable and out of place working to solve biomedical ethical problems. They should not. *Medicine and the clinician provide key information that assists in making informed ethical decisions, but the decision itself is ethical (moral), not clinical.* The distinction between clinical and ethical aspects of biomedical decision making is critical and is one managers must not forget. Managers will gain confidence with greater experience and exposure to biomedical ethical issues. Their participation is needed because increased medical staff–administration interaction results in a more effective and efficient organization, and because all biomedical problems have administrative dimensions. Thus, the manager's involvement is critical.

Managers do not supersede clinicians but are important to preventing or solving a wide range of biomedical ethical problems through actions, including serving on institutional ethics committees and institutional review boards and participating in resource allocation decisions. In addition, managers are key in developing the processes and operationalizing the policies, procedures, and rules that implement the organization's philosophy.

As noted in the section on administrative ethics issues, managers need not take postgraduate courses in philosophy or ethics to identify the presence of potential problems, although such courses might be helpful. Primarily, identifying potential ethical problems requires sensitization, an inquiring mind, and a reasonably well-developed personal ethic. Questions such as the following help identify biomedical ethical problems:

- Is there a clearly enunciated value system reflected in the organization's culture?

- Is there an institutional ethics committee to resolve ethical issues?
- Is this patient being treated as I would wish to be?
- Is the patient protected from unnecessary risk?
- Does the consent process adequately inform the patient about the treatment contemplated?

As in any problem solving, asking the right questions may be the most important part of the process.

A key role for managers is stimulating the medical staff and other caregivers to develop the expertise to prevent or effectively address biomedical ethical problems. To do so, caregivers must be availed of procedures and rules to follow. Here, the manager's role as a catalyst is much the same as that played in traditional administrative activities. Regrettably, codes of administrative ethics provide limited guidance in addressing biomedical ethical issues.

SOLVING PROBLEMS

Unresolved ethical problems exact the same destructive effect on an organization as do problems involving personnel, finance, or the medical staff. Therefore, it is imperative that managers use a methodology for solving them. This poses difficulties, however, because few managers are formally trained in ethics. Ethical issues may seem more subtle than management problems, and because managers tend to be pragmatic, they are less inclined to grapple with nuances. Sometimes ethical problems are combined with and overshadowed by administrative issues. Furthermore, managers may consider ethical issues less important than other problems, perhaps because they do not comprehend their potentially devastating effect. These obstacles are surmountable, however.

In 1910, the American educator and philosopher John Dewey wrote in *How We Think* that problem solving comprises three stages: identifying the problem, identifying the alternatives, and determining which alternative is best. Implicitly or explicitly, successful managers use a similar process. The stages of the process include identifying the problem in terms of both the current manifestation (which may be only a symptom) and the underlying cause; developing alternative solutions and the decision criteria to judge them acceptable, unacceptable, or optimal; preparing an implementation plan for the solution selected; and developing a means to evaluate the solution, once implemented.

Philosophers use a similar methodology, *moral reasoning*, to analyze ethical problems. Its components are surprisingly similar to the manager's problem-solving methodology:

- *Analyzing*—separating the overall structure of a problem in a particular case into its major components
- *Weighing*—assessing the strengths and weaknesses of various alternatives that could be used in solving the problem by balancing them against one another
- *Justifying*—providing a compelling and sufficient moral reason that appeals to an established moral principle, such as "always tell the truth" [any such principle must be compatible with the organization's philosophy and the manager's personal ethic]
- *Choosing*—selecting one or more of the available alternatives, preferably on the basis of a position that can be and has been shown to be justified
- *Evaluating*—reexamining the choices and their justifications, identifying unanswered questions, and relating decisions about one particular case to similar cases[2]

Problem solving is rooted in two broad models, the rational and the heuristic. Defining the problem is addressed differently by each. The rational model (sometimes identified with programmed decisions) assumes that one is faced with a specific problem and focuses primarily on a search for the optimal solution. Operations research, for example, is primarily a quantitative expression of the rational model to a wide range of management issues. In the hospital, it includes problems such as work scheduling—for example, developing a computer program that maximizes the preferred work schedule of a large number of nurses, or a program evaluation and review technique (PERT) chart used to schedule construction of a new building. These and similar techniques help an organization establish effective patterns for problem solving.

The heuristic model (sometimes identified with nonprogrammed decisions, or a learning model) acknowledges that some problems may be more diffusely defined, poorly structured, and are often not routine. It uses an iterative process of dealing with problem definition, as well as solution. Heuristic general problem-solving techniques have been suggested for training administrators. Heuristic problem-solving approaches that are quantitative and computer-based have been advocated.[3]

The distinctions between the rational and heuristic models suggest that solving ethical problems is heuristic. First, however, process and substance components must be separated, and ethical problems that recur and have similar features must be distinguished from those that are unique and unlikely to recur. Process components are more amenable to analysis and solution by the rational model than are substance (content/issue) components. Ethical problems that recur and have similar features are also more amenable to using the rational model. Even here, however, implementing the process may uncover unique or subtle problems of substance, such as the relative authority of different individuals in the decision-making process. The two problem-solving theories are not mutually exclusive, and the heuristic model often benefits from using a rational model for some analysis. Thus, problem solvers should never exclude either model.

Graduate programs in health services administration and business administration teach the process of problem solving. Such methodologies are useful in solving ethical problems and are similar to the generic problem-solving model in Figure 4. The model is shown in two dimensions but should be conceptualized with time as the third dimension. In this respect, the model is like a corkscrew: While the process cycles from problem analysis to evaluation of results, the whole activity is moving through time.

In Figure 4, problem analysis begins when the manager objectively or intuitively finds something amiss. This occurs when actual results deviate from desired or expected results or a situation occurs that demands an organizational response. Examples of developments requiring management's attention include a rapid decrease or increase in outpatient admissions, increased turnover among staff in a department, more uneaten food returned from patient rooms or the cafeteria to dietary, or an announcement that competing emergicenters are opening or closing. Some of these potential problems are foreseen through analysis of routinely collected data; others are apparent only after they occur. Obvious and defined problems will be more amenable to the rational than the heuristic model.

Similarly, the ethical dimensions of some situations are apparent. If a patient is diagnosed as being in a persistent vegetative state (PVS), an ethical problem having both clinical and administrative dimensions exists. An ethical problem is also present when the organization lacks an effective consent process. In such situations, heuristic problem solving is not the most effective methodology.

A potential administrative and biomedical ethics problem needs a solution only when the problem solver determines that it must be solved. Sometimes, before an ethical problem can be resolved, it ends (e.g., the patient in PVS cannot be resuscitated after cardiac arrest). The problem is gone, but it has not been solved.

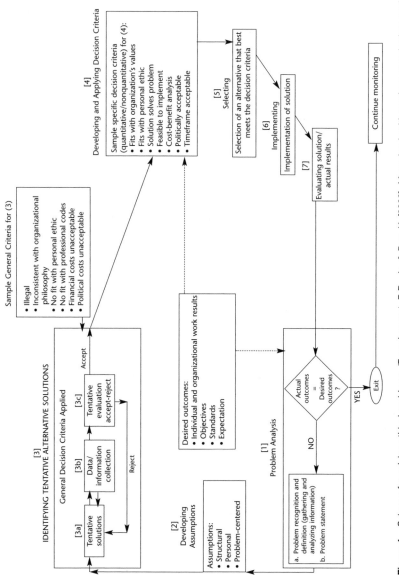

Figure 4. Schema for solving ethical problems. (From Longest, B.B., Jr., & Darr, K. [2008]. *Managing health services organizations and systems* [5th ed., p. 279]. Baltimore: Health Professions Press; adapted by permission.)

Sample General Criteria for (3)

- Illegal
- Inconsistent with organizational philosophy
- No fit with personal ethic
- No fit with professional codes
- Financial costs unacceptable
- Political costs unaccceptable

[4]
Developing and Applying Decision Criteria

Sample specific decision criteria (quantitative/nonquantitative) for (4):
- Fits with organization's values
- Fits with personal ethic
- Solution solves problem
- Feasible to implement
- Cost-benefit analysis
- Politically acceptable
- Timeframe acceptable

[5]
Selecting

Selection of an alternative that best meets the decision criteria

[6]
Implementing

Implementation of solution

[7]

Evaluating solution/ actual results

Continue monitoring

[3]
IDENTIFYING TENTATIVE ALTERNATIVE SOLUTIONS

General Decision Criteria Applied

[3a]
Tentative solutions

[3b]
Data/ information collection

[3c]
Tentative evaluation accept-reject

Accept

Reject

Desired outcomes:
- Individual and organizational work results
- Objectives
- Standards
- Expectation

[2]
Developing Assumptions

Assumptions:
- Structural
- Personal
- Problem-centered

[1]
Problem Analysis

a. Problem recognition and definition (gathering and analyzing information)
b. Problem statement

Actual outcomes = Desired outcomes ?

NO

YES

Exit

Berry and Seavey[4] argued that problem definitions "are fundamentally subjective [and] . . . are not objective, concrete realities; they are perceptions of reality." This statement is correct as it bears on perceptions of cause and effect but must be qualified when applied to other situations. For example, several unexplained deaths in a nursing facility are a fact and will be defined by a manager as a problem that needs solving. Perceptions (subjectivity) vary in determining the cause or in identifying the underlying situation (problem) that may be the cause. Views of problems and their solutions are affected by the positions held and responsibilities of the individuals involved. Nursing service will likely provide a different explanation of the deaths than will management.

Context is more important in solving problems that are primarily ethical than when solving management problems with few ethical dimensions. The context of ethical problems is the organization's philosophy and mission interpreted and applied by a manager who is a moral agent with a personal ethic. Once an ethical problem has been recognized and defined as a problem needing a solution, it must be understood. The information about its extent and character may be available in existing data, or special efforts may be required to obtain it. Managers solving ethical problems will experience data deficits similar to those they confront when solving other problems.

Rectangle 2 in Figure 4 asks managers to identify three types of assumptions: those about the context of the problem, those about themselves, and those about the problem itself. The Baby Boy Doe case undoubtedly affected staff, and it is reasonable to assume that in similar cases, staff will become depressed and angry and morale will decline. One may also assume that a few staff members will be so upset that they will resign, turn to a union, or refuse to work in the nursery. Assumptions such as these require judgment by managers and may result in a decision to ignore the situation (i.e., not define it as a problem requiring a solution), which is what occurred in the case of Baby Boy Doe. The hospital accepted the parents' directives and determined there was either no problem that required a solution or that the solution was to do nothing. Such a result is dependent on the organization's philosophy and the individual manager's personal ethic. Choosing to do nothing may be a solution, but only if it solves the problem as stated and meets the decision criteria better than other alternatives. Doing nothing must never be unchosen or occur by negligence.

Preliminary review of options occurs in Rectangle 3, in which tentative alternative solutions are identified and assessed. Here, decision makers may brainstorm creative solutions. Managers solving administrative or biomedical ethical problems must be mindful of the organization's philosophy as well as their own personal ethic. Unless the constraints of the context can be changed, solutions falling outside them must be discarded. Arbitrarily ignoring or applying these constraints creates inconsistencies and discontinuities that eventually cause serious problems for the organization and the manager. Other, more general criteria are also applied in such instances.

Alternative solutions that pass this preliminary screening are subject to detailed assessment. This assessment compares each option against specific decision criteria. Examples of these criteria are shown in Rectangle 4 of Figure 4: time available to solve the problem, real costs of all kinds (e.g., political, financial, reputation), opportunity costs, feasibility of implementation, adequacy of solving the problem, and benefits derived. Applying more specific criteria results in better solutions and outcomes. A primary benefit of greater specificity in the process is that managers must review, analyze, and be as precise as possible, both in defining the problem and in selecting the alternative that best solves it. This exercise is useful because it hones management decision making. A more sophisticated approach is to weight or assign relative values to decision criteria, since some are more important than others.

Before and after selecting an alternative, the manager must consider implementation and evaluation. A common failing is that great effort is put into developing a solution and beginning implementation. Then, managers are distracted by other problems. The result is that the solution flounders before it is fully implemented. Implementing the solution should receive as much attention as selecting it. Evaluation must be included in the solution so that difficulties can be identified and timely corrective action taken. Corrective actions are a subset of the problem-solving process and may involve the same or similar steps.

This ethical problem-solving methodology is useful for decision making by one manager, by a group of managers, by governing body committees, or by special-function committees, such as institutional ethics committees, institutional review boards, or infant care review committees. It is effective for solving one problem, considering guidelines for a class of problems, or developing a process to bring a similar methodology to bear on solving individual problems or groups of problems. Regardless of the source of decision making, once the process is established and policies (which have gone through a similar problem-solving process) have been formulated and implemented, operating procedures and rules will be established. This means that an issue such as consent has been considered and that the ethically acceptable policies, procedures, and processes have been identified and implemented. The desired result is that many ethical problems will be prevented. Exceptions and special attention will be necessary when the facts differ sufficiently from the assumptions implicit in the policy and procedures derived from it.

In this regard, it is unnecessary to distinguish administrative from biomedical ethical problems. Because both types will occur, policies should be adopted prospectively. Procedures and rules derived from the policies will address the majority of predictable, recurring ethics problems. That is why, for example, a governing body adopts a conflict of interest policy applicable to itself and management. Despite the usefulness of policies and procedures, problems occur in interpreting and applying them and unique ethical issues arise. It bears repeating that the problem-solving model discussed previously is usable on two levels: general policy development and consideration of specific situations or cases.

In most ways, implementing solutions to administrative or biomedical ethical problems is the same as for management problems, though some distinctions are noteworthy. One is that ethical issues are often emotional. Examples are evidence that a manager has acted unethically (administrative ethics), or that a patient's view of life and death has been violated or challenged (biomedical ethics). Thus, managers and staff who work to solve ethical problems must exercise greater sensitivity to human factors and must understand that they are not dealing with units of production or ordinary services. Another distinction is that administrative and biomedical ethical issues may have the potential for legal consequences. Although all health services organizations should apply a standard that is much higher than the minimum set by the law, mistakes do occur, and occasionally, there are problems that bring in lawyers. Yet another distinction is that negative public relations consequences may occur inside and outside the organization.

DEVELOPING A PERSONAL ETHIC

Health services managers begin their careers as adults who have an implicit personal ethic. In developing that ethic, managers have been affected by numerous influences beyond their own introspection, including family and friends, religious principles and teachings, secular education, and the law. It is in this context that adults become managers and that a personal ethic about management emerges. Some managers' personal ethic may be only an intuitive sense of right and wrong, with no identifiable source or explicitly defined code of conduct.

Developing a personal ethic necessitates introspection and self-examination. Questions such as the following are helpful: "Who am I?," "How do I view certain actions or activities?," "What do I consider unethical?," and "What is morally right or wrong?" Understanding and grappling with questions such as these are critical as managers search for the "right" answer to ethical problems. Both nascent and experienced health services managers use numerous sources to develop and refine their personal ethic. Chief among them are professional codes of ethics; organization values and culture; educational socialization; and the association and pressure of peers, subordinates, and superiors.

In selecting the principles to be included in a personal ethic, managers should apply the criteria of comprehensiveness, consistency, and coherence and ask themselves the following questions:

- Do the principles apply to the broadest possible range of ethical issues?
- How useful and applicable are they in solving ethical problems?
- Do they use the scientific method in terms of exactness, systemization, and predictability?
- Are the ethical concepts clear and consistent?
- Are they in conflict with or consistent with other knowledge or life experiences?
- Are they reasonably adaptable to a changing world?

Although the criteria of comprehensiveness, consistency, and coherence are not applied with the rigor employed by a moral philosopher, they should be used when developing, judging, or reconsidering a personal ethic and when analyzing the ethics of others or disputing their reasoning or conclusions. In developing and reconsidering one's personal ethic, it is useful to paraphrase Plato, who said that the unexamined life is not worth living.

The moral philosophy of casuistry has special relevance in the manager's efforts to hone a personal ethic. Casuistry's emphasis on cases and the reiterative nature of cases and similar events provide special assistance in terms of a personal ethic. Virtue ethics has a unique role here too. The virtues noted in Chapter 1 should be included in a personal ethic, and reexamining whether one is a virtuous manager will reinforce or highlight a need for further attention.

In addition to the manager's personal ethic, the organization's philosophy is vital to ethical decision making. It is tempting to say that the personal ethic is and ought to remain the most important factor. However, one cannot ignore the realities of bureaucratic life. Some sectarian health services organizations seek complete congruence between a manager's personal ethic and the organization's ethic by hiring no one above mid-level management who is not an adherent to that faith. The wisdom of such a policy is examined in later chapters. Suffice to say that in modern, complex health services organizations, a significant and undesirable potential for discontinuity exists between the philosophy of the organization and that of its managers. However, the extent to which these philosophies must be identical, or even congruent, is unclear. It is likely that the organization's philosophy and the values expressed in its culture will have a greater effect on development of the personal ethic of a younger, less experienced manager. Like everyone, managers can become set in their ways.

CONCLUSION

In solving problems, successful managers implicitly or explicitly use a methodology similar to that outlined in Figure 4. Effectively solving ethical problems requires the same attention and a similar approach. Managers cannot ignore ethical problems, and they must be prepared to participate in solving them. It is critical, however, to separate the technical and clinical dimensions from the ethical. This does not mean that health services managers supersede physicians or other clinical staff when biomedical ethics are present. It does mean that in an effort to operationalize the principles and virtues discussed in Chapter 1, managers must participate effectively in solving all types of ethical problems. It is the nature of the job that managers serve as team leaders and catalysts. Serving as the organization's conscience is consistent with the manager's role as moral agent in a position of ethical leadership. In terms of administrative ethics, the manager's role is preeminent, but not to the exclusion of physicians.

Successful managers have a well-developed personal ethic and a clear perspective on administrative and biomedical ethical issues. This ethic has been defined by drawing from a wide variety of sources. A personal ethic cannot be chiseled in stone; it will evolve over time. Although one's basic view of the world is likely to remain relatively stable, experience, maturation, and technological developments will affect one's personal ethic.

NOTES

1. Paul B. Hofmann. (1995, November/December). Performing an ethics audit. *Healthcare Executive 10*(2), p. 47.
2. Frank Harron, John Burnside, & Tom Beauchamp. (1983). *Health and human values* (p. 4). New Haven, CT: Yale University Press.
3. David E. Berry & John W. Seavey. (1984, March/April). Reiteration of problem definition in health services administration. *Hospital & Health Services Administration 29*(2), p. 58.
4. *Ibid.*, p. 59.

Guiding Ethical Decision Making

Asignificant problem with applied administrative and biomedical ethics is that numerous written and unwritten factors influence management behavior. These factors are a blend of intellect, experience, education, and relationships. The common result is a too-often ill-defined personal code of conduct. A poorly defined personal ethic combined with tolerance for varying views may cause managers to believe that there is no one best answer to questions of administrative and biomedical ethics. Lacking a well-defined personal ethic, managers have no lodestar to guide them as they seek to answer the basic question of normative ethics, "What ought I to do?" The mind-set of a personal ethic helps them to filter out vague, contradictory guidance, and to lead and shape rather than being led and shaped.

Key to a defined, robust personal ethic is self-analysis and introspection. Questions such as "Who am I?," "What is my bottom line?," and "For how long, if ever, will I tolerate certain behaviors?" must be asked by managers who wish to understand and hone their personal ethic. Plato asserted that the unexamined life is not worth living. This is also true of a personal ethic.

Managers of health services organizations are ex officio community leaders. This prominence raises for managers (and more generally the profession) questions of the demarcation between private and professional lives. Private conduct that breaches the profession's code of ethics and the culture of the organization may result in disciplinary action. Beyond the tension between managers' private and professional lives is that between a manager's personal ethic and the organization's philosophy. The philosophy and mission of the organization guide development and implementation of policies, procedures, and rules. An important issue for individuals and organizations is the need for congruence between the organization's philosophy and the manager's personal ethic.

Chapters 3 and 4 suggest development and content of an organizational philosophy and examine its importance in the delivery of services. Codes of ethics and their role in guiding health services managers and helping them develop a personal ethic are examined. The dynamic between the organization's philosophy and the manager's personal code is analyzed as well.

Assistance for managers and organizations in solving ethical problems is discussed in Chapter 5. Specialized committees that focus on different categories of ethical problems and other assistance are suggested. As leader and moral agent, the manager acts to prevent, identify, and solve ethical problems.

CHAPTER 3

DEVELOPING ORGANIZATIONAL VALUES, VISION, AND MISSION

Managers confront a variety of moral and symbolic issues in health services organizations. This chapter focuses on the organization's need to identify and adopt values and principles—a philosophy. It is within the context of this philosophy that a vision and a mission are developed. The vision statement presents the goals the organization seeks to achieve. The mission statement describes its specific activities. Defining the philosophy prospectively minimizes conflicts among competing values. The sequence of philosophy–vision–mission is the theoretical ideal. The reality is that more likely the mission is defined first or that it evolves from historical activity in the context of an implicit, rather than explicit, philosophy. The concept of "visioning" in health services organizations was first used in the 1980s and continues to the present. It is the rare health services organization that does not have a framed copy of its values, vision, and mission hanging in the lobby. This chapter describes the importance of identifying the moral values and principles that provide a context for the vision and mission statements and the necessity of reflecting these values across the organization.

Mission (and vision) is necessarily limited by, and is a function of, the physical location, size, resources, and other aspects of the organization's internal and external environments. These factors can usually be affected only over time. A significant change in them requires review of the mission, many of whose elements directly relate to the moral values and principles identified by the organization's governance and management. The decision of a nongovernmental acute care hospital not to perform abortions, for example, is derived from a determination that such services are incompatible with its moral values and principles. Offering abortion services raises other questions, the answers to which must be consistent with the organization's position on abortion. For example, is performing

abortions compatible with legally required efforts to provide medically indicated treatment to live aborted fetuses? Some organizations avoid these
questions and the attendant ethical implications by simply adhering to the
law—they offer all legal services. This equates legality and morality. Such
an approach only partially solves the problem, however, because the law
is poorly developed in a number of areas in which administrative and biomedical ethical problems arise.

Although a governing body may adopt a statement of philosophy with
certain values and principles, this is no indication that the staff agrees.
Generally, staff in organizations pay limited attention to such matters; the
health services field is no exception. Many staff may not know the organization's philosophy, despite reasonable efforts to communicate it. Even
if the philosophy is understood, many members make no commitment to
it. If little attention is paid to the organization's stated moral values and
principles (philosophy), it is not surprising that even less attention is paid
to what should have been said but was not. For such staff, the organization is but a place to work. They do their work and are unconcerned about
what the governing body and senior management say is the context for or
the goals of service delivery. Absent significant discontinuity—when even
sabotage is possible—it is rare for staff to overtly challenge what is being
done. If challenged, the results tend to be negative rather than positive in
outcome and effect.

Consideration must be given to how much more effective the organization could be were it built on a clearly understood system of shared
values and goals. Adequately communicated to and accepted by staff, a
resource-supported goal as simple as "getting the caring back into curing"
could reap rewards for the organization through improved efficiency and
patient care and relations. Moving staff in the same direction—a direction
known in advance and recognized as important in the organization—will
positively affect staff attitude, productivity, and effectiveness.

DEVELOPING AN ORGANIZATIONAL PHILOSOPHY

The starting point for an organization to prevent and, if necessary, solve
ethical problems is its philosophy. The statement of philosophy identifies
values and principles reflecting the moral right and wrong for the organization, thus distinguishing the acceptable from the unacceptable. It is
helpful if the philosophy statement is sufficiently precise that performance
in achieving it can be measured. At minimum, the statement of philosophy
must be consistent with the law.

The statement of philosophy is different from the mission statement and should be developed separately. The philosophy statement provides a context for the mission statement; the mission statement is subordinate to it. Some organizations include references to values in their mission statements. A mission statement that "the corporation owns and operates hospitals to provide care for the sick and injured" provides no information about the moral context of care. A mission statement that "the hospital provides care for the sick and injured in the context of humanitarian principles" is imprecise but provides a clearer values or moral context than the first.

Health services organizations with no specific, written philosophy nonetheless have an identifiable de facto or operational philosophy. The aggregate decisions and actions taken by the governing body and management reflect implicit, if ill-defined, philosophical bases. Management actions may be contradictory or inconsistent, and this suggests another negative aspect of not determining prospectively a comprehensive organizational philosophy. This lack of continuity and consistency will lead to incompatible, even contradictory, policies, procedures, and rules. The effect is diminished efficiency. Equally important is that the mixed, even contradictory messages that staff members receive will confuse and frustrate them, with a resulting decline in patient focus and quality.

The importance of identified and shared values in organizations is now widely understood, if less frequently operationalized. In the early 1980s, however, it was a new concept, one that was synthesized by Peters and Waterman in their study of successful American corporations.[1] The quote attributed to IBM's former president Thomas J. Watson, Jr., is instructive: "The basic philosophy of an organization has far more to do with its achievements than do technological or economic resources, organizational structure, innovation, and timing." That statement's context was the focus on customer service so important to IBM's reputation and financial success at the time. If consumers and service are important to IBM, which has many characteristics of a products-based organization, consider the importance of customers and service in healthcare. The centrality of shared values is shown in Figure 5, the 7-S Framework, developed by McKinsey & Company.

Deal and Kennedy[2] also identified the characteristics of successful companies:

- They stand for something—that is, they have a clear and explicit philosophy about how they aim to conduct their business.

- Management pays a great deal of attention to shaping and fine-tuning these values to conform to the economic and business environment of the company and to communicating them to the organization.
- These values are known and shared by all the people who work for the company—from the production worker right through to the ranks of senior management.

Building on the importance of shared values or philosophy that make up a culture, Deal and Kennedy[3] identified the essential elements of a culture: 1) understanding and fitting into the business environment—the single greatest influence in shaping a corporate culture, 2) values—the basic concepts and beliefs of an organization, 3) heroes who personify the culture's values and are role models for employees, 4) rites and rituals that show employees the kind of behavior expected of them, 5) ceremonies that provide visible and potent examples of what the company stands for, and 6) the cultural network—the primary (but informal) means of communication within an organization that is the "carrier" of the corporate values and heroic mythology.

In further explaining corporate cultures, Kennedy[4] noted the following:

> Culture isn't a single thing. It's not a budget; it's not a plan; it's not the shape of a building. It is an integrated pattern of all the things that go on in an organization on a day-to-day basis. Each company has its own unique culture, values, and standards communicated internally by style, dress, expectations, and assumptions.
>
> New people in the workplace find out what is expected of them because their peers take them aside and say, "Look, don't wear jeans here. Come in to work on time, or you do this or that." They lay out some of the unwritten rules of behavior that are required for entrance into your workplace. That's how culture transmits itself to each new generation of persons. They don't come in and invent a whole new style of organization. They come in and learn from those around them what's going on in the organization and how they are expected to behave.

An organization's values are inextricably linked to its culture. To transform the organization so that its culture is a living reflection of values that facilitate the mission and vision, management must know which values are present in the culture. This presents somewhat of a chicken-and-egg situation. Regardless, management must biopsy the culture. This can be compared to a financial audit, except it is the organization's values that are being audited. Direct measures such as observation, staff surveys, exit interviews of departing staff members, and focus groups can be used. Proxy

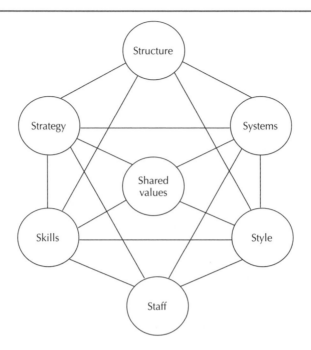

Figure 5. The McKinsey 7-S Framework. (From McKinsey & Company, Inc. Reprinted by permission.)

measures of culture include patient satisfaction surveys and service area surveys. Regardless of how it is done, however, management cannot effectively transform the organization's culture until its present content and course are known.

The barriers to establishing strong corporate cultures in any organization are a particular problem in health services organizations. For hospitals, barriers include:[5]

- Hospitals must serve diverse medical needs of heterogeneous populations.
- The number of external variables (forces outside the organization that affect it) is much greater for hospitals than it is in ordinary business enterprise.
- Hospital outcomes are difficult to define and to measure.
- It is difficult to nurture the keen proprietary sense of individual endeavors among leadership and management staff at all levels.
- Hospital board members are not active participants in its culture.
- Hospital physicians are a subculture, and peer acceptance and recognition, participation in professional activities, and stature based on

professional contribution and expertise are more important than the rewards of belonging to a particular hospital.

- Elaborate peer reward systems in nursing are complicated by a deep search for professional identity.

- Support staff and especially allied medical personnel increasingly tend to have a professional identification independent of the hospital.

- Another special subculture in hospitals is the administrators, who are caught between the role of facilitating the delivery of medical care and that of running a cost-effective "business"; as a result, they often isolate themselves from other subcultures.

Beyond these factors, and implicit in them, is the need for managers to view their relationships with staff and patients in a consistent fashion. Paying lip service to the organization's avowed goal of patient care but in fact focusing on economic or other nonpatient considerations is a contradiction that will not be lost on staff, who will respond to real incentives rather than platitudes. Not only must the decisions and actions of leaders be consistent with organizational values, but staff must *perceive* that they are consistent, lest the leader be judged a hypocrite. If values and how they are understood evolve over time, managers must solicit feedback to identify any disconnect between what they are saying and what employees are hearing.[6]

Management must know and understand the culture and values in its organization. Just as important, management must know how the culture and values mesh with or diverge from those the organization wishes to develop. The organization can mold a culture, but it can move neither faster than nor in directions that are opposed to or misunderstood by internal stakeholders. This congruence is critical. The organization's philosophy and derivative vision and mission statements are the primary points of reference for its corporate culture and subordinated activities. All efforts to develop excellence are a function of these statements.

A logic is evident in the link between the strength of a culture and organizational performance. The first piece of logic is that of goal alignment—a strong culture causes staff to metaphorically march to the same drummer—the pheromone of the organization. Second, a strong culture aids in performance by creating an unusual level of motivation among staff—shared values and behaviors make staff feel good about working for an organization; the resulting commitment or loyalty makes them strive harder. Third, a strong culture aids in performance because it provides needed structure and controls without relying on a bureaucracy, which can diminish motivation and innovation.[7]

Closely linked to the concept of organizational philosophy and corporate culture is management's view of the organization's staff. McGregor's Theories X and Y, Maslow's hierarchy of needs, and the 14 points enumerated by W. Edwards Deming echo the importance of management's view of its employees, which is likely to be similar to how patients are viewed by a health services organization. Dysfunction is rife in an organization that treats employees as adversaries or as a means to an end and distrusts them while it urges staff to treat patients with dignity and respect. Employees see the hypocrisy and respond negatively. Peters and Waterman[8] sounded this theme, quoting Thomas J. Watson, Jr.: "IBM's philosophy is largely contained in three simple beliefs. I want to begin with what I think is the most important: our respect for the individual. This is a simple concept, but in IBM it occupies a major portion of management time."

Culture as Pheromone

The values of an organization are reflected in its culture. If they are positive, these values will bind the organization together. The resulting congruence of values will enhance operational and mission effectiveness.

Insects communicate, attract, and repel using pheromones. Bees and ants are the best-known organized insect societies that use unique pheromones to perform many of the tasks needed to survive and thrive. Bees are probably the most widely studied and best understood of organized insect societies.

In many ways, the *api regina*, or queen bee, is the bee colony. She is the center of attention and has a retinue of attendant bees whose sole task is to feed, groom, and support her work. The queen is critical to the hive; only she can lay the eggs that enable the colony to survive and thrive. But the queen bee performs another essential task; she binds the colony into an organized society. Each *api regina* emits a unique pheromone. This pheromone is spread throughout the hive by the movement of bees' wings. It allows the bees to recognize the queen and one another. Guard bees at the entrance to the hive recognize those attempting to enter by their scent and know that they belong to the hive. The bees that come from another hive to "rob" a hive's honey are driven away. When there is danger, the bees emit an alarm pheromone and the colony immediately acts to defend itself.

Worker bees newly emerged from the comb in which they develop from egg to larva to pupa perform nurse and housekeeping tasks for several days until they are strong enough to become field bees and forage for nectar. Young worker bees have very active wax glands. The liquid wax they secrete is used to build comb in the classic hexagonal shape. The queen lays her eggs in this comb. Other comb is used to store pollen, beebread, and the nectar that is processed into honey. When the honey is ready, the comb containing it is sealed with a wax cover. The natural antibacterial properties of honey allow it to be stored indefinitely.

Their tasks are instinctive; no control or direction is apparent. The average summer life expectancy of a worker bee is about 45 days. Thus, their development must occur in rapid order. When strong enough to fly, nurse and house bees become field bees who forage for nectar-producing flowers, bring the nectar to the hive in their honey stomachs, and add enzymes so that the minute amounts of nectar can be processed into the honey, which is food for the hive and so pleasing to human palates. In gathering nectar, bees pollinate the flowers of plants and trees that produce a wide variety of food for human consumption. About 30% of the U.S. food supply could not be produced without pollinating insects, especially the honeybee.

Of what relevance to the modern health services organization is the pheromone that binds a bee colony? Simply put, the organization's value system is a metaphor for the queen's pheromone. Health services organizations do not have an *api regina* (although some situations might suggest otherwise). But organizations do have a managerial hierarchy with similar characteristics. By their example, managers—especially those who are senior—exude a values pheromone. Those who work in the organization identify one another by their personal value systems—their personal ethic—and this ethic connects them with other staff and largely reflects the value system of the organization. A positive value system enables the organization (the colony) to thrive and produce the output that enables its success. In the case of honeybees, the honey will sustain the hive. In a health services organization, it is the delivery of patient care, for which the organization receives the revenue that enables it to thrive. A health services organization with high-quality services enjoys satisfied customers who return for treatment and recommend it to others.

Content of a Philosophy Statement

Organizational Content The values and principles stated in an organization's philosophy establish a moral framework for its vision and mission. The philosophy provides a context and operative values—it gives delivery of health services a life, a meaning—and recognizes that these values are unique and represent more than delivering a product or rendering a service. Policies, procedures, and rules are derived from the mission statement and make the organization operational. The approaches taken by health services organizations are varied. Typically, those that are faith based have a greater focus on values and ethical principles. The commitment to values and ethical principles is not, however, exclusive to faith-based organizations. The Joint Commission on Accreditation of Healthcare Organizations (The Joint Commission) recognizes the importance of an ethics framework and identifies specific elements.[9]

Sutter Health is a large, West Coast health services system. Its values include honesty and integrity, excellence and quality, innovation, affordability, teamwork, compassion and caring, and community.[10] Its mission, vision, and values are reproduced in Appendix A. These values reflect ethical principles and some of the virtues enunciated in Chapter 1.

Trinity Health is a faith-based health services system that provides services across the continuum, from acute to long-term care and hospice. It has the classic trilogy of mission, vision, and values. Core values include respect, social justice, compassion, care of the poor and underserved, and excellence.[11] Trinity Health's mission, core values, and vision statement are reproduced in Appendix A.

The George Washington University Medical Center includes a teaching hospital, schools of medicine, nursing, and public health, and a physician group practice. Its mission is teaching with creativity and dedication; healing with quality and compassion; and discovering with imagination and innovation. Its vision is to improve the health and well-being of our local, national, and global communities. The specific elements of the institution's vision appear in Appendix A.[12]

MountainView Regional Medical Center is a midsized hospital in Las Cruces, New Mexico. Its mission identifies a caring environment, its healthcare team, and service excellence. Stated values include safety, compassion, teamwork, and efficiency.[13] The MountainView mission and values statements are reproduced in Appendix A.

Mayo Clinic is a large, multi-specialty group practice that operates hospitals and a medical school, conducts research, and engages in postgraduate medical education. Its primary value is "The needs of the patient come first." Core principles include practice, education, research, mutual respect, commitment to quality, work atmosphere, societal commitment, and finances.[14] Its mission, values, and principles are reproduced in Appendix A.

Sunrise Senior Living is a nonsectarian for-profit organization that provides a gamut of services to seniors. Its core values include passion, joy in service, stewardship, respect, and trust.[15] Its mission, principles of service, and core values are reproduced in Appendix A.

Relationship with Patients   One cannot imagine a health services organization that does not identify its role vis-à-vis patients in the context of respect for persons, beneficence, nonmaleficence, and justice, as well as the virtues discussed in Chapter 1. These values mandate delivery of medical services to patients with respect and in a manner that enhances human dignity. Staff members must know their responsibilities and duties toward patients in this regard. Patients are the reason why the organization exists, and all efforts are directed at meeting patient needs by safely delivering high-quality services.

Williams and Donnelly[16] asserted that accountability to the patient takes precedence over all other duties and relationships in health services organizations. They were pioneers when they had the temerity to assert that accountability to patients demanded that hospitals inform them if they had been harmed by medical misadventure. These views are mainstream today; in fact, the expectation is even broader. The Joint Commission requires that organizations provide information about unanticipated outcomes of care, treatment, and services to patients. Its standards spell out how licensed independent practitioners (typically, these are physicians) or their designees are involved when unanticipated events occur.[17] This requirement continues to be controversial, if not as radical as in the 1980s. Informing patients and their families, as appropriate, of problems during treatment is the ethically (morally) right course. In addition, there is increasing evidence that informing patients and their families, as appropriate, about medical misadventures makes them less likely to seek legal redress because they believe the organization is being honest and that they are being treated fairly. However, this may not make believers of governing bodies, managers, and physicians. Intellectually, they may agree with the ethics of this degree of accountability, but many will react with measured skepticism because the legal system demands an adversarial approach. Apologies are being addressed in the states. In 2010, 12 states considered bills to make expressions of regret and the like inadmissible in court.[18] This issue receives further attention in Chapter 8.

The economic hazards of implementing such a philosophy are significant, especially in organizations with a voluntary medical staff. Regrettably, the organization that becomes supportive of patients and disregards its physicians risks alienating the physicians, who provide its economic livelihood. The organization will likely have angry physicians. One answer to this seeming dilemma is to immerse physicians in the corporate culture, thus making its organizational philosophy and value system part of their perspective. Hence, physicians will see substandard clinical treatment as endangering the corporate culture and will work with the organization—to the ultimate benefit of the patient.

The view expressed by Williams and Donnelly, and now by The Joint Commission and several states, is consistent with the high degree of trust that the public places in health services organizations, and it is an appropriate measure of the duty organizations should meet in turn. The public has every right to expect that the organization and its managers will treat them with respect and dignity and will seek to right any wrongs. For many patients, this results in a changed relationship with the organization. Sometimes employee zealousness diminishes the perception of respect.

Last Chance

As she was making one of her occasional rounds to patient floors, CEO Frances Long was surprised to see the director of development for River Bend Hospital, Mark Oxley, leaving the intensive care unit (ICU). Oxley has been responsible for development, including fund-raising, for almost four years. He is very effective and has increased donations from a few hundred thousand dollars per year to well over one million. In passing, Long spoke briefly to Oxley but wondered to herself, "What could he be doing in the ICU?"

Long remarked to the ICU nurse supervisor that she had been surprised to see Oxley there. The nurse supervisor told her that she knew Oxley because he came to the ICU regularly; he spoke to patients and their family about remembering River Bend in a bequest or other means of donating money or assets to the hospital. Long asked for more details and the nurse supervisor described some positive, but also some negative, events that involved Oxley and family members. The supervisor told Long that most ICU patients are too ill to talk to Long, and this meant that most conversations were with family members. One family member likened Oxley's conversation with her terminally ill father as that of a vulture circling over a dying animal. Other family members were more positive; they were pleased with the care at River Bend and told Oxley that they would consider making a donation.

Soliciting donations in the ICU seemed tawdry to Long. River Bend always needed donations, but she wondered if Oxley's behavior went beyond the bounds of ethical behavior. Certainly, it exceeded the bounds of good etiquette.

Oxley's behavior is not appropriate because it treats patients (and their families) as objects, not persons worthy of respect. Long must counsel Oxley that he should review the mission and values of River Bend Hospital—which should address the expectations in the situation described—and approach his tasks of fund-raising within that context. He must do so in a way that does not negatively affect patients and their families.

Relationships with Staff   Like patients, employed and nonemployed (typically physicians) staff are entitled to be treated with respect and loyalty. Staff are the organization's most important asset because, ultimately, they determine the manner in which services are delivered. Like patients, staff must not be treated as a means to an end. The ethical aspects of these relations are most apparent in the organization's policies. Examples include reasonable and equitable performance appraisals and evaluation standards known in advance and fairly applied; forthright efforts to eliminate capriciousness, arbitrariness, and prejudice in human resources decision making; due process in grievances and disciplinary proceedings; and determination of the attributes and capabilities required for each position and then matching staff with them.[19] These considerations of ethics in employee relations also evidence good management. Employees who believe that they work in an ethical environment are six times more likely to be loyal to their employer than those who believe their employer is unethical. Employees must have the organization's values communicated to them and see that the actions of management fit with those stated values.[20]

Employees are in an unequal position of power with the organization and supervisors: the employment relationship limits their freedom of action. Consequently, for example, a manager who borrows money from employees is unethical. Such an action jeopardizes management's credibility, but more important, it reflects a lack of respect for employees, who are being used as a means to an end. Employees are also used in such a manner if they must undertake high-risk activities (e.g., caring for patients with highly infectious diseases) with poorly developed procedures and processes or inadequate training, supplies, and equipment. This example is a rare instance in which the duty of beneficence toward the patient is superseded by the virtues of loyalty and justice to staff, and also by the principle of nonmaleficence, a decision supported by a utilitarian calculus.

Physicians are the economic lifeblood of health services organizations. In most instances, they are there at the organization's sufferance, as either employees or independent contractors. In either relationship, the presence of these high-profile professionals complicates the organization's interactions with patients and other staff. If, for example, quality of care issues arise, the organization must meet its obligations to protect patients and further their interests by intervening, as necessary, in the physician-patient relationship. The resulting political and economic problems likely to arise for governance and management mean that intervention occurs only reluctantly and less often than it should.

Employees and medical staff should participate in developing the organization's philosophy and its vision and mission statements. Increased congruence between the philosophies of organization and staff benefits all involved; most important, it benefits patients. Rapport between the organization and its staff is essential to developing a strong, positive corporate culture.

Relationship with the Community   In some geographic areas, community (service area) and patients (or potential patients) are synonymous. The organization's philosophy should specify its relationship to the community: What is its obligation to provide less-than-cost or free care to Medicaid patients or to those who cannot afford to pay? What is its obligation to provide controversial services such as abortion? Prospectively answering questions such as these causes the organization to consider important issues about itself and the role it can play. This probing assists in honing an organizational philosophy and provides an opportunity for introspection and staff involvement in establishing and strengthening a corporate culture.

Going the Extra Mile[21]

The senior managers of a home health agency (HHA) serving five rural counties were indicted (and later convicted) of Medicare fraud. The HHA served more than 1,000 patients and had more than 225 employed staff and independent contractors. During initial criminal proceedings against the senior management, their further actions caused the HHA to go into bankruptcy. The payroll was weeks behind. By the end of the next 2-week pay period, the staff had not been paid for a month. Many were home health aides earning less than $9.00 an hour. Most of the staff were parents.

A senior supervisor met with the staff and told them of the HHA's problems. As a group, they decided to continue caring for all the patients. Some managers loaned their staff money, even though it violated company policy. Within a few weeks, the bankruptcy judge released the payroll, and a semblance of normality returned. Continuity of patient care was maintained.

What a compelling case! The HHA staff had developed a strong culture of beneficence, nonmaleficence, loyalty, and honor—principles and virtues lacking among the corrupt senior management. Their actions reflect proudly on the highest traditions of the health services field. Loaning money to staff in violation of the company policy was morally justified, given the exigencies of the situation and the honorable purposes for which it was done. The staff and supervisor should be given kudos for their shared actions.

Relationship with Other Institutions   Revising the organizational philosophy is difficult but necessary as the external environment changes. The organization must deal forthrightly and honestly with other entities, even actual or potential competitors. This ethic fits with effective competition—it simply means the organization competes honestly, with no hint of fraud or deception. In the past, there were few incentives for health services organizations to cooperate, but significant changes in the delivery of health services and economic pressures will force them into networks or systems. Major differences in moral philosophies inhibit cooperative efforts, a problem that may be insurmountable when sectarian and nonsectarian organizations contemplate a merger or joint efforts.

DEVELOPING A MISSION STATEMENT

Vision statements are aspirational and inspirational. As such, they sketch what the organization would like to become. They set a direction for the organization and broadly state its role and activities.

The mission statement is the applied portion of the vision statement. It operationalizes the means by which the vision is accomplished. The mission statement may originate in the articles of incorporation, the documents filed to establish the health services organization as a legal entity. The statement of objectives or the purposes for which the corporation was formed are useful in developing a mission statement. The need for the mission statement to be consistent with and reflect the organization's philosophy has been amply described. A simple mission statement is that a community hospital association will:

- Establish, operate, and maintain a hospital
- Engage in educational activities related to treating the sick and injured
- Engage in health-promotion and disease-prevention activities
- Promote and perform scientific research related to care of the sick and injured
- Engage in other activities designed to promote the general health of the community

More elaborate are the objectives (mission statement) of Sterling County Hospital,[22] in which elements of an organizational philosophy are included:

- To recognize man's unique composition of body and soul and man's basic right to life. Sterling County's concept of total care, therefore, embraces the physical, emotional, spiritual, social, and economic needs of each patient
- To affirm that the primary objective of our health services is to relieve suffering and to promote and restore health in a Christian manner that demands competence, mercy, and respect
- To generate and cultivate a source of allied health manpower by orienting and supporting personnel development in the areas of individual skills, knowledge, and attitudes
- To participate in the development of health services that are relevant to the total community needs by meaningful area-wide and regional planning and in a partnership for health concept

These mission statements show what the two organizations seek to accomplish. An important distinction is that the first has no values context, nor are its activities linked to a larger value system. The second statement has a more philosophical context.

Organizations state their missions differently. A pediatric medical center states that it will serve any child, regardless of ability to pay. Such a mission statement incorporates the philosophy that treating the child is primary; economics are secondary. Sectarian health services organizations cite their religious creeds; nonsectarian organizations typically link their activities to humanitarian motives. The publicly owned Sterling County Hospital is unique by having a religious reference in its mission statement. Sample organizational philosophies and vision and mission statements are shown in Appendix A.

RECONSIDERING THE ORGANIZATION'S PHILOSOPHY

A competitive environment will significantly affect the way many health services organizations born of eleemosynary (charitable) motives view themselves. Competition and reports of large profits will change how others, especially patients and communities, view them. Aggressive competition is at variance with the philosophy and historical mission of many organizations that serve the sick and injured and do so from a sense of duty and charity rather than from a desire to establish new product lines, increase their market share, or maximize net income over expense. The organization that does not possess the stamina, resources, or mind-set to reconsider its philosophy and mission may become uneconomic and cease to exist.

An Acceptable New Image?

Sebastian Hospital was founded by a Christian congregation in 1891. Its philosophy and mission statements include a strong commitment to care for the sick and injured regardless of ability to pay. This mission posed no problems during its first 90 years. Even after the community purchased the hospital in 1950, it continued to function in much the same fashion. Sebastian successfully weathered a controversy about abortion in 1973. The compromise solution limited where in the hospital abortions would be performed and how staff would be assigned.

Increasing cost pressures during the 1970s and diagnosis-related groups in the early 1980s caused substantial financial problems. A switch to all-payer prospective payment, which would prohibit cost shifting, was imminent. In addition, there was pressure for corporate reorganization. Planning consultants first recommended enterprises such as a physician office building, a parking facility, and a motel. Some of these suggestions complemented the primary mission. The trustees saw other suggestions as tangential. Another new type of enterprise was proposed: a joint venture with members of the medical staff.

The administrator was concerned that Sebastian's 100-year focus would change dramatically. It was one thing to manage a facility competently but quite another to be razzle-dazzle entrepreneurs. Would the caring reputation that Sebastian had achieved so successfully disappear in a blaze of marketing efforts and joint ventures? The administrator wondered whether Sebastian was hopelessly out of step with its environment.

This case illustrates the dilemma confronting many not-for-profit hospitals. The same or similar problems affect most health services organizations in the sense that they must rapidly adapt to what seem to be revolutionary environmental changes. Interinstitutional competition is less problematic when a community has one of each type of institutional provider. Even in these cases, however, organizations are beginning to offer competing services. It is common that hospitals compete with their medical staff members as both offer highly remunerative outpatient ancillary and diagnostic services. The loss of revenue to hospitals may mean the difference between economic life and death. Such economic tensions diminish the ability of not-for-profit organizations to carry out their historic missions.

Initially viewed with disdain by managers because it conjured up images of individuals with questionable parentage selling unneeded services of little value, marketing has become an accepted, even necessary, part of health services delivery. The preference is still to focus on health promotion and disease/accident prevention and treatment, but marketing is the buzzword; organizations that fail to heed it risk their very survival.

Competition per se is not at variance with a charitable mission. The context has changed and the stakes have increased, but managers should view such changes as a challenge—an opportunity to do what they have been doing even more effectively. Successful corporate restructuring and effective marketing allow the organization to develop revenue streams that enable it to provide charitable services.

A more insidious problem, and one fraught with conflicts of interest, occurs in certain joint ventures between health services organizations, such as hospitals, and their medical staffs. Physicians who earn income by referring patients to providers in which they have an ownership interest or a profit-sharing arrangement have an ethical conflict of interest. States began to prohibit physician referral to such facilities or mandate disclosure to patients. Organized medicine took note of such conflicts of interest in 1985.[23] Since then, several federal laws have set limits on physician self-referral for federal program beneficiaries.

A different philosophical dilemma faced St. Joseph Hospital, which was established in 1870 and owned over its history by various orders of Catholic sisters. In 1971, it was sold to the Creighton Regional Health Care Corporation, a not-for-profit corporation with a lay governing body. It operated St. Joseph as a Roman Catholic teaching hospital for Creighton University. In 1984, a contract was signed with American Medical International (AMI), a for-profit hospital system, under which AMI would acquire St. Joseph Hospital and operate it as a full-service Roman Catholic teaching hospital. Based on this transfer of ownership, the Catholic Health Association (CHA) terminated St. Joseph's membership because "the Hospital is not operated, supervised, or controlled by or in conjunction with the Roman Catholic Church in the United States."[24] The term *full-service* is operative here. The controversy surrounding the decision suggested that other important, unstated reasons were questions about the morality of the profit motive in health services and that other AMI hospitals performed abortions. Critics of CHA's action argued that a profit motive was compatible with St. Joseph's mission and that its bondholders were paid several million dollars of interest—an action indistinguishable from paying dividends to stockholders. St. Joseph continues to be unaffiliated with CHA.[25]

The case of St. Joseph Hospital is important because the CHA acted when a member hospital became incompatible with its philosophy and mission. Regardless of how one judges CHA, its decision was based on a specific philosophy—a crucial underpinning for any organization. The values issues arising from the merger of faith-based and nonsectarian health services organizations can be significant. This is especially true if there are limitations on types of medical services that can be provided (e.g., certain reproductive services in hospitals affiliated with the Roman Catholic Church). Put most starkly, the issue is whether the demands of non-adherents can trump the organization's philosophy (values). It is argued that in a pluralistic society, quasi-public organizations such as hospitals do not have the luxury of limiting services needed and demanded by the public. Providing such services, however, necessarily causes the organization to violate its values or its institutional moral agency—that which personal providers, such as physicians, would call conscience. When a change in ownership eliminates certain reproductive choices, the result is commonly finessed by establishing a freestanding center that has limited, if any, connection with the faith-based organization.

UNDERSTANDING PATIENT BILLS OF RIGHTS

Patient bills of rights (PBOR) provide guidance about the appropriate ethical relationship between the patient and the organization and its staff. Titles vary, but PBOR have been published by such organizations as the American Hospital Association (AHA), The Joint Commission, the U.S. Department of Veterans Affairs (VA), and the American Civil Liberties Union (ACLU). In addition, health services organizations have developed their own statements. PBOR developed by private organizations reflect the law on confidentiality and consent, for example, but are not legally binding. Philosophical differences among the various PBOR are significant.

The AHA first adopted a PBOR in 1973.[26] In 2003, the AHA PBOR was replaced by a brochure titled "The Patient Care Partnership: Understanding Expectations, Rights, and Responsibilities." This plain-language document informs patients about their rights and responsibilities during their hospital stay. There are sections on high-quality hospital care, a clean and safe environment, involvement in one's care, protection of one's privacy, preparing the family for when the patient leaves the hospital, and helping with bill and insurance claims. Specific statements address knowing the identity of doctors, nurses, and other involved in one's care, including their training status; informing the patient if anything unexpected happens during hospitalization; consent; and information regarding power of attorney and advance directives. This statement is patient oriented; it has little institutional bias.[27]

The ACLU's PBOR[28] was drafted as a model law for the states to enact. A much more demanding set of patients' rights distinguishes it philosophically from the AHA's bill. The ACLU bill views the patient as an autonomous individual entitled to full involvement in the care process. For example, the bill mandates that each patient must have access to a 24-hour-per-day patient rights advocate, who may act on behalf of the patient and assert or protect the rights set out in the model bill. In addition, patients have a right to all the information in their medical records and a right to examine and copy them. The ACLU bill details the information to be provided when consent for treatment is obtained. The ACLU PBOR's expectations in protecting patient rights are unconventional, but its provisions are worth considering.

The Department of Veterans Affairs' "Patient and Nursing Home Resident Rights and Responsibilities"[29] and The Joint Commission's "Patient Rights"[30] lie philosophically between the AHA's and ACLU's PBOR. The VA's PBOR recognizes that some patients may have lengthy stays in nursing facilities or hospitals, and there are provisions on the right to wear one's own clothing, keep personal items, and refuse visitors. Specifically mentioned are choosing whether to participate in research, participating in treatment decisions, and, importantly, the right to be informed of all outcomes of care, including potential injuries. Advance directives are identified only by implication. In the 1990s, The Joint Commission standards included the patient's responsibility to cooperate with caregivers. For 2011, its standards emphasize patient rights that organizations are expected to perfect, such as informed consent; providing information about caregivers; patient wishes relating to end-of-life decisions; the duty to respect, protect, and promote patient rights; and a right to gain access to protective and advocacy services. Provisions address ethical issues in research and clinical trials. The Joint Commission's view of the organization's ethical obligation to patients is moving closer to the ACLU's.

Documents such as PBOR developed by health services organizations set an ethical tone for relationships with patients and serve as a nonformal source of law in a dispute. The usefulness of such documents is limited by the organization's willingness to adopt one already available or to develop its own, and, more important, to implement the PBOR by making its contents known to patients and monitoring processes that demonstrate its application.

PBOR statutes have been enacted in 23 states. All establish a grievance policy, four protect a private right of action, and one stipulates fines for violations.[31] PBOR that are state mandates change the dynamics considerably; complying with the law becomes the minimum level of performance. Further, these enactments may change the psychological relationships among patient, staff, and organization. This is not to say that there will less attention paid to the ethics of patients' rights, but that the PBOR enacted by statute may not reflect the values of the organization. Nonetheless, the ethical organization obeys the law.

STRATEGIC MANAGEMENT

The organization's philosophy also affects strategic management (planning). The philosophy must be articulated if objectives are to be consistent and set appropriately. The organization's view of its social responsibility should be reflected in its organizational philosophy and vision and mission statements. Only then should strategic management occur.

An organization's philosophy, vision, and mission state the ideal—ends thought to be unattainable in their idealized version but progress toward which is believed possible.[32] The mission statement must be usable to measure performance, define the organization's business, be unique to the organization, and be relevant to all stakeholders, and it should be exciting, challenging, and inspiring. In contrast, the vision is a verbal picture of what the organization's stakeholders want it to be.[33] In this respect, perhaps the most difficult aspect of developing an organization's strategy is determining the balance between social responsibility and economic performance.[34] The perspective that the health services organization is a social enterprise with an economic dimension may no longer apply; in fact, the external environment may have caused the obverse to be true. Resolving this dilemma and the resulting problems will be increasingly difficult. Although the governing body is primarily responsible for developing a philosophy as well as vision and mission statements, senior management prepares and operationalizes the strategic plan. All participants must ensure that there is consistency between the organization's philosophy and its specific policies, procedures, and rules.

ACHIEVING CONGRUENCE OF PHILOSOPHIES

Several questions should be asked about the relationship between the manager's personal ethic and the organization's philosophy: To what extent must organizational philosophy and the personal ethic of a manager mesh? If the organization is to be a community of shared values, must all managers be in full agreement with the philosophy? As a class, are managers sufficiently professional to be effective in an organization when they may not agree fully with its values? What degree of congruence is needed? A literal interpretation of Deal and Kennedy's work suggests that philosophical divergence is to be discouraged; all values must be shared by all employees, including managers.

Some sectarian health services organizations require that managers at mid-level and above be adherents to the religion of the sponsoring group. Apparently, they judge their philosophy and mission so unique that only coreligionists can effectively manage their organizations. Some moral philosophies are unique, but this requirement seems largely unsupportable. If this policy also breeds conformity and diminishes innovation, it becomes counterproductive.

The organization's interview and preemployment processes should explain its philosophy and determine the applicant's personal ethic about health services and their delivery. This information permits both parties to judge their philosophical congruence, which should occur whether or not the applicant is a coreligionist, because even those of the same faith often have divergent views. Similarly, nonsectarian organizations may not want to employ individuals whose ethic constrains them from participating in services such as electroconvulsive therapy. In such cases, this information can and should be known prospectively.

It is key that persons may reach the same conclusions about an organization's activities and its relationship with patients using a moral philosophy independent of the organization's religious doctrine. These managers would be as effective in achieving the same goals as others in the organization because they share the same values and the same philosophy. The ultimate measure is the congruence between the organization's philosophy and the results of a manager's decision making, although there are other indications. Someone claiming to be morally neutral is potentially the most inimical to an organization seeking to implement a philosophy and strengthen its corporate culture.

CONCLUSION

This chapter examined the importance of a philosophy, or values, in determining and guiding an organization's vision and mission. From them are derived policies and procedures, the stuff from which the abstract and sometimes elusive aspects of an organization are operationalized. Developing a strong corporate culture is the result of shared values. Shared values are crucial in easing discontinuity and achieving corporate effectiveness. However, individuals who disagree must be willing to speak out, and it is problematic if the organization becomes an environment of "group think," which leads to a dangerous level of peer-enforced conformity.

A variety of sources assists in developing an organization's philosophy, including religious affiliation/orientation and humanist/humanitarian motives. Employee and patient bills of rights are also important. Whatever sources an organization uses, the principles of respect for persons, beneficence, nonmaleficence, and justice, as well as complementary virtues, are essential.

NOTES

1. Thomas J. Peters & Robert H. Waterman, Jr. (1982, reissued 1997). *In search of excellence: Lessons from America's best-run companies* (p. 15). New York: Macmillan Library Reference.
2. Terrence E. Deal & Allan A. Kennedy. (1982, reissued in paperback 2000). *Corporate cultures: The rites and rituals of corporate life* (p. 22). New York: Perseus Books Group.
3. *Ibid.*, pp. 13–15.
4. Allan A. Kennedy. (1985, October). Corporate values/corporate culture. In *Excellence in management: Lessons learned from other industries* (pp. 5–7). Report from a special conference for the American College of Hospital Administrators Fellows.
5. Terrence E. Deal, Allan A. Kennedy, & Arthur H. Spiegel, III. (1983, January/February). How to create an outstanding hospital culture. *Hospital Forum 27*, pp. 21–28, 33–34.
6. Amy C. Edmondson & Sandra E. Cha. (2002, November). When company values backfire. *Harvard Business Review 80*(11), pp. 18–19.
7. John P. Kotter & James L. Heskett. (1992). *Corporate culture and performance* (p. 18). New York: The Free Press.
8. Peters & Waterman, pp. 15–16.
9. Joint Commission Resources. (2011). *Ethics framework.* Retrieved January 3, 2001, from http://www.jcrinc.com/Chapter-1-Defining-Main-Components/Developing-and-Implementing-an-Ethical-Infras/Ethics-Framework/.
10. Sutter Health. (n.d.). *Our commitment.* Retrieved November 1, 2010, from http://www.sutterhealth.org/about/comben/commitment/index.html.
11. Trinity Health. (n.d.). *Mission, values, vision.* Retrieved November 1, 2010, from http://www.trinity-health.org/AboutUs/MissionValuesVision/index.htm.
12. George Washington University Medical Center. (n.d.). *Our mission.* Retrieved January 5, 2011, from http://www.gwumc.edu/about/ourmission.
13. MountainView Regional Medical Center. (n.d.). *Mission and values.* Retrieved January 6, 2011, from http://www.mountainviewregional.com/About/Pages/Mission%20and%20Vision.aspx.

14. Mayo Clinic. (n.d.). *Mayo Clinic mission and values*. Retrieved November 1, 2010, from http://www.mayoclinic.org/about/missionvalues.html.
15. Sunrise Senior Living. (n.d.). *Mission, principles of service and core values*. Retrieved November 1, 2010, from http://www.sunriseseniorliving.com/the-sunrise-difference/principles-and-values.aspx.
16. Kenneth J. Williams & Paul R. Donnelly. (1982). *Medical care quality and the public trust*. Santa Monica, CA: Bonus Books.
17. Joint Commission on Accreditation of Healthcare Organizations. (2004). Ethics, rights, and responsibilities. In *Accreditation manual for hospitals*. Oakbrook Terrace, IL: Author.
18. National Conference of State Legislatures. (2010). *Medical professionals apologies 2010 legislation*. Retrieved January 3, 2011, from http://www.ncsl.org/?tabid=21347.
19. Bonnie J. Gray & Robert K. Landrum. (1983, July/September). Difficulties with being ethical. *Business 33*, pp. 28–33.
20. Study: Ethical climate closely linked to employee commitment. (2000, August 18). *ACHe-news*.
21. This case was developed from an incident related to the author by Dorothy H. Mitchell, RN, MSHA, Brunswick, Georgia, May 2003.
22. Ed D. Roach & Bobby G. Bizzell. (1990). Sterling County Hospital. In Jonathon S. Rakich, Beaufort B. Longest, Jr., & Kurt Darr (Eds.), *Cases in health services management* (2nd ed., p. 144). Baltimore: Health Professions Press.
23. Editorial. (1985, September). Dealing with conflicts of interest. *New England Journal of Medicine 313*, pp. 749–751.
24. Richard L. O'Brien & Michael J. Haller. (1985, July). Investor-owned or non-profit? *New England Journal of Medicine 313*, pp. 198–201.
25. Information on the Catholic Hospital Association available at http://www.chausa.org/home/, and on the Creighton University Medical Center at http://www.creightonhospital.com/en-us/aboutus/pages/default.aspx (retrieved December 16, 2010).
26. American Hospital Association. (1992, October 21). *A patient's bill of rights*. Retrieved November 18, 2003, from http://www.hospitalconnect.com/aha/about/pbillofrights.html.
27. American Hospital Association. (n.d.). *The patient care partnership: Understanding expectations, rights, and responsibilities*. Retrieved March 12, 2011, from http://www.aha.org/aha/issues/Communicating-With-Patients/pt-care-partnership.html.
28. George J. Annas. (2004). *The rights of patients: The authoritative ACLU guide to the rights of patients*, 3rd ed. New York: New York University Press, pp. 14–16.
29. U.S. Department of Veterans Affairs. (2006). *Patient and nursing home resident rights and responsibilities*. Retrieved January 5, 2011, from http://www.patientadvocate.va.gov/rights.asp.
30. The Joint Commission on Accreditation of Healthcare Organizations. *Patient rights*. Retrieved January 4, 2011, from http://e-dition.jcrinc.com/Browse.aspx?P=2&C=53&Seq=11.
31. Michael K. Paasche-Orlow, Dan M. Jacob, Mark Hochhauser, & Ruth M. Parker. (2008). National survey of patients' bill of rights statues. *Journal of General Internal Medicine 24*(4), pp. 489–494. The authors note that average

U.S. adults read at an 8th-grade level, yet PBOR usually require advanced college reading. This raises a crucial aspect of effectively implementing PBORs.

32. Russell L. Ackoff. (1981). *Creating the corporate future.* New York: John Wiley & Sons.
33. Russell L. Ackoff. (1999). *Re-creating the corporation: A design of organizations for the 21st century* (pp. 83–84, 87). New York: Oxford University Press.
34. James Webber. (1982, April 1). Planning. *Hospitals 56,* pp. 69–70.

CHAPTER 4

CODES OF ETHICS
IN HEALTH SERVICES

Many factors influence human behavior and interaction. Among the most basic are those arising from the individual's legal relationships with society—those increasingly pervasive laws, ordinances, regulations, and court decisions. Other formal sources of law, such as the bylaws of a corporation, apply only to a specific entity. The link between formal sources of law and ethics was described in the Introduction. In addition, there are nonformal sources of law, such as standards of justice, public policies, moral convictions, customary laws, and notions of individual equity. Both formal and nonformal sources of law are used by health services organizations. Codes of ethics adopted by professional associations are important because they state goals and aspirations, guide members, and serve as a reference point to discipline those who deviate from the norm.

In 1978, the U.S. Congress created the Office of Government Ethics (OGE) in the executive branch to prevent conflicts of interest on the part of government employees and to resolve those that occur.[1] The law requires financial disclosure and restricts activities after leaving government service, accepting gifts from outside sources, and "extracurricular" earned income, honoraria, and employment. Remote or inconsequential financial interests are not thought to affect integrity and are therefore exempt. OGE's primary source of information is the employee's annual financial disclosure statement. Similarly, states provide ethical and legal guidance for their employees.[2]

Self-regulation is a hallmark of the learned professions, historically, law, medicine, and the clergy. Their ethics are reflected in bar discipline, principles of medical ethics, and ecclesiastic law. As law and medicine, as well as newer professions, sought regulation (economic protection) through legislation, or as regulation was forced on them, many of their ethical principles were incorporated into statutes or regulations, or, for lawyers, court-adopted rules of professional conduct.

Groups seeking professional status adopt codes of ethics. Codes are common in health services, and managerial, clinical, and technical groups have them. Their language is usually general, and performance standards are typically so vague as to make fair enforcement impossible. In the latter regard, the profession of law is a notable exception. A wag would say that this is as it should be, because lawyers seem plagued by ethics problems. The American Bar Association (ABA) is a private association that has developed Model Rules of Professional Conduct. These rules, as well as codes of conduct developed by state bar associations, reflect the profession's ethics. These statements of professional ethics take on the weight of judicial sanction because a state's highest court uses them to develop its rules of professional conduct for lawyers licensed in the state. Furthermore, these rules are used to sanction errant lawyers. For example, as officers of the court, lawyers have a duty to inform the appropriate professional authority if they know that another lawyer has violated the rules of conduct in a way that raises a substantial question as to the lawyer's honesty, trustworthiness, or fitness as a lawyer in other respects.[3] The state's highest court typically appoints a board of professional responsibility to enforce its rules and to review and investigate complaints, which are heard by a special panel of judges. Adverse action by this panel results in penalties ranging from admonition or probation to suspension or revocation of the lawyer's license to practice law.

It is clear, however, that even with reasonably stringent enforcement, a code of ethics can only guide the behavior and decisions of individuals who want to do the right thing but need help determining what that is. Individuals trying to get away with something are always on the fringes of a profession, and principles of ethical conduct (and legal requirements) only encourage them to become more devious to avoid being caught. Even in the absence of a code, some actions inevitably raise questions of character.

Mr. B

Mr. B sought a job as a health services consultant. He contacted two firms and was interviewed by both. One offered him a position. Mr. B verbally accepted the offer, even though it meant moving his family. Several days later, as a courtesy, he called the second firm to tell them he had taken a position. The managing partner said, "Gee, that's really too bad. I was going to offer you a job in your area and pay you $5,000 more than you got from the other firm."

Mr. B has an ethical problem. There is no written agreement, but he verbally accepted the first offer—he gave his word. Were Mr. B to call the first firm and explain what happened, they would likely release him. After all, who wants a disgruntled employee? This action does not affect his ethical obligation to take the job he accepted, however. Having given his word, Mr. B made a commitment that he is morally bound to keep. The virtue of promise keeping applies here. Only if Mr. B can show morally overriding considerations, such as great hardship to his family, can he avoid his commitment.

CODES FOR MANAGERS

In addition to what is considered minimally acceptable, codes also state the vision of the profession. The goals stated in the vision may be unachievable. The profession must work toward them, nonetheless, because progress is possible. These aspects of codes of ethics are similar to the philosophy and vision statements developed by organizations.

In the sister field of business, the corporate scandals of the late 20th and early 21st centuries highlighted the importance of business ethics. These scandals caused educators to reconsider the place of teaching ethics in business programs and to give their graduates a better grounding in values that may prevent similar problems in the future. Accredited schools of business must provide ethics education in both the general knowledge and skills portion of the accreditation standards for undergraduates, and the management-specific portion of the standards for undergraduate and graduate students.[4] Like any business skill, the importance of reinforcing application of appropriate values in business has been known for decades; experts agree that ethics can be taught *and* learned, and that moral development takes place in everyone.[5] The implications? Classroom and continuing education in ethics for health services managers is essential, despite the skepticism of some.[6]

Health Services Executives

First among health services management professional associations is the American College of Healthcare Executives (ACHE), known before mid-1985 as the American College of Hospital Administrators. In 2010, the ACHE had more than 38,000 members.[7] The ACHE has had a Code of Ethics since 1939, 6 years after its founding. Initially, it was linked to the code of ethics for hospitals developed by the American Hospital Association

(AHA). Ensuing iterations made the ACHE code distinct; it also became more explicit than the AHA code. A major revision of the ACHE code occurred in 1987, and significant changes were again made in 2003.

The latest iteration of the code was adopted in 2007. The preamble establishes a context for the code and continues the concept introduced in 1987 that the health services manager is a moral *advocate* (*moral agent* was used in 1987) who must evaluate the possible outcomes of any decisions. It is suggested but not explicitly stated that healthcare executives are morally responsible for their decisions. Noteworthy is the executive's obligation to act in ways that will merit the trust, confidence, and respect of healthcare professionals and the public, and that, therefore, they "should lead lives that embody an exemplary system of values and ethics." This expectation melds the public and private lives of healthcare executives, and it is reinforced by a code provision that directs healthcare executives to refrain from participating in any activity that demeans the profession's credibility and dignity.

The 2007 iteration has five sections that detail the healthcare executive's responsibilities to the profession, to patients or others served, to the organization, to employees, and to the community and society. A sixth section charges affiliates who have reasonable grounds to believe that another affiliate has violated the code with a positive duty to communicate such facts to the ethics committee. A lengthy section on conflicts of interest in earlier iterations has been replaced by a modest and largely inadequate dictate to "disclose financial and other conflicts of interest."

In 2003, the section on the executive's responsibilities to the organization was substantially expanded. Added were the need to report negative information, prevent fraud and abuse and aggressive accounting that may result in disputable financial reports, act to minimize clinical and management errors and disclose them when they occur, implement an organizational code of ethics and monitor compliance, and provide ethics resources to staff to address organizational and clinical issues. These important additions were retained in the 2007 iteration.

The code pays little attention to the role of managers in resolving biomedical ethical issues. It does, however, include the need to establish a process that both resolves values conflicts among patients (and their families) and staff and ensures patient autonomy and self-determination. An important continuing lapse is attention to the independent moral duty that healthcare executives owe to patients. For example, the code has yet to define the limits of loyalty (fidelity) to the organization and the point at which it is superseded by an ethical duty to the patient. This is a vital facet of the manager as moral agent (advocate) and an essential element of the code as a living document that builds professional self-respect and esprit de corps.

Disciplinary actions under the code are highly structured and emphasize thoroughness and fairness. The ethics committee receives complaints alleging unethical conduct. The process includes initial screening of the complaint by the committee chair, informing the respondent (the affiliate) of the allegations, investigating the allegations, and the issuing of a recommendation from the committee to the board of governors. The respondent may appeal the committee's adverse findings and recommendations. The first appeal is to the board of governors. If unsuccessful, a second appeal is made to an ad hoc committee appointed by the board of governors. This committee has the authority to affirm the decision of the board of governors or to impose a lesser sanction. All information developed in the process is privileged.[8]

This lengthy grievance process is consistent with the expectations of procedural and substantive due process usually found in private associations. Judicial review is possible, but courts are reluctant to intervene in the actions of private associations. Expulsion is the maximum disciplinary action available to the ACHE or any private association. Because affiliation is not linked to licensure, expulsion is significant only if colleagues and potential employers consider membership in the ACHE important and identify expulsion as a measure of the individual's professional character. If they do, the former affiliate's employment and career opportunities become more limited. Enforcement makes codes of ethics vital, living documents that offer greater usefulness to members as they confront ethical issues and work to solve them.

The ACHE supplements its code by issuing policy statements that suggest a standard of behavior and offer specific guidance for members. Many address ethical issues: establishing an ethical environment for employees, decisions near the end of life, impaired healthcare executives, and health information confidentiality.[9] The 2007 ACHE Code of Ethics is reproduced in Appendix B.

Nursing Facility Administrators

The American College of Health Care Administrators (ACHCA) has approximately 2,500 members, the majority of whom are managers of long-term care facilities.[10] Its 2003 code is reproduced in Appendix B.

Members are obliged to meet four "expectations," which are divided into prescriptions and proscriptions.[11] The expectations state that members shall: 1) hold paramount the welfare of persons for whom care is provided; 2) maintain high standards of professional competence; 3) strive, in all matters relating to their professional functions, to maintain a professional posture that places paramount the interests of the facility and its residents; and 4) honor their responsibilities to the public, their profession, and relationships with colleagues and members of related professions. The prescriptions and proscriptions are analogues. Examples of issues presented include addressing the quality of services; maintaining confidentiality of information about recipients of care; providing continuing education; handling conflicts of interest; and fostering increased knowledge, supporting research, and sharing expertise.

Like the ACHE, the ACHCA expects members to provide information to its standards and ethics committee of actual or potential code violations and to cooperate with inquiries into matters of professional conduct related to the code of ethics. The latter requirement suggests a disciplinary dimension, but neither enforcement nor appeals processes are included. The code's preamble states that the ultimate responsibility for applying standards and ethics falls to the individual. The ACHCA code pays even less attention to biomedical ethical issues than does the ACHE code—an important lapse for both groups.

Public Health

The American Public Health Association (APHA) is the professional association for public health practitioners. The APHA has no code of ethics, but its website links to several sources that provide ethical guidelines for practice and research in public health.

The best source of ethical guidance for public health practitioners is found in the "Principles of the Ethical Practice of Public Health," developed by the Public Health Leadership Society and published in 2002. It reads as follows:[12]

1. Public health should address principally the fundamental causes of disease and requirements for health, aiming to prevent adverse health outcomes.
2. Public health should achieve community health in a way that respects the rights of individuals in the community.
3. Public health policies, programs, and priorities should be developed and evaluated through processes that ensure an opportunity for input from community members.
4. Public health should advocate and work for the empowerment of disenfranchised community members, aiming to ensure that the basic resources and conditions necessary for health are accessible to all.

5. Public health should seek the information needed to implement effective policies and programs that protect and promote health.

6. Public health institutions should provide communities with the information they have that is needed for decisions on policies or programs and should obtain the community's consent for their implementation.

7. Public health institutions should act in a timely manner on the information they have within the resources and the mandate given to them by the public.

8. Public health programs and policies should incorporate a variety of approaches that anticipate and respect diverse values, beliefs, and cultures in the community.

9. Public health programs and policies should be implemented in a manner that most enhances the physical and social environment.

10. Public health institutions should protect the confidentiality of information that can bring harm to an individual or community if made public. Exceptions must be justified on the basis of the high likelihood of significant harm to the individual or others.

11. Public health institutions should ensure the professional competence of their employees.

12. Public health institutions and their employees should engage in collaborations and affiliations in ways that build the public's trust and the institution's effectiveness.

A separate section explains each principle. It is unclear how and by whom (or what) success (or failure) is judged. There is no attention to the ethical implications of good management and the need to use resources wisely. Apparently, individual managers and/or their organizations make these judgments. No enforcement mechanisms for the principles are identified.

CODES FOR CAREGIVERS

Physicians

Codes of ethics in medicine date from the 18th century B.C. and the Code of Hammurabi, which established fee schedules for physicians and veterinarians. It imposed harsh punishments if a physician harmed a patient, including the loss of a physician's hands if treatment resulted in the loss of a patient's eye or life.

A very different code developed from the teaching and work of Hippocrates (circa 460–370 B.C.). A ruler imposed the Code of Hammurabi, but the Hippocratic philosophy governing relationships among physicians and between physicians and patients was developed by Greek physicians, one of whom may have been Hippocrates, for their own use. The Hippocratic oath has never received public sanction or force of law. It established standards of conduct, some of which are found in contemporary codes of medical ethics, as well as in state licensing and regulation of physicians.

The Hippocratic oath contains a largely obsolete section describing expected relationships between physicians and their teachers and students. Other provisions no longer used include restrictions on performing surgery, assisting in abortion, and only applying dietetic measures in healing. Hippocratic prohibitions on assisting in suicide and refraining from sexual misconduct with patients and others in the household, as well as broad restrictions on confidentiality of information learned during treatment, are found in contemporary codes, explicitly or implicitly.

The American Medical Association (AMA) was founded in 1847. Its first code of medical ethics was based on the work of Sir Thomas Percival, English physician, philosopher, and writer. Revisions of the AMA's code, Principles of Medical Ethics, occurred in 1912, 1957, 1980, and 2001.[13] The revision of the 1980 principles added precision to professional ethics for physicians. The changes were not as dramatic as those between the 1957 and 1980 versions, however. The 1980 version eliminated proscriptions on advertising and voluntarily associating with practitioners who have no scientific basis for treatment. In addition, the 1957 principles had a strong element of paternalism—physicians were expected to act in ways *that they considered to be in the patient's best interests.* Eliminating that provision reflected a major philosophical shift for the AMA. In commenting on the changes between the 1957 and 1980 versions of the principles, Veatch[14] observed, "It is the first document in the history of professional medical ethics in which a group of physicians is willing to use the language of responsibilities and rights," rather than that of benefits and harms.

The 2001 iteration (reproduced in Appendix B) continues to emphasize providing competent medical care, honesty in all professional interactions, and safeguarding patient confidences. Changes from the 1980 version include adding *rights,* with the expectation that physicians will provide medical care with "respect for human dignity and rights," will "maintain a commitment to medical education," and will participate in activities contributing to "the betterment of public health." New principles VIII and IX state that "a physician shall, while caring for a patient, regard responsibility to the patient as paramount," and that "a physician shall support access to medical care for all people," respectively. Principle II has been reworded to state that AMA members "shall . . . strive to report physicians deficient in character or competence, or engaging in fraud or deception, to appropriate entities."[15] Critics of organized medicine argue that this continuing, vital duty has been widely ignored.

The AMA's Council on Ethical and Judicial Affairs assists members in interpreting the principles by publishing opinions on issues such as experimentation, genetic engineering, abortion, and terminal illness. These opinions usefully supplement the Principles of Medical Ethics. The 1993 statement, "Fundamental Elements of the Patient–Physician Relationship," complements the AMA's principles by focusing on the rights of patients (see Appendix B).

Just as it is clear that health services managers and their organizations benefit from increased attention to ethics, there is also evidence that physicians (and their patients) can benefit from education in ethics, professionalism, and moral reasoning: "[Orthopedists] with higher moral reasoning and levels of professionalism . . . perform better clinically [and] also have fewer malpractice claims."[16]

Nurses

The American Nurses Association (ANA) code of ethics was first formally adopted in 1950, although precursors date from the "Nightingale Pledge" of 1893.[17] The preface to the 2001 iteration of the Code of Ethics for Nurses (reproduced in Appendix B) states that the code includes humanist, feminist, and social ethics; adherence to ethical principles; and the cultivation of virtues. It also asserts that

> The ethical tradition of nursing is self-reflective, enduring, and distinctive. . . . *The Code of Ethics with Interpretive Statements* provides a framework for nurses to use in ethical analysis and decision-making. The Code of Ethics establishes the ethical standard for the profession. It is not negotiable in any setting nor is it subject to revision or amendment except by . . . the ANA.[18]

Noted in a description of the code's evolution are doing no harm (nonmaleficence), benefiting others (beneficence), loyalty, honesty, social justice, and the autonomy of patient and nurse.[19]

Code expectations run a gamut that includes principles to guide practice, primary commitment to the patient, individual accountability, duties to self and others, improving healthcare, advancing the profession, collaboration, and obligations to the profession. Many of the code's nir sions are specific. An interpretive statement follows each ⊤ ⸜ nurses are obligated to counter or expose problem⸢ⸯ promotes, advocates for, and strives to protect th of the patient." The interpretive statement discu the context of privacy, confidentiality, research, sta questionable and impaired practice.[20] Nursing has ti

In the recent past, nurses have been consistently perceived as the most honest and ethical professional group. In 2009, they outpolled physicians 83% to 65% and were rated highest of any group identified in the survey.[21]

CODES FOR ORGANIZATIONS

Hospitals

The AHA, the most important trade association for hospitals, last revised its guidelines for ethical conduct in 1992.[22] The guidelines are divided into community role, patient's care, and organizational conduct. Members are expected to improve community health status and deliver high-quality, comprehensive services efficiently. The importance of coordinating with other health services organizations is emphasized. Some provisions are specific: the need for informed consent; confidentiality; and mechanisms to resolve conflicting values and ethical dilemmas among patients and families, medical staff, employees, the organization, and the community. Members should try to accommodate the religious and social beliefs and customs of patients whenever possible. The guidelines identify the expectations regarding employee policies and practices and the accommodation of religious and moral values held by employees and medical staff. Conflicts of interest are defined. Neither disciplinary nor grievance proceedings are included.

Long-Term Care Facilities

The American Health Care Association (AHCA) is the national association of state associations of long-term care facilities, primarily nursing facilities. Its code of ethics was developed for use by the AHCA as an organization, but it is intended to serve as a model for its state members and, in turn, their facility members. The AHCA's organizational values, as identified in the preamble, include concern for individuals in need, quality service, service to the community, integrity and honesty, fairness, accountability, respect for employees, and stewardship. Topics in the body of the code include moral responsibility, good business practices, making difficult choices, acting responsibly, the obligation to provide quality service, dealing with conflicting values, the use of information, responsible advocacy, potential conflicts of interest, respect for others, and fairness in competition.[23] AHCA's code is not a tool for certification and there are no sanctions for failing to meet its standards. Some states require nursing facilities receiving Medicaid funds to follow a patient bill of rights based on that of AHCA.

The American Association of Homes and Services for the Aging (AAHSA) is the national association that represents not-for-profit or government-sponsored organizations that provide housing, health, community, and related services to meet the needs of older adults. AAHSA's ethics are reflected in its "Membership Covenant," which was first adopted in 1991. Its current covenant, adopted in 2001, includes a set of beliefs and a set of values.[24] The beliefs focus on quality of care and services; the value of elders in society; the special role of not-for-profit organizations; the role of legal, ethical, and professional standards in member organizations; offering programs and services based on contemporary research; and the leadership role of the AAHSA. Specific stewardship responsibilities include continuous quality improvement, public disclosure and accountability, consumer and family rights, workforce excellence, community involvement, ethical practices, and financial integrity. The membership covenant has no reporting or disciplinary process.

PHILOSOPHICAL BASES FOR CODES OF ETHICS

Codes of ethics for the health professions blend various moral philosophies and ethical theories. To a varying extent, the principles of respect for persons, beneficence, nonmaleficence, and justice, as well as several of the virtues, are found in all codes.

The ACHE and ACHCA codes blend consequentialism (teleology), deontology, and virtue ethics but emphasize the latter two. Respect for persons and beneficence predominate. The statements on confidential information, for example, are grounded in deontology and virtue ethics, not in consequences. As noted, the duty to report violations was added to the ACHE code in 1987. In 2003, it required that "an affiliate of ACHE who has reasonable grounds to believe another affiliate has violated this *Code* has a duty to communicate such facts to the Ethics Committee."[25] In 2003, the ACHCA code contained a similar provision.

The preamble of the 2001 Principles of Medical Ethics of the AMA provides the context of its amended view of physician duty and respect for patients: "A physician must recognize responsibility to patients first and foremost, as well as to society, to other health professionals, and to self."[26] This philosophy is absent in the Hippocratic oath and the 1957 AMA principles, which emphasized paternalism. This change carries important implications for resource allocation by suggesting that physicians must consider the societal or broader effects of individual treatment. This admonition is based on justice rather than beneficence (which focuses on patients) and adds a dimension of utilitarianism—to consider the greatest good for the greatest number.

As noted, the underpinnings of the ANA's Code of Ethics for Nurses include several moral philosophies. The code remains grounded in deontology, however, which is duty based. Within this context, respect for persons, nonmaleficence, beneficence, and justice undergird relationships with patients, and the virtues of self-improvement, collaboration, and integrity are stressed.

APPLYING CODES OF ETHICS

Use and Enforcement

As noted, codes of ethics should be living documents that are used and applied by an association. General education about code provisions is the first step. In addition, the professions must provide members with regular information about the code's interpretation, application, and enforcement. However, more attention should be given to making health services administrative or institutional codes living documents that are useful in guiding decisions. Encouraging and responding to this interest remain important challenges to the professional associations. It is encouraging that the majority of managers in leadership positions have used the ACHE code to teach others about expected behaviors and to counsel colleagues.[27]

Educating, counseling, and propagating professionalism among members are vital uses for codes. They assume even greater importance and usefulness when they are enforced. Unenforced, they are platitudes, seemingly intended primarily for public consumption. Enforceable codes are precise and include interpretation of provisions. Absent sufficient detail to guide members, enforcement results in arbitrary decision making and a lack of fairness. As noted, private associations are unlikely to be held to constitutional requirements of due process, but it is nonetheless fair (just) that they meet such a standard. This theme should underlie an association's relationships with members. Enforcement with feedback to members provides additional knowledge and understanding for the profession and makes the code a living document. This crucial attribute uses casuistry in building a body of cases and experience.

When health services professionals are licensed, disciplinary actions are usually a matter of public record. Reports of disciplinary actions against the licenses of physicians and other caregivers appear occasionally in the press. Among health services managers, only nursing home administrators are licensed—the result of significant historical problems in nursing facilities. Scandals elsewhere in health services could lead to demands for licensure of managers, an approach less desirable and likely no more effective than self-regulation. This scenario highlights the importance of the profession's voluntary efforts and the need to enforce usable, living codes of ethics.

Separating Private and Public Actions

Health services managers are quasi-public figures; the public's interest in them and their organizations is a function of the latter's prominence in the community. A manager's public role is greater in small communities, in which the organization, especially an acute care hospital, is economically, politically, and socially significant. This prominence means that health services managers are community leaders ex officio. They are in a fishbowl whether or not they desire it. Managers of major health services organizations in urban areas are also de facto community leaders. Health services managers must be prepared to accept this trust and use the public's confidence to improve community health. Such a role demands exceptional performance.

Private citizens have a broad zone of privacy. Persons who become community leaders diminish their zone of privacy, and greater prominence diminishes privacy further. Younger, less experienced managers have difficulty understanding that persons in positions of prominence cannot escape public scrutiny. These managers jealously guard their privacy and generally consider what happens in their personal lives to be irrelevant to their performance as managers. Would that this were so. Their role in the organization and the public's expectations deny them this luxury. New to the next generation of health services managers are the temptations of the social media. Increasingly, potential employers are reviewing social media postings by applicants to see if what is stated or shown there raises questions of competence or moral turpitude that might be disqualifying. Persons whose lives are an open book should expect the information to be used by anyone with access to those online services.

Three dimensions affect the dynamic between public and private lives: 1) the corrupt moral standard that the right or wrong of an action is unimportant—the question is whether one is caught; 2) the organization's culture and the community standard of behavior and morality; and 3) administrative effectiveness. "It's okay if you don't get caught" or "It's okay, everybody's doing it" are unacceptable bromides for health services managers. The following simple examples highlight the effect of such views. Most employees would be embarrassed to be seen photocopying personal papers at their place of employment or to have their superiors note personal long-distance telephone calls made at the organization's expense. Wasted time, personal use of office supplies and equipment, and personal telephone calls will not result in disciplinary action by either a professional association or the organization (except in extreme cases). Such actions must be regulated by the individual's personal ethic. Members of the profession must consider that small infractions are governed by the principles developed in Chapter 1, as well as by their personal ethic.

The organization's philosophy and the community standard of morality are important because they affect managers' views of what is acceptable, thus tempering the manager's personal ethic. The micro-community that is the organization develops a culture whose mores and standards are unique, demanding, and ignored at one's peril.

Organizational Culture

It Just Isn't Done!

Several university faculty were invited to have lunch with 20 middle- and senior-level managers of a data processing firm. The group was enthusiastic and highly motivated; most were younger than age 40. Lunch was a break in a long day of seminars and meetings. When the waiter asked for drink orders, no one from the firm ordered an alcoholic beverage. Instead, they ordered milk or soda. One of the faculty remarked about this unusual behavior and was told there was an unwritten company policy that no member of the staff should go back to work after having an alcoholic beverage.

This attitude may seem straitlaced, and it is certainly different from the "two-martini lunch" once described as the norm in business. Yet this "rule" reflected the group's self-view (culture), and substantial peer pressure would likely be directed at anyone who disregarded it. On both a macro- and a micro-level, this is the type of influence that health services managers can bring to bear for the good of patient and profession.

Administrative effectiveness is a question for the manager's manager, who determines whether problems have fatally flawed someone's ability to lead. Managers with badly tarnished reputations lose their effectiveness. Managers who are ridiculed, whose character deficits are blatant and widely known, or for whom respect is eroded or gone must be dismissed.

An example of private behavior considered unacceptable in a health services manager is driving while intoxicated (DWI). Regardless of the view held by professional associations, governing bodies are intolerant of managers charged with DWI, even though such behavior for a housekeeper would go unnoticed. Problems such as DWI run counter to the organization's view of the manager qua leader and its philosophy, which will be unwritten for problems such as alcohol and drug abuse, illicit sexual activity, and spouse abuse. Illegal activities are unethical per se. They are not explicitly prohibited because they run so counter to good character.

A further reason such behavior is unacceptable is that the governing body has no wish to be embarrassed by an errant manager. An organization faced with scandal will separate itself from the source. This reaction reflects the instinct for organizational survival as well as indignation and moral revulsion. Instilling an awareness of the importance of ethical behavior in others is a continuing challenge in organizations.

It may seem unfair that managers are held to a higher standard than the larger community. Employees and the public expect more of leaders than of followers. The health services management profession correctly expects its members to avoid the temptations and problems affecting those outside it.

This a Laughing Matter?

One afternoon, Joan Zimmerman, the chief operating officer of a large hospital, encountered two younger members of her management staff conversing in hushed tones. As she approached unnoticed, they burst into laughter. One of the two blushed and turned his eyes downward as Zimmerman greeted them and asked lightheartedly about the source of their amusement. Neither spoke. Sensing there was something she should know, Zimmerman pressed for an answer. The awkward situation was interrupted by Zimmerman's pager, which asked her to call the operator immediately. Later, one of the two managers asked to see her. He related an amazing story about the female director of a support department with a high turnover rate. In routine exit interviews conducted by human resources, several young male employees said they were leaving because they could no longer endure the sexual harassment by the department's director, who insisted that the young men have sex with her. Employees who refused were given the worst schedules and treated badly in other ways.

Zimmerman was told that the problem had existed for some time and was an open secret in the hospital. She was shocked and distressed that she had not been told.

This case has several dimensions. First, sexual harassment is against the law. Second, sexual harassment breaches the principle of respect for persons.

Third, the unfair treatment of staff by the department head breaches the principle of justice. Finally, the department director has failed to live the virtues of self-control, temperance, and integrity.

The immediate problem is to investigate the allegations against the department director and take disciplinary action, if appropriate. Also of concern is that younger managers were amused, not offended. Their reaction may show immaturity rather than approval or true amusement; regardless, it is a problem that needs attention. Managers lead by words and actions; actions are far more important.

Two other issues must be addressed. The first is that Zimmerman was unaware of the problem. The second is the lack of action taken by staff and managers who knew of the allegations, which, if true, cast a shadow over the organization. First among staff who should have been more alert and taken action are those in human resources (HR). Turnover in a unit should be investigated by HR and appropriate action taken. Exit interviews are a common means to obtain information about matters needing such attention.

Zimmerman must make clear to all staff that such behavior is intolerable. It breaches the trust reposed in managers, breaches their fiduciary duty to the staff and the organization, and is inconsistent with any viable organizational philosophy. If true, the alleged actions of the support department director diminish the regard in which all managers in the organization are held, and, ultimately, diminish organizational effectiveness. Cynicism can become a cancer that will destroy the organization.

CONCLUSION

Most codes of ethics provide only general guidelines. Even specific provisions require interpretation and the courage to apply them. Interpretation is crucial, because even great detail cannot address the nuances and intricacies of all circumstances. A highly detailed code would be excessively legalistic; applying it would be impractical and nightmarish.

Of the professional groups in health services management, the ACHE has the most detailed code. This detail enhances its usefulness to guide health services managers, whether or not they are ACHE members. In most respects, however, the code is too general to provide performance standards.

Codes in the health services field carry only the sanctions available to the professional association, of which expulsion is the maximum disciplinary action. This limitation is unlikely to affect the individual's legal right to engage in the profession.

In addition to the expectations of ethical codes, state law regulates most clinicians. Licensure statutes—or *practice acts*—incorporate ethical principles similar to their private associations, and licensing boards are usually composed of individuals from the profession being regulated. This tends to give the group's ethical precepts the force of law; breaching them could lead to license suspension or revocation. It is noteworthy that the proceedings of public regulators are distinct from those of private associations or professional groups. A license is a condition of membership in the professional association, but membership in the association is not required for licensure—an appropriate distinction between private and public action.

For groups such as hospital managers, the lack of licensure increases the importance of self-regulation. The public looks to such professionals as important in safeguarding health services delivery. Unless self-regulation is effective and maintains the public's confidence, licensing or another form of governmental regulation will result.

Another pragmatic consideration is what contributes to managers' success. Historically, integrity was identified as the personality trait most important for success, more important than any other skill or factor.[28] Integrity's importance undoubtedly continues. This additional stimulus to be ethical and above reproach in all aspects of their lives should cause health services managers to be vigilant about themselves and their colleagues. These are significant reasons for maintaining the public's trust in health services managers and their organizations.

More important than pragmatism to encourage ethical behavior is that it is the right thing to do—it is a principle for life and the profession. The slightest hint of impropriety in personal behavior must be avoided. What a tragedy for the late Hyman G. Rickover, father of the nuclear submarine fleet and a retired U.S. Navy admiral, with an astounding 64 years on active duty, to be forced to admit that be took gifts from defense contractors. Rickover claimed that the gifts were trinkets and that taking them did not affect his judgment. The Secretary of the Navy insisted that the gifts were worth tens of thousands of dollars. Whatever the facts, these revelations badly, and sadly, tarnished a distinguished career. It is just such situations that health services managers must assiduously avoid. Failing this, managers damage the public trust, risk their careers and reputations, and violate the principles of any personal ethic worthy of the name.

NOTES

1. U.S. Office of Government Ethics. (n.d.). *Background and mission*. Retrieved February 22, 2011, from http://www.usoge.gov/about/background_mission .aspx.
2. Anita Cava, Jonathan West, & Evan Berman. (1995, Spring). Ethical decision-making in business and government: An analysis of formal and informal strategies. *Spectrum 68*(2), pp. 34–35.
3. American Bar Association. (n.d.). *Rule 8.3: Reporting professional misconduct*. Retrieved April 14, 2004, from http://www.abanet.org/cpr/mrpc/rule_8_3.html.
4. Association to Advance Collegiate Schools of Business. (n.d.). *Frequently asked questions: Why won't AACSB international require a course in ethics for all business programs?* Retrieved November 12, 2010, from http://www.aacsb.edu/ resources/ethics-sustainability/faq.asp.
5. Peter Arlow & Thomas A. Ulrich. (1983, Spring). Can ethics be taught to business students? *Collegiate Forum*, p. 17; Archie B. Carroll. (2003, February 17). Can ethics be taught? *UGA News Service*. Retrieved November 14, 2003, from http://www.uga.edu/columns/030217/news12.html; Ameet Sachdev. (2003, February 14). Ethics moves to head of class. *Chicago Tribune*. Retrieved February 23, 2011, from http://articles.chicagotribune.com/2003-02-14/ business/0302140374_1_ethics-and-leadership-training-advance-collegiate -schools-business-schools.
6. Dan Seligman. (2002, October 28). Oxymoron 101. *Forbes*, pp. 160, 162, 164.
7. American College of Healthcare Executives. (2010). *ACHE annual report, 2010*. Retrieved February 23, 2011, from http://www.ache.org/abt_ACHE/ annual_report/10_annual_report/ACHE_Annual_Report_10.pdf.
8. American College of Healthcare Executives. (n.d.) *ACHE grievance procedure*. Retrieved October 8, 2010, from http://www.ache.org/abt_ache/grievance .cfm.
9. American College of Healthcare Executives. (2003). *ACHE ethical policy statements*. Retrieved March 16, 2011, from http://www.ache.org/policy/index_eth ics.cfm.
10. Whitney O'Donnell, member services coordinator, ACHCA, personal communication, January 4, 2011.
11. American College of Health Care Administrators. (n.d.). *Advocacy: Code*. Retrieved March 1, 2011, from http://www.ache.org/abt_ache/facts.cfm.
12. Public Health Leadership Society. (2002). *Principles of the ethical practice of public health: Version 2.2*. Retrieved March 16, 2011, from http://www.apha.org/ NR/rdonlyres/1CED3CEA-287E-4185-9CBD-BD405FC60856/0/ethicsbro chure.pdf.
13. Tanya Albert. (2001, January 1). AMA's Principles of Medical Ethics may be infused with new "lofty ideas." *American Medical News*. Retrieved August 18, 2003, from http://www.ama-assn.org/amednews/2001/01/01/prsa0101.htm.
14. Robert M. Veatch. (1980, June). Professional ethics: New principles for physicians? *Hastings Center Report 10*, p. 17.
15. American Medical Association. (2003). *Newly adopted principles of medical ethics, June 2001*. Retrieved March 16, 2011, from http://www.ama-assn.org/ama/

pub/physician-resources/medical-ethics/code-medical-ethics/principles-medi
cal-ethics.shtml.

16. DeWitt C. Baldwin, Jr., & Wilton H. Bunch. (2000, September). *Moral reasoning, professionalism, and the teaching of ethics to orthopaedic surgeons.*
Clinical Orthopaedics and Related Research 378, pp. 97–103.

17. American Nurses Association. (2001). *Code of ethics for nurses with interpretive
statements.* Retrieved January 4, 2011, http://www.nursingworld.org/MainMe
nuCategories/EthicsStandards/CodeofEthicsforNurses/Code-of-Ethics.aspx.

18. *Ibid.;* extract reprinted by permission.

19. *Ibid.*

20. *Ibid.*

21. Jeffrey M. Jones. (2009, December 9). U.S. clergy, bankers see new lows in
honesty/ethics ratings. *Gallup.* Retrieved December 16, 2010, from http://
www.gallup.com/poll/124628/clergy-bankers-new-lows-honesty-ethics-rat
ings.aspx.

22. American Hospital Association. (1992). *Hospital management advisory: Ethical
conduct for health care institutions.* Chicago: Author.

23. American Health Care Association. (2003). *Code of ethics.* Retrieved March 16,
2011, from http://www.ahcancal.org/about_ahca/MembersOnlyDocs/AHCA
_code_of_ethics.pdf.

24. American Association of Homes and Services for the Aging. (2001). *AAHSA
membership covenant.* Retrieved March 16, 2011, from http://www.aahsa.org/
WorkArea/DownloadAsset.aspx?id=9847.

25. American College of Healthcare Executives. (2003). *Code of ethics.* Retrieved
October 31, 2003, from http://www.ache.org/abt_ache/code.cfm.

26. American Medical Association. (2003, July 15). *E-principles of medical ethics.*
Retrieved March 16, 2011, from http://www.ama-assn.org/ama/pub/physi
cian-resources/medical-ethics/code-medical-ethics/principles-medical-ethics
.shtml.

27. William A. Nelson & Paula P. Schnurr. (2003, November/December). Affiliates comment on code of ethics. *Healthcare Executive 18*(6), pp. 54–55.

28. Walter J. Wentz & Terence F. Moore. (1981). Administrative success: Key in-
gredients (special issue). *Hospital & Health Services Administration 2,* pp. 85–93.

CHAPTER 5

ORGANIZATIONAL RESPONSES TO ETHICAL ISSUES

T hus far, little has been said about how organizations organize to solve administrative and biomedical ethical problems. The starting point is the organization's philosophy, which reflects its values and establishes moral direction and a framework for the vision and mission. The philosophy is subject to the minimum set by external constraints such as criminal and civil laws and their derivative regulations and court cases. For example, federal guidelines to protect human subjects are a starting point for the organization's relationship with patients participating in federally funded clinical research.

The personal ethic of the manager, as employee and leader, both influences and is influenced by the organizational philosophy. In addition, the manager organizes the organization and allocates resources to prevent and solve ethical problems. Such problem solving occurs in the context of the organizational philosophy but is affected by the manager's personal ethic, which should be more specific and comprehensive than the organizational philosophy. This dynamic reinforces the importance of the personal ethic, lest the manager lose an essential attribute of leadership—clear moral direction.

Since the 1970s, health services organizations have established various means to solve ethical problems; most prominent are institutional ethics committees (IECs), institutional review boards (IRBs), and infant care review committees (ICRCs). IECs can provide a broad range of assistance on administrative and biomedical ethical issues. IRBs are specialized IECs that focus on research ethics. They are more helpful in preventing and solving problems in biomedical ethics than administrative ethics. ICRCs review the care of infants with disabilities.

INSTITUTIONAL ETHICS COMMITTEES

The progenitors to IECs were abortion selection committees (which determined, prior to *Roe v. Wade* [1973], if a pregnant woman's health or life were sufficiently at risk to justify an abortion) and medical morals committees in Roman Catholic hospitals (which assessed certain treatment decisions in light of Church teachings).[1] Later, in the 1960s, committees selected recipients of renal dialysis at a time when there were many more medically suitable patients than available machines.

The 1976 court decision regarding Karen Ann Quinlan directed the establishment of an "ethics" committee that was to review her prognosis. Such committees confirmed prognoses and helped determine whether to continue life-sustaining treatment. Prognosis committees were often called "God squads" because they determined when treatment would be withdrawn so the patient died from the underlying disease process(es).

The role of IECs in the 21st century is expected to be much broader. An early source of information about IECs was a national survey completed for the President's Commission for the Study of Ethical Problems in Medicine and Biomedical and Behavioral Research, which was published in 1983.[2] Smaller hospitals did not have an IEC, and such bodies were not ubiquitous in large hospitals. Hospitals with teaching programs were most likely to have IECs. It was estimated that there were fewer than 100 such bodies nationwide. The Quinlan case had encouraged hospitals to establish IECs.

The number of IECs grew rapidly in the early 1980s. By 1985, surveys done by the National Society of Patient Representatives found that 59% of hospitals had them. The Baby Doe controversies in the early 1980s caused many hospitals to establish specialized IECs to address the ethical problems of newborns with profound disabilities. The growth in numbers of new IECs slowed in the late 1980s, however.[3] This lack of growth was confirmed by 1993 estimates that nationally, almost 60% of hospitals had IECs; state and regional ethics networks put the number at 65%–85%.[4] By contrast, a 1993 survey by the Catholic Health Association found that 92% of members responding had an IEC.[5] Already by 1990, it was suggested that hospital ethics committees had matured and must reconsider their roles to determine whether they should be involved in new ways and in other aspects of organizations.[6] In the 1990s, IEC involvement in case consultation seemed to decline; IECs were more likely to be involved in issues of appropriateness of technology, patients' rights, relationships among healthcare providers, and conflicts of social values.[7] Another survey of acute care hospitals found that 86% of IECs play a role in ongoing clinical decision making through ethics consultation; all IECs among respondents to the survey were involved in developing institutional clinical policy. The survey found that 4.5% of IECs wrote policy on managed care.[8] In the 21st century, the emphasis on ethics case consultation has increased significantly. The source for case consultation is the IEC, which acts as the "mother ship." The specifics of case consultation are discussed later in this chapter.

Nonacute health services are moving from hospitals to other types of settings. Growth in the need for and use of IECs will be greatest in nursing facilities, health maintenance and managed care organizations, and integrated delivery networks. A survey by the American Association of Homes and Services for the Aging found that the numbers of ethics committees among its members had increased from 29% in 1990 to 45% in 1995 and that many others were in the planning stage. The committees review cases and consult, make and review policy recommendations, and educate and advise staff and administration. Of organizations with committees, 86% surveyed found them useful.[9]

IECs in nonacute care organizations are likely to develop differently, depending on their unique activities and roles. It has been suggested that, unlike physicians on IECs in hospitals, physicians on IECs in nursing facilities play a minor role and that administrative staff are much more important. Average staff education levels in nursing facilities tend to be lower, which may exacerbate cultural and class differences between staff and patients. Because nursing facilities are heavily regulated, it is also likely that a considerable focus will fall on legal rather than ethical issues.[10] An important context for ethics committees is the 1992 requirement of the Joint Commission on Accreditation of Healthcare Organizations (The Joint Commission) that hospitals have a mechanism to resolve ethics issues.[11] This requirement is usually met by having an IEC.

Organization

Complex health services organizations such as acute care hospitals would benefit by establishing an ethics committee with two subcommittees, one that addresses administrative ethical issues, the other biomedical issues. An alternative is to have two ethics committees, one for administrative ethical issues and one for biomedical ethical issues. Specialization is desirable because a committee prepared to address administrative ethics problems may be inadequately prepared to address biomedical ethics problems. Greater specialization is needed within the broad categories of administrative and biomedical ethics (e.g., ICRCs). Committee proliferation or overlap should be avoided, but the various types of ethical problems must be addressed effectively. Because of the need to solve both general, organization-wide problems and specific, sometimes very technical problems, the committee with subcommittees model is encouraged. Given that few hospitals follow the specialized ethics committees model, however, the IEC will be discussed here as one entity that addresses both administrative and biomedical ethical issues.

Veatch[12] argued that the different ethical tasks undertaken by IECs are mutually exclusive because they emphasize different ethical principles. He recommended organizing ethics using the following models:

1. *An autonomy model*—implements decisions of competent patients whose wishes are known
2. *A social justice model*—grapples with broad issues such as organizational healthcare policy, resource allocation, and cost effectiveness
3. *A patient benefit model*—makes decisions for patients unable to make decisions for themselves

Ethics committees that use autonomy models are accountable to the patient, whereas ethics committees that use a social justice model must be accountable to the organization (or the community). The first and third models emphasize biomedical ethical issues. The second model could address administrative as well as biomedical issues, if it were determined desirable to address the two types in one committee.

Before considering ethical problems, an IEC must develop a statement of its ethic, the context for which is the organizational philosophy. The IEC's ethic does not determine how to solve each type of problem. It is a statement of general principles that guide deliberations and determine its recommendations. This exercise is essential to the effectiveness of the IEC because it identifies and minimizes differences in the personal ethic of members. Only by understanding and enunciating its own ethic can the IEC appreciate how its values differ from those of a patient, for example, an essential understanding if patient autonomy is to be respected.

Roles of IECs

Since their early, focused beginnings, IECs have broadened their activities greatly.

General Roles IECs have two general roles. One is to assist in developing or reconsidering the organizational philosophy (to move the organization toward a more desired culture) and the derivative vision and mission statements. The experience and range of interdisciplinary membership will likely produce results that are better reasoned and more thorough. Education is the second role. The IEC's composition and the experience of its members make it a reservoir of knowledge and expertise; the typical case-based approach reflects casuistry, which was discussed in Chapter 1. These resources should be made available to the governing body and staff. Such attributes add a level of sophistication to the organization and improve the quality of administrative and biomedical ethical decision making.

Generic Activities   IECs undertake generic activities such as policy development, education, case review, and guidance for individuals upon request. Specific activities could include developing consent forms and policies, identifying criteria for macro-resource allocation, and providing guidance on issues related to whistle-blowing, developing do-not-resuscitate (DNR) and patient consent procedures, addressing involuntary discharge, considering patient safety issues, and advising on withholding or withdrawing life support. Another possible role is to help establish and maintain a culture of patient safety.[13]

Ethics Issues   Currently, IECs focus almost exclusively on biomedical ethical problems and devote little time to administrative ethical issues, such as conflicts of interest, or to consulting on policy formulation and macroallocation decisions. Such a narrow range of activities is regrettable because it diminishes the potential value of IECs. The principal benefits of IECs in biomedical ethics include facilitating decision making by clarifying important issues, shaping consistent policies about life support, and providing opportunities for professionals to air disagreements. IECs appear not to have been effective at increasing the ability of patients' families to influence decisions or at educating professionals about issues relevant to life-support decisions.

Ethics Consultation   Ethics consultation is an important activity for IECs that involves its members in advising and assisting to resolve patient-centered biomedical ethics problems. Ethics consultation is similar to clinical consultation. Consultation is performed by clinical and nonclinical members of the IEC with special interest and preparation in biomedical ethics. The IEC develops and recommends policy regarding ethics consultation to administration. It also serves as a sounding board for problems that develop during ethics consultation.

Clinicians who provide ethics consultation are a bridge between the ethicist and clinical staff attending the patient. These clinicians are a resource for the ethicist and vice versa. In ethics consultation, IEC members are on call and are supplemented, as needed. A variant uses a primary consultant assisted by other members of the IEC. The primary consultants and those assisting them have varying backgrounds, but all are trained in ethics and participate in case reviews, ethics instruction, and regular meetings of the staff. An early example of an ethics consultation service was developed at the University of Virginia in the late 1980s.[14]

In the early 1980s, the President's Commission found that IECs were involved in few cases and were dominated by medical professionals to the exclusion of patients and, frequently, family members.[15] After a spurt of involvement in the mid-1980s and early 1990s, case consultation declined. Yet, the problem of patient representation, control, and attendance (by family members) has continued, and this has renewed interest in the importance and need for case consultation. Ethics consultation is commonly available at all larger hospitals. Top goals of ethics consultation include intervening to protect patient rights, resolving real or imagined conflicts, changing patient care to improve quality, and increasing patient/family satisfaction.[16] Attendance of patients by family members raises significant questions of patient autonomy, especially regarding resource allocation and consent. A medical center study of reasons for ethics consultation found that by far the most common involved issues related to surrogate decision makers. This category was followed by DNR/end-of-life issues, living donor transplant, patients refusing medically indicated care, and challenging or disruptive patients. Last, by a considerable margin, was consultation for medical futility of care,[17] which suggests that such concerns have been overstated.

Cultural Diversity   Organizations with culturally diverse stakeholders must have staff and IEC members who are sensitive to various views about medical services. This is especially true for significant events such as dying and death.

Last Wishes

A Native American was admitted to Memorial Hospital's emergency department in grave condition. His cardiac insufficiency was terminal. He was able to communicate his wishes, verified by his friend, that extreme measures not be used and that he be allowed to die naturally and peacefully. Death was expected within hours or a few days. His friend explained to nursing staff that in their religion a dying person's spirit could only enjoy eternal bliss if the person died in the open and the spirit could go to the sky, unfettered by the walls and ceilings of a building. Nursing staff wanted to meet the dying man's wishes but were uncertain what to do. They could not take the patient outdoors until he was in the final moments of the dying process. They monitored him closely. When they determined that he had died—even though a physician had not pronounced him dead—they put him on a gurney, covered him, and took him outside through the service entrance. After a few moments away from the building, they returned his body to the nursing unit. His friend came back to the hospital a short time later. He thanked the staff for letting the dead man's spirit "go to the sky."

Nursing staff was able to accommodate the patient's wishes without compromising his care or that of other patients. They acted appropriately, if outside traditional bounds of the nurse–patient relationship. Meeting patients' spiritual needs, generally, has been identified as important to faster response to treatment and reduced likelihood of depression. Failure to meet spiritual needs increases the risk of death and poor mental health and reduces quality of life. Despite this, clinicians receive little or no training in the subject.[18]

Membership

The President's Commission found that biomedical IECs were interdisciplinary. Physicians were most common, averaging about 5 members per committee. Committees averaged one member of the clergy. Members found on fewer than half the committees were attorneys, laypersons, social workers, and physicians in graduate education programs (residents). Administrators served on only about half the committees. The commission found no strong community link, something that governing body members and individuals from the organization's service area could provide. Community members bring a vital perspective to decision making.[19] The commission found that managers were underrepresented, perhaps because they lacked interest in clinical matters. It was suggested in the early 1990s that nurses were also underrepresented, both in terms of their numbers in health services organizations and in the number of biomedical ethical problems they encounter.[20] Current information about IECs suggests that physicians continue to be the most common members. Nurses are no longer underrepresented; 71% of hospitals have nurse members performing ethics consultation. One study found that about half of all committee members were physicians and nurses.[21] Social workers, chaplains, administrators, and attorneys are other professionals likely to be involved in ethics consultation. Most receive training through formal direct supervision by a more experienced committee member. About two-thirds of hospitals reported having administrators involved, which suggests appropriately greater involvement by that group as well.[22]

Relationships

To a significant extent, an IEC's effectiveness will be a function of its location in the organization. The IEC could be a standing committee of the governing body, the medical staff, or administration. Concerns that physicians will dominate IECs cause some experts to suggest that they should be a governing body or administration committee. Members should be chosen for their ability to analyze ethical issues in an unbiased manner and not because they represent a constituency.

IEC relationships vary depending on its activities (role), which may be general or specific. General activities span the organization, and, as noted, include refining the organizational philosophy, ethics education, macroallocation decision making, and policy development (e.g., conflict of interest policy). Common specific-level activities are case and microallocation consultations and situational analyses. An example of a specific activity is determining whether a particular decision is consistent with the organizational philosophy.

The IEC should be proactive in developing and revising the organizational philosophy and in considering the ethical implications of macroallocation of resources. Similarly, the IEC should take the initiative in reviewing the consent process. The committee may choose a more passive role for some issues, however, and wait to be consulted in specific instances of conflicts of interest and misuse of confidential information, or in specific biomedical ethics problems.

Except as noted above, IECs are most likely to be effective when they wait to be consulted, rather than when they interpose themselves in decisions about specific ethical problems. As consulting bodies, IECs only make recommendations to decision makers. Ethics consultation recommendations may be optional or mandatory. Following the advice given by an IEC may be optional or mandatory. Table 1 shows the combinations.

One study found that most physicians (72%) thought consultations yielded information that would help with future ethical issues. Many other physicians hesitate to ask for an ethics consultation. Common reasons cited were that consultations were too time-consuming, that they might make the situation worse, that consultants were unqualified or unhelpful, and that solutions were not consistent with good practice.[23] Physicians are

Table 1.   Matrix of possible roles for institutional ethics committees (IECs)

Involvement of IEC in decision making	Acceptance and use of advice provided by IEC
Optional	Optional
Optional	Mandatory
Mandatory	Optional
Mandatory	Mandatory

unlikely to accept an ethics consultation that is mandatory–mandatory. Furthermore, mandated involvement is not desirable for situations in which the physician is willing to develop alternatives and communicate them to the patient and others concerned. Even if physicians are unwilling to involve an ethics consultation, there are benefits to making the analysis and recommendation available to decision makers.

The Institutional Ethics Committee

The chief executive officer of Community Health Plan (CHP) had been approached by a group from "north of the river." This area of the city was economically depressed and over the previous decade had lost many of its health services delivery organizations and physicians to the suburbs. It seemed to be in a downward spiral, with no end in sight. Decreasing numbers of insured patients meant that organizations were increasingly unable to serve the area. The city-owned hospital had made several ill-fated attempts to serve the area north of the river with a clinic system, but its efforts were scandal-ridden. The clinic system became a political football with little credibility in the community.

The representatives from north of the river were community leaders, none of whom appeared to have political ambitions. They seemed genuinely willing to do whatever they could to assist in securing high-quality health services for their community. They proposed that CHP establish and provide clinical staff for three storefront clinics in the area. The community leaders stated that they would find volunteers to remodel the facilities and work in clerical jobs.

The CEO presented the proposed initiative to the IEC, which included members of the governing body, managers, and physicians and other caregivers. In making the presentation, the CEO stressed the health plan's historical role in providing services to those in need, its not-for-profit status, and its continuing modest surplus. The members listened patiently, but the minute the CEO finished, all of them seemed to speak at once. Several members opposed the proposal and made the following points about the suggested venture:

1.   The area north of the river was the city's responsibility. Providing care to the needy is not something a small, not-for-profit health plan like CHP should attempt.

2. The organization's primary obligation was to enhance benefits for its enrollees and not to become involved in new schemes. New services had been requested by several of their physicians and many plan members.

3. The modest surplus the plan had accumulated over several years could be easily consumed by the proposed venture. The chief financial officer noted that an increase in reinsurance premiums was expected in the next quarter.

4. If the plan pulled the city's political chestnuts out of the fire by providing even stopgap assistance, the city would never get its house in order and develop the system needed north of the river.

Several members spoke in favor of working with the community north of the river and made the following points:

1. Helping the north-of-the-river community was the right thing to do. The people living there deserved healthcare services. Someone noted that the plan's own start came about when several physicians in the community fought the prevailing attitude among their peers about the prepaid practice of medicine.

2. Those opposing the proposal were putting dollars ahead of people's health. They must be willing to assist those who are less fortunate.

3. Plan members would support such an initiative if it were properly explained to them.

4. The positive publicity could further the plan's interests by increasing the number of enrollees.

It seemed to the CEO that this was a no-win situation. The organizational philosophy was not well developed and the proposal was a major step. Should something be done to help the north-of-the-river community? The IEC members had raised valid points that merited further discussion.

This case describes issues arising from decisions about macroallocation of resources. Problems here are more complex because CHP is being asked to volunteer assistance and to do so from its own modest surplus. Relevant theories of justice in allocating resources include retribution or compensatory justice (distributing resources to make up for past wrongs); just deserts (help would go to those who had not earned it and CHP's leadership had no right to risk the plan's solvency, which was something the membership paid to achieve); egalitarianism in access to health services, and whether it was government's responsibility to provide it to the community north of the river; and utility as a prospectively determined element of beneficence.

A significant problem for CHP was that it did not consider this aspect of its relationship with unique subsets of the community in formulating its organizational philosophy and vision and mission statements. It would do well to develop these prospectively in a comprehensive fashion rather than address them ad hoc. Resource allocation receives further attention in Chapter 13.

Summary

IECs are useful in many ways. Overall, their effects should improve administrative and biomedical decision making. However, one cannot assume that the mere presence of an IEC preordains its success. As with all undertakings, IECs should be evaluated so that performance can be improved.[24]

IECs present significant potential problems. Organizational concerns, especially legal ramifications and avoiding public embarrassment, can easily overwhelm concerns about patient goals.[25] At the extreme, it has been suggested that because IECs represent organizations, they cannot be objective; as a result, when a dispute arises, they will take management's side to avoid risk, and thus fail in their vital role as patient advocates.[26] Management must ensure that IECs are not subverted in this manner.

INSTITUTIONAL REVIEW BOARDS

Health services managers may think research and experimentation are exclusive to academic health centers, in which rigorous protection and standards of review are applied. Many health services organizations, however, engage in research, some of which may not even be known to nonclinical managers.

Ethical Principles in Research

Contemporary codes of research ethics emphasize the subject's voluntary, informed consent. The modern emphasis on consent in research began in 1900 when a Prussian state government commission identified unambiguous consent as essential.[27] The research subject's mental competence receives less attention than does consent. A provision in the Nuremberg Code (1949) states that subjects should be able to halt the experiment if they no longer wish to continue. This proviso places a heavy burden on the subject, who may become incapacitated by the experiment itself or by an unrelated medical problem, or who may be intimidated by the setting or individuals involved. Subjects also usually lack the technical expertise to understand when their safety is threatened. This weakness was partially corrected in the Declaration of Helsinki (1964, revised 1975 and 1989), which recommends establishing an independent committee to review and approve the experimental protocol.

In 1978, the National Commission for the Protection of Human Subjects of Biomedical and Behavioral Research issued *The Belmont Report: Ethical Principles and Guidelines for the Protection of Human Subjects of Research*, which identified the ethical principles and guidelines for research involving human subjects. Its most influential contribution was the enunciation of three basic precepts: 1) respect for persons (met through an informed consent process), 2) beneficence (weighing risks and benefits), and 3) justice (fair selection of subjects). The *Belmont Report* provided important guidance on the boundaries between research and clinical medicine.[28] In fact, its principles and guidelines are reflected in the type of committee required by the U.S. Department of Health and Human Services (DHHS).

All research codes and guidelines permit nontherapeutic research and recognize that volunteers for whom the experimental treatment offers no potential diagnostic or therapeutic benefit are needed for certain research. The utilitarian language present in all codes balances the risk to the subject (in nontherapeutic research) with the benefit to society. Conversely, emphases on voluntary and informed consent suggest a Kantian philosophy and reflect the principles of nonmaleficence and respect for persons, as well as the virtues of fairness, honesty, and trustworthiness. This perspective is embedded in the DHHS regulatory framework ("Protection of Human Subjects"; Public Welfare, 45 C.F.R., 2001).

A primary problem with research codes other than federal regulations is that they inadequately separate the physician's roles as healer and researcher. The ethical burden on physicians is heavy because the duality of interests of physician-researchers puts them at high risk of encountering an actual conflict of interest. What is good for the research subject as patient may diminish the integrity of the experimental design. This problem is exacerbated in nontherapeutic research because the risk to the subject is not balanced by potential benefits. American Medical Association (AMA) guidelines recognize the dilemma and stress adequate safeguards for the welfare, safety, and comfort of the subject and written consent after full disclosure.[29]

Establishing Institutional Review Boards

To protect human subjects, health services organizations conducting federally funded research should establish an IRB, which is an independent committee comprising scientific and nonscientific members that complies with federal law.[30] IRBs conduct initial and continued review of research involving human subjects. Committees with similar activities are considered IRBs as well.

In the health services field, the DHHS and the Food and Drug Administration (FDA) are the most important federal entities that require an IRB to review, approve, and maintain oversight of research studies. The DHHS requirements for IRBs and protection of human subjects are applicable to research funded (i.e., supported or conducted by and regulated under a specific research statute) by 17 federal agencies and departments that have adopted the "common rule" or "federal policy" for the protection of human subjects.[31] Examples of federal agencies that use DHHS requirements are the Department of Defense, the Department of Veterans Affairs, the Environmental Protection Agency, the National Science Foundation, and the Consumer Product Safety Commission.

Research that involves human subjects and is either wholly or partly funded by the federal government must be reviewed by an IRB with a process that meets DHHS criteria. Although technically not required, research funding applications typically include assurances that the organization will comply with DHHS IRB requirements for human subjects (and other DHHS requirements for the protection of human subjects) for *all* its research, federally funded or not.[32]

The FDA regulates the interstate sale of drugs, biologicals (i.e., vaccines), and medical devices and has the same requirements as DHHS. Unlike the DHHS, however, compliance with the FDA's guidelines, including the use of IRBs, is necessary regardless of the funding source. A few states (e.g., New York) regulate medical research, but in most cases, either the DHHS or FDA regulates health-related research.

The FDA does not regulate surgical experimentation. For example, the FDA did not judge that coronary artery bypass surgery or radial keratotomy (ophthalmic surgery) were safe and efficacious or that they should be generally available. Neither does the FDA regulate innovative clinical care, which is defined as new uses of existing treatments, drugs, biologicals, and devices. *Innovative care* is distinguished from standard clinical activity, and its use requires more than the review and consent procedures for standard therapies. Absent government regulation, the organization's managers and clinical staff are essential in monitoring the activities of clinicians who develop innovative uses of drugs or treatments or who attempt new surgical procedures.

It is not easy for hospitals, most of which have no ongoing research programs, to define experimentation and innovative therapy. Nonetheless, definitions are important, not only because they determine whether there is a need to meet legal requirements or to form an IRB, but also because the organization must ensure that its own, presumably more rigorous, procedures for consent and protection of the patient are followed. The following case illustrates the problem.

This Is Experimenting?[1]

An internal auditor conducted an audit of supplies used in biopsies. The data for kidney biopsies revealed significant discrepancies: The use of biopsy packs exceeded the number of procedures by 50%. The auditor was puzzled, but double-checking requisitions and utilization data showed them to be correct. Theft was unlikely.

The auditor made informal inquiries and spoke to technicians in the cytology laboratory. One agreed to speak confidentially about the additional kidney biopsies. The technician told the auditor that one of the nephrology fellows was using a second biopsy pack to take additional tissue during kidney biopsies. The tissue was sent to cytology for special studies ordered by the fellow. The technician said the fellow was testing a new theory about treating end-stage renal disease.

Is this research? Yes. The nephrology fellow's activities meet the definition of research as systematic investigation designed to develop or contribute to generalizable knowledge. Taking additional tissue or using part of the specimen in the manner described is experimentation, although the act of obtaining it is not experimental. By trying to prove or disprove a theory, the nephrology fellow is performing research. However, taking the additional tissue requires consent separate from that for the routine, initial biopsy. There is no evidence a second consent was obtained. Taking more tissue or performing a second biopsy puts the patient at additional risk, without any actual or potential diagnostic or therapeutic benefit. The organization and its managers have an absolute duty to prevent unauthorized research, and policies and procedures regarding such a practice are essential. Innovative treatments, too, must be closely monitored. With innovative treatment, the level of concern increases with the degree of risk. Adequate consent is essential for both experimentation and innovative therapy.

There are ethical considerations in the economics of this case, too. The second study adds to the laboratory's workload. If third parties are paying for these charges (or costs), and are told they are part of a patient's diagnosis or treatment, the organization is acting dishonestly toward the payer.

Organizational policies must distinguish standard clinical care from experimental procedures. Obtaining a few extra milliliters of amniotic fluid during amniocentesis causes moderate additional risk. Taking unused urine routinely collected for other purposes or performing analyses on the expelled placenta pose no risk to the patient but require consent nonetheless. Minor or nonexistent risks do not justify ignoring patients' rights and the duties owed to them. DHHS and FDA regulations recognize minimal research risk and permit special review procedures. Protocols for research in these categories can receive expedited review and approval from the IRB.

Defined as attempting new means, methods, and techniques, medicine has always engaged in research; without it, medical knowledge would stagnate. Protecting the rights and welfare of human subjects remains problematic, however.

Fever All Through the Night

Beverley Atchison, vice president for administration, finished reading the minutes of the utilization review committee. Atchison noted that a lengthy discussion had occurred with regard to the seemingly overlong stay of a pediatric patient. In fact, the attending pediatrician had appeared before the committee to explain the length of stay and her unique treatment regimen.

The case involved a child with a fever of unknown etiology. Routine tests after hospitalization showed no pathology. The physician explained that she had read about fever therapy in the literature and was impressed with its possibilities. Therefore, she decided to determine its appropriateness in cases of fever of unknown etiology. She ordered Tylenol if the fever went above 102.5 degrees Fahrenheit. Otherwise, there was to be no intervention.

The pediatrician stated that the efficaciousness of fever therapy was proven because after 3 days the child made a full recovery. The regimen raised numerous questions among the committee members, however.

This regimen is innovative; it could even be experimental. The case raises two ethical issues: Did the child's parents receive information about the treatment adequate to give informed consent? This question bears directly on how the hospital determines that informed consent is obtained in such cases. Because the therapy was innovative, special consent and review procedures should have been used. If fever therapy is determined to be experimental rather than innovative, the second issue is whether the research was therapeutic or nontherapeutic. Experimental treatment that may benefit the subject is therapeutic—the subject is also a patient. Nontherapeutic research involves healthy subjects or patients with medical problems other than those that might benefit from the experimental treatment. Nontherapeutic research must receive closer attention because the subject will not benefit and may be at increased risk.

Had this innovative (perhaps experimental) therapy been presented to an IRB for review and approval, additional safeguards would have been required. An IRB reviewing pediatric research must be persuaded of the justification for the therapy's risks and benefits. The IRB must find that the activity falls into one of four categories: 1) research not involving greater than minimal risk; 2) research involving greater than minimal risk but presenting the prospect of direct benefit to the individual subjects; 3) research involving greater than minimal risk and having no prospect of direct benefit to the individual subjects, but likely to yield generalizable knowledge about the subject's disorder or condition; or 4) research not otherwise approved but that represents an opportunity to understand, prevent, or alleviate a serious problem affecting the health or welfare of children.[33]

Notable in the fever therapy case is the nursing staff's apparent lack of concern about the unusual orders. The nursing code emphasizes protecting the patient and requires the nurse to intervene if the patient is unnecessarily put at risk. Timely reporting should have occurred through the nursing hierarchy. This aspect of the case suggests a much more widespread need to protect patients and further their interests.

Membership and Purpose

Organizations may choose the members of their IRB, but federal regulations (and perhaps state law) govern composition of the membership, the nature of the review that is conducted, and the conflicts of interest of IRB members.[34] IRBs review research proposals for conformity with the law, standards of professional conduct and practice, and institutional commitment and regulations. IRBs acceptable to the DHHS have a minimum of five members with varying backgrounds (at least one whose professional interests are scientific and one whose interests are nonscientific) and who are capable of reviewing research proposals and activities of the type commonly performed by the organization.[35]

An IRB that is acceptable to the DHHS must apply the following requirements in reviewing research activities:[36]

- Minimize risks to subjects.
- Determine that risks to subjects are reasonable relative to anticipated benefits, if any.
- Select research subjects equitably.
- Obtain informed consent from each prospective subject or each subject's legally authorized representative.
- Appropriately document informed consent.

- Monitor the data collected to ensure the safety of subjects.
- Protect the privacy of subjects and maintain the confidentiality of data.

There must be additional safeguards when subjects are likely to be vulnerable to coercion or undue influence. Examples include children, prisoners, pregnant women, persons with mental retardation, or those who are economically or educationally disadvantaged. Several provisions identify the information needed for informed consent.

The FDA uses the same basic elements of consent as the DHHS but applies special provisions when the subject is in a life-threatening situation that necessitates use of the test article and the subject cannot provide legally effective consent, time is insufficient to obtain consent from the subject's legal representative, or no alternative method of generally recognized therapy that provides an equal or greater likelihood of saving the subject's life is available.

Requirements

Regulations issued in 1981 eliminated the requirement that any organization receiving DHHS funding had to use DHHS guidelines in *all* research, regardless of funding source. This marked a shift in the role of the federal government in protecting human subjects and in research, generally. The change also magnified the responsibilities of managers and researchers and put greater reliance on the organization's policies and procedures and on managers' personal ethic in judging the research. Problems such as those in the Willowbrook case, which is discussed below, are likely to increase state regulation of research.

As a practical matter, organizations with multiple research funding sources, one of which is the federal DHHS, are likely to use the same DHHS-qualified IRB for all research protocols. It is easy to slip, however, and managers must be alert to potential ethical problems in formal research programs as well as in isolated instances of innovative therapy or surgical experimentation.

A mix of moral philosophies and values is found in the DHHS regulations. Beneficence and its subsidiary, cost–benefit analysis, determine the benefits of research. Conversely, a Kantian (deontological) perspective and the principles of nonmaleficence and respect for persons underlie the requirements for consent, privacy, and confidentiality. The virtues of honesty, trustworthiness, and integrity are appropriate here, too.

It has been argued that nondiagnostic and nontherapeutic research on children and adults who are considered legally incompetent should be prohibited.[37] Congress *has not* given the FDA authority to require extensive testing on children. The ethical, economic, political, legal, and scientific problems of research involving children are so daunting that researchers have been reluctant to address the issue. Despite efforts by Congress and the FDA to encourage testing of pharmaceuticals and biologicals on children, little research involving children is done, and most prescriptions for children are based on physician trial and error.[38] It has been estimated that 50%–75% of drugs used in pediatric medicine have not been studied adequately to provide appropriate labeling information.[39] As noted, nontherapeutic research on children is permitted. A risk–benefit ratio is applied, and no child can be placed in unnecessary jeopardy. Assent from both the child and parents or legally authorized representatives are required.

Hepatitis for Children with Mental Retardation?[40]

Willowbrook State Hospital, an institution for the care of people with mental retardation in Staten Island, New York, housed more than 5,000 residents in 1971.

Dr. Saul Krugman was a consultant in pediatrics and infectious diseases. When he began work at Willowbrook in the early 1950s, he discovered that major infectious diseases, including hepatitis, measles, shigellosis, parasitic infections, and respiratory infections, were prevalent. Conditions at Willowbrook were like those found at similar facilities elsewhere in the United States. Dr. Krugman and his colleagues undertook a study of these diseases, including research on a measles vaccine and hepatitis.

In 1956, Dr. Krugman, Dr. Joan Giles, and Dr. Jack Hammond began studies on hepatitis. The final phase of the research (1965–1970) involved 68 children ages 3–10. The researchers injected an infected serum to cause hepatitis in the residents of their research unit. The objective was to gain a better understanding of hepatitis and possibly develop methods of immunizing against it. The research was approved by the Armed Forces Epidemiological Board, one of the funders of the research; the executive faculty and the Committee on Human Experimentation of New York University, where Dr. Krugman held a faculty position; and the New York State Department of Mental Hygiene.

The researchers defended their decision to expose the children to strains of hepatitis on the following grounds:

1. They were exposed to the same strains that were endemic to the facility.
2. They were admitted to a special, well-equipped, and well-staffed unit and were isolated from exposure to other infectious diseases prevalent in the institution. The health risk was thus lower for those in the experiment than for those in the hospital at large, in which multiple infections occurred.
3. They were likely to have a subclinical infection followed by immunity to the particular hepatitis virus.

The researchers emphasized that only children whose parents gave informed consent participated in the experiment.

A storm of adverse publicity arose when the experiment was made public in 1967 by a New York state senator, who charged that children were being used as human guinea pigs. Nevertheless, the research continued. In 1971, the group's work produced spectacular results, when Dr. Krugman and co-workers were able to immunize a small group of children against serum hepatitis (hepatitis B [HBV]). The preliminary results were hailed as a scientific breakthrough. In defending the research, Dr. Krugman reported that the injections that induced hepatitis in the research group were given only after employing great thought and professional discretion and only with the informed consent of the parents. He stated that the doses were small and that the inoculations usually produced the infections without making the children sick. (After 12 years of legal and regulatory controversy, Willowbrook State Hospital closed at the end of 1987, when a federal court approved a final settlement.)

Although Dr. Krugman and his colleagues made a convincing case for undertaking and continuing the research, the Willowbrook case illustrates several ethical problems. The consent obtained from parents or surrogates was given under duress—they almost certainly believed that children who were part of the group purposely infected with HBV would fare better than children living among the population at large, in which conditions were much worse. Such considerations make it difficult to apply the principles of beneficence and nonmaleficence.

The general benefit of being in the special unit is an argument that should receive some credence. The children were somewhat protected from other diseases prevalent at Willowbrook and received treatment for the sequelae of HBV. In addition, it can be argued that this research is therapeutic; even though the children did not have HBV, they were almost certain to become infected with it. Children in the unit were also likely to be less harmed in other ways than would children in Willowbrook, thereby generally meeting the principle of nonmaleficence. The real problem, however, is that the children were being used as a means to an end, despite a potential for great social benefit if the research were successful.

The research protocols had been approved by prominent and appropriate review bodies and the research continued for 16 years (1956–1971). Assuming effective consent from parents or legally authorized representatives, federal guidelines would have permitted this nontherapeutic research. At the same time, however, the organizational philosophy through its managers could have applied a more demanding standard—using the virtues of justice, compassion, and integrity—to the point of prohibiting the research. In fact, research that is not clearly therapeutic for children and others unable to give voluntary and competent consent is so fraught with ethical problems that it is rarely undertaken. Regrettably, this conundrum has resulted in a dearth of certain types of clinical knowledge, especially that of the therapeutic effects of drugs and biologicals on children—which, as noted, is ultimately to their detriment.

A question of justice in allocating state funds is raised by the horrific conditions at Willowbrook. Is it fair that human beings are treated so? In the absence of an increase in state appropriations, however, the principles of respect for persons, beneficence, and nonmaleficence must be applied within financial limits.

The research conducted on children at Willowbrook seems to be from another era—one with far less attention paid to protecting human subjects, especially children. Yet, three decades later an even more unacceptable example of research involving children occurred in Baltimore, and involved the Kennedy Krieger Institute, an affiliate of Johns Hopkins University. The EPA-funded study, with state and city governmental sponsors and collaborators, sought to find inexpensive alternatives for reducing or eliminating the risks of lead paint in homes. A large number of families with healthy young children were placed in rental housing with various levels of lead risk abatement. Parents were not told of the full extent of the risk; upon discovering it, they sued.[41] Maryland's highest court faulted the Johns Hopkins Hospital IRB and ruled that "in Maryland a parent . . . cannot consent to the participation of a child or other person under legal disability in nontherapeutic research or studies in which there is any risk of injury or damage to the health of the subject."[42]

Exempt Research and Research Warranting Expedited Review

Six categories of research are exempt from DHHS requirements. Examples are research conducted in established or normally accepted educational settings involving normal educational practices; research involving use of educational tests, survey and interview procedures, or observation of public behavior; and research involving the collection or study of existing data, documents, records, and pathological or diagnostic specimens. Limits are specified.[43]

DHHS regulations identify research warranting expedited review as a category to which different provisions apply. Expedited review allows special procedures for approval of certain types of research that pose no more than minimal risk to human subjects. The review is conducted by the IRB chair, or by one or more experienced reviewers designated by the chair. In reviewing the research, the reviewer exercises all of the IRB's authority. Research may be disapproved only in accordance with the nonexpedited procedure.[44] Subject to limitations, research categories appropriate to expedited review include clinical studies of drugs and medical devices; collection of blood samples; collection of biological specimens such as hair and nail clippings and deciduous teeth; collection of data through noninvasive procedures; research using materials collected for other purposes; collection of data from various types of recordings; research on individual or group characteristics or behavior; and continuing review of research previously approved by the IRB.[45] Expedited review greatly facilitates several kinds of research.

Falsification of Research Data

A unique dimension to problems in research occurred in the late 1970s and early 1980s.[46] John Darsee, a fellow in cardiology at Emory University and Harvard University and a brilliant physician of unusual talent, perpetrated an amazing fraud. Darsee was found to have falsified large quantities of research data on the genetic and biochemical factors affecting heart disease. Some of these data had been published in leading medical journals. Other data were being used for papers in process. Many of the articles listed prominent physician-researchers as coauthors, some of whom later asserted they had no knowledge that they had been identified as such.

Darsee's champions supported him until the evidence of his deception proved overwhelming. Darsee's detractors argued that his supporters were too easily charmed by his personality and talents. When researchers and administrators at Emory and Harvard learned of the fraud, they withdrew his papers and abstracts that had been submitted for publication. The only course for articles already published was to urge readers to disregard them. It is claimed that no patients were harmed because of Darsee's clinical work, a claim verifiable only by reviewing medical records. Much more potential harm, however, lies in the fact that Darsee's list of publications includes more than 100 articles and abstracts. Readers unaware of the fraud cannot know which publications contain false data.

The organizations involved were forthright after the fraud was discovered. What happened violated both the ethics of research and the proscriptions imposed by funding organizations (e.g., the National Institutes of Health). The most pointed questions, however, concern the adequacy of surveillance, not only of Darsee but also of all physicians in training who engage in research and collect research data. Subsequent self-assessment at Emory led to new safeguards in reviewing the work of physicians in training and in monitoring the use of names of teaching staff as coauthors. Research findings are also reviewed much more extensively since the Darsee affair. Despite the safeguards, some people argued that "[they] won't prevent the generation of fraudulent data, but under this system someone like Darsee couldn't send out articles at the rate of one a week without raising suspicions."[47] Healthy skepticism regarding research integrity is wise. One study of research misconduct stated

> Nearly one generation after the effort to reduce misconduct in science began, the responses by NIH scientists suggests that falsified and fabricated research records, publications, dissertations, and grant applications are much more prevalent than has been suspected to date. Our study calls into question the effectiveness of self-regulation.[48]

Another investigation suggested that falsifications and fabrications are symptomatic of wider problems, such as plagiarism, conflicts of interest, failing to meet human subject requirements, misuse of confidential information, failing to present data that contradict one's own previous research, and failing to report others' use of flawed data or questionable interpretation of data.[49]

Summary

Regulations such as those imposed by the DHHS focus responsibility on the organization and its IRB. Irrespective of legal requirements, the organization's managers are charged with independent duties under the principles of respect for persons, beneficence, nonmaleficence, and even justice (e.g., equitable selection of research subjects) in order to protect the patient. The virtues of honesty, integrity, and trustworthiness are applicable as well. Managers must establish and maintain systems and procedures to prevent unauthorized research and to provide the necessary extra protection when innovative treatment or surgical research are proposed or undertaken. The Darsee affair raises a unique set of potential problems in teaching and research institutions, the most important being staff awareness about the parameters of acceptable practice and the courage to act on those observations.

INFANT CARE REVIEW COMMITTEES

ICRCs are another type of specialized IEC. They focus on the biomedical ethical problems of infants with life-threatening conditions. The Child Abuse Amendments of 1984 (PL 98-457) directed the DHHS to encourage

the establishment of ICRCs in health facilities, especially those with ter-
tiary-level neonatal units. The DHHS identified the following guidelines
for ICRCs:

> (1) educate hospital personnel and families of disabled infants with
> life-threatening conditions; (2) recommend institutional policies and
> guidelines concerning the withholding of medically indicated treat-
> ment from infants with life-threatening conditions; and (3) offer
> counsel and review in cases involving infants with life-threatening
> conditions.[50]

The guidelines make it clear that the DHHS considers it prudent to establish an ICRC but that the organization decides whether to do so. Chapter
10 provides the background for the original Baby Doe regulations and the
Child Abuse Amendments.

Certain aspects of the ICRC's membership and administration recommended in the guidelines are notable. Members should include individuals
from varied disciplines and perspectives because a multidisciplinary approach provides the expertise to supply and evaluate pertinent information.
The committee should be large enough to represent diverse viewpoints
but not so large as to hinder its effectiveness. Recommended membership
includes a practicing physician (e.g., pediatrician, neonatologist, pediatric
surgeon), practicing nurse, hospital administrator, social worker, representative of a disability group, lay community member, and member of the
facility's medical staff, who is the chairperson.[51] The recommendation to
include a representative of a disability group on the ICRC runs counter
to the principle that members of such committees should not represent
specific groups.

The DHHS suggested that the ICRC have adequate staff support,
including legal counsel; that the ICRC recommend procedures to ensure
that both hospital personnel and patient or resident families are informed
of its existence, functions, and 24-hour availability; that the ICRC self-ed-
ucate about pertinent legal requirements and procedures, including state
law requiring reports of known or suspected medical neglect; and that the
ICRC maintain records of deliberations and summary descriptions of cases
considered and their disposition.[52]

Many groups, including the AMA, the American Hospital Association
(AHA), and various medical specialty associations, objected vociferously
to the original Baby Doe regulations and sought to block implementation.
The Child Abuse Amendments and regulations, however, were supported
by health services trade associations, which ran the gamut from institutional and personal providers to specialized groups. In fact, the associations

were instrumental in developing the law and regulations. The AHA enthusiastically backed the new law, and few hospitals will have philosophical problems complying with it.[53]

SPECIALIZED ASSISTANCE

This section outlines assistance for organizations and their managers and clinical staffs in solving administrative and biomedical ethical problems. Analogues to IECs and specialized committees such as IRBs and ICRCs that can assist managers to identify and solve administrative ethical problems are not as well developed but should be given further nurturing and attention.

Ethicists

A less formal approach than the ethics consultation provided through an IEC may be found in larger hospitals, but it should not be limited to them. This option employs ethicists on a full- or part-time basis. Ethicists are often doctorally qualified philosophers who may be faculty at a university or medical school and who consult with clinical staff on biomedical ethical issues.

Organizations needing the assistance of an ethicist can look beyond universities and medical schools and consider persons with specialized preparation in ethics and its application in health services delivery. This makes the ethicist a clinically oriented, problem-solving extension of an IEC.

Dispute Resolution

Treatment options and decisions regarding them often cause disputes among stakeholders, such as patients, families, and clinicians. The various types of ethics committees (e.g., IECs, IRBs, ICRCs) may be able to resolve disputes, but being part of the organization may raise questions of objectivity. If objectivity is a problem, arbitration and mediation should be considered to resolve disputes. Arbitration involves a neutral person—the arbitrator—to whom the parties give the authority to make a decision that they agree to accept. Mediators are neutral persons who work with the parties to reach a mutually acceptable result; mediators have no authority to make or impose a decision. Competent neutrals can minimize the power imbalances present in health services settings, especially when non-clinicians are involved in the dispute.[54] One objective of improved dispute resolution is to weld a multidisciplinary group into a cohesive and mutually supportive team so that they can resolve their differences and maintain the quality of patient care. Formal dispute resolution could also assist the various types of ethics committees. It is overly optimistic to believe that the act of establishing an interdisciplinary ethics committee necessarily means that it will be successful.

CONCLUSION

This chapter examined committees established to address ethical issues. Typically, these committees include IECs as well as IRBs and ICRCs, which are specialized ethics committees. In addition to hospitals, ethics committees can provide assistance in a wide range of health services organizations, including nursing facilities, managed care organizations (MCOs), and hospices, all of which experience ethical problems similar to those found in hospitals. The greatest growth is likely in nonhospital settings. Hospice and nursing facilities, for example, confront issues related to dying and death, and MCOs face issues of resource allocation and physician incentive plans. Ethics committees in all settings will be involved in solving complex ethics issues, some of which (e.g., organizational philosophy) may come under mandatory review.

Ethics consultations and ethicists can be involved on a more discretionary basis to assist in identifying and analyzing the moral obligations, rights, responsibilities, and considerations of justice that bear on a general issue or on the ethical issues in a specific case.[55] They can assist physicians and are more likely to be used than are biomedical ethics committees, which physicians may view as cost ineffective. Beyond considerations of efficiency, it may be more palatable for physicians to consult with a single ethicist than to seek guidance from a committee. Ethicists can serve a similar function for managers by assisting them in identifying and solving administrative ethics problems and working with an administrative IEC.

Economic pressures resulting from cost cutting by third-party payers—particularly government—and new competitive pressures are affecting all health services organizations, but especially acute care hospitals. Managers may be tempted to use economic justification for decisions that implicitly, or even explicitly, affect quality of care negatively. The conflict between economic interests and quality considerations lies near the surface in most relationships with patients. The technical nature of health services and the average consumer's limited ability to judge results make it imperative that individuals associated with healthcare delivery expend every effort to further the quality of care and protect the interests of patients.

NOTES

1. Judith Wilson Ross, John W. Glaser, Dorothy Rasinski-Gregory, Joan McIver Gibson, & Corrine Bayley. (1993). *Health care ethics committees: The next generation* (p. 1). Chicago: American Hospital Publishing.
2. President's Commission for the Study of Ethical Problems in Medicine and Biomedical and Behavioral Research. (1983). *Deciding to forego life-sustaining treatment: A report on the ethical, medical, and legal issues in treatment decisions* (p. 443). Washington, DC: U.S. Government Printing Office.
3. D. Holthaus, M.T. Koska, P. Eubanks, & T. Hudson. (1989, November 20). Right to die: An executive report. *Hospitals 66*(22), p. 34.
4. Ross et al., p. ix.
5. Joanne Lappetito & Paula Thompson. (1993, November). Today's ethics committees face varied issues. *Health Progress*, p. 34.
6. Cynthia B. Cohen. (1990, March/April). Ethics committees. *Hastings Center Report 20*, pp. 29–34.
7. Lappetito & Thompson, p. 34.
8. Glenn McGee, Arthur L. Caplan, Joshua L. Spanogle, & David A. Asch. (2001, Fall). A national survey of ethics committees. *American Journal of Bioethics 1*(4), pp. 60–64.
9. American Association of Homes and Services for the Aging. (1995, July). *Summary report: Survey on ethics involvement in aging services*. Washington, DC: Author.
10. Ross et al., p. 8.
11. Francis Bernt, Peter Clark, Josita Starrs, & Patricia Talone. (2006, March/April). Ethics committees in Catholic hospitals. *Health Progress*, pp. 18–25.
12. Robert M. Veatch. (1983, July). Ethics committees proliferation in hospitals predicted. *Hospitals 57*(13), pp. 48–49.
13. Mark E. Meaney. (2004, Summer). Error reduction, patient safety, and institutional ethics committees. *Journal of Law, Medicine, & Ethics 32*, pp. 358–364.
14. John C. Fletcher, Margo L. White, & Philip J. Foubert. (1990). Biomedical ethics and an ethics consultation service at the University of Virginia. *HEC Forum 2*(2), pp. 89–99.
15. President's Commission, p. 448.
16. Ellen Fox, Sarah Myers, & Robert A. Pearlman. (2007). Ethics consultation in United States hospitals: A national survey. *American Journal of Bioethics 7*(2), pp. 13–25.
17. David J. Ramsey, Mary Lou Schmidt, & Lisa Anderson-Shaw. (2010, January/February). Online ethics discussion forum facilitates medical center clinical ethics case reviews. *JONA'S Healthcare Law, Ethics, and Regulation 12*(1), pp. 15–20.
18. Harold G. Koenig. (2003, July/August). Meeting the spiritual needs of patients. *Satisfaction Monitor.* Retrieved March 12, 2011, from http://www.ourjourneyof hope.com/resources/meeting-the-spiritual-needs-of-patients.pdf.
19. Marilyn M. Mannisto. (1985, April). Orchestrating an ethics committee: Who should be on it, where does it best fit? *Trustee 38*(4), pp. 18–19.

20. Ross et al., p. 5.

21. Bernt et al., p. 20.

22. Fox et al., p. 17.

23. Gordon DuVal, Brian Clarridge, Gary Gensler, & Marion Danis. (2004, March). A national survey of U.S. internists' experiences with ethical dilemmas and ethics consultation. *Journal of General Internal Medicine* 19, pp. 251–258.

24. Linda S. Scheirton. (1993). Measuring hospital ethics committee success. *Cambridge Quarterly of Healthcare Ethics 2*, pp. 495–504.

25. Mannisto, pp. 17–20.

26. Amy Haddad & George Annas. (1994, July). George Annas quoted in "Do ethics committees work?" *Trustee 47*(7), p. 17.

27. Abbey S. Meyers. (2000, January 30). A lot of rules, too many exceptions. *Washington Post*, p. B3.

28. National Commission for the Protection of Human Subjects of Biomedical and Behavioral Research. (1979, April 18). *The Belmont report: Ethical principles and guidelines for the protection of human subjects of research.* Retrieved March 13, 2011, from http://ohsr.od.nih.gov/guidelines/belmont.html.

29. American Medical Association. (Updated June 1994 and June 1998). *Opinion 2.07—Clinical investigation.* Retrieved January 3, 2011, from http://www.ama-assn.org/ama/pub/physician-resources/medical-ethics/code-medical-ethics/opinion207.shtml.

30. Public Welfare, 45 C.F.R. § 46 (2001), and Food and Drugs, 21 C.F.R. § 56 (2001).

31. Mark Barnes & Sara Krauss. (2000, August 31). Conflicts of interest in human research: Risks and pitfalls of "easy money" in research funding. *BNA's Health Law Reporter 9*(35), p. 1383.

32. *Ibid.*

33. Michelle K. Russell-Einhron & Tom Puglisi. (2001). *The PricewaterhouseCoopers IRB reference book* (pp. 199–200). Washington, DC: PricewaterhouseCoopers.

34. Barnes & Kraus, p. 1382.

35. Public Welfare, 45 C.F.R. § 46.107 (2001).

36. Public Welfare, 45 C.F.R. § 46.111 (2001).

37. Paul Ramsey. (1970). Research involving children or incompetents. *The patient as person* (p. 252). New Haven, CT: Yale University Press.

38. Peter B. Budetti. (2003, August 20). Ensuring safe and effective medications for children. *Journal of the American Medical Association 290*(7), pp. 950–951.

39. Rosemary Roberts, William Rodriguez, Dianne Murphy, & Terie Crescenzi. (2003, August 20). Pediatric drug labeling: Improving the safety and efficacy of pediatric therapies. *Journal of the American Medical Association 290*(7), pp. 905–911.

40. Articles from several issues of the *New York Times* were used to prepare the Willowbrook case and provide background information: January 11, 12, and 13, 1967; March 24, 1971; April 18, 1971; January 11, 1972; May 25, 1981; January 8, 1984; April 19, 1985; and March 3, 1987.

41. Manuel Roig-Franzia & Rick Weiss. (2001, August 21). Md. appeals court slams researchers. *Washington Post*, p. B1; Manuel Roig-Franzia. (2001, August 25). My kids were used as guinea pigs. *Washington Post*, p. A1.

42. Grimes v. Kennedy Krieger Institute, 366 Md. 29, 782 A.2d 807 (2001).

43. Office for Protection from Research Risks. (1997, December 23). *Summary of basic protections for human subjects.* Retrieved August 17, 2003, from http://ohrp.osophs.dhhs.gov/humansubjects/guidance/basics.htm.

44. Public Welfare, 45 C.F.R. § 46.110 (2001).

45. Office for Human Research Protections. (1998, November 9). *Categories of research that may be reviewed by the institutional review board (IRB) through an expedited review.* Retrieved March 13, 2011, from http://www.hhs.gov/ohrp/policy/expedited98.html.

46. Claudia Wallis, Sue Wymelenberg, & Renie Schapiro. (1983, February 28). Medicine: Fraud in a Harvard lab. *Time.*

47. *Ibid.*

48. Sandra L. Titus, James A. Wells, & Lawrence J. Rhoades. (2008, June). Repairing research integrity. *Nature 453*(19), pp. 980–982.

49. Brian C. Martinson, Melissa S. Anderson, & Raymond Dearies. (2005, June). Scientists behaving badly. *Nature 435*(9), pp. 737–738.

50. Final Rule, Child Abuse and Neglect Prevention and Treatment Program, 45 C.F.R. §1340 (1985).

51. Services and Treatment for Disabled Infants; Model Guidelines for Health Care Providers to Establish Infant Care Review Committees, 50 Fed. Reg. 14,893 (1985).

52. *Ibid.*

53. *Summary: Survey of infant care review committees.* (1984). Paper presented at the Annual Meeting of the American Academy of Pediatrics, Chicago.

54. Jerry P. Roscoe & Deirdre McCarthy Gallagher. (2003, Spring). Mediating bioethical disputes: Time to check the patient's pulse? *Dispute Resolution Magazine 9*(3), pp. 21–23.

55. John C. Fletcher, Norman Quist, & Albert R. Jonsen. (1989). *Ethics consultation in health care.* Chicago: Health Administration Press.

Section III

Administrative
Ethical Issues

Virtually all administrative problems that arise in managing health services organizations and programs have ethical dimensions. These ethical problems are qualitatively distinct from those encountered in the business world.

Business ethics literature burgeoned in the 1980s, and courses in business policy and ethics are now common in graduate and undergraduate business programs. For-profit enterprise has no tradition of an independent duty or obligation beyond that established by law; appropriately, emphasis is placed on profitability and caveat emptor (let the buyer beware). Business ethics literature examines concepts such as honesty, integrity, and benevolence; duties of employees to one another and the organization; and duties of organizations to employees. These aspects are similar to those that health services managers apply. Absent, however, is the concept of respect for persons, which emphasizes autonomy, fidelity, and confidentiality. Further, beneficence is not a focus in business ethics. The principle of justice is found only at the periphery of business ethics. The differences between business and health services are cited not to criticize business but to distinguish the two fields of endeavor, whose foci and purposes are, simply put, quite different.

The public's view and that of the health services field have been that health services managers have a higher calling, one that goes well beyond the financial bottom line. Codes of ethics in health services define this calling and the intrinsic duties of managers. This definition arose from the link with medical and nursing professionals and the not-for-profit status common to health services. Acute care hospitals have historical links with religious orders; Samaritan motivation created unique relationships. The totality of this higher calling emphasizes the caring and the curing aspects of health services. It reflects society's sense that the sick are a unique group, one with special status; they need protection and are not to be exploited. Despite occasional harsh criticism, especially of financial management and the quality of care, the Samaritan image of health services organizations is largely intact.

Administrative ethics issues that confront health services managers cover a gamut, from conflicts of interest to governing body and medical staff relations to an independent duty toward patients. Such problems can be subtle. They may appear in several guises but are identifiable and solvable by alert, conscientious managers. The ethical issues and concerns of managers in their relationships with the organization, staff, patients, and community are considered in Chapters 6, 7, and 8. Considered, too, are the effects of infectious diseases such as acquired immunodeficiency syndrome/human immunodeficiency virus (AIDS/HIV), hepatitis B, and hepatitis C on these relationships, and the special duties and responsibilities that they raise.

Section III identifies and examines administrative ethical issues. By and large, they are distinct from the biomedical ethical issues considered in Section IV. Differences between administrative and biomedical ethical issues are important, but the two often blur in practice. Patient consent provides an example of these differences. Administrative ethics of consent likely affect patients as groups rather than individuals, and they affect managers' relationships with the organization, peers, profession, and community. Biomedical ethics of consent usually affect individual patients or specific types of patients. The two merge in the ethical duty of the organization to assure itself that patients have freely given informed consent to clinicians for treatment. Administrative and biomedical ethical problems actually or potentially affect one another. The primary focus of each type of ethical problem differs, however.

CHAPTER 6

CONFLICTS OF INTEREST AND FIDUCIARY DUTY

onflict of interest is a common administrative ethical issue in health services organizations. A conflict of interest can arise when someone has a duality of interests or duties. This duality of interests occurs when duties are owed to two or more persons or organizations, and meeting the duty to one makes it impossible to meet the duty to the other. A classic example of a duality of interests that will lead to a conflict of interests occurs when a decision maker—such as a director (trustee) or manager—is also a decision maker on the same question for an organization with which the health services organization does business. The manager cannot meet the duties owed to both organizations—the duties conflict with each other. Conflicts of interest also arise for clinicians. Conflicting duties owed to different patients by the same physician, for example, are an important reason to separate the organ transplant team from the physician who is treating the potential donor. Other dual interests that can result in conflicts of interest arise when a duty owed to the organization by a physician are in conflict with those owed by the physician to patients or colleagues, or when patients with the same diagnosis and physician but in different payment categories receive different care in the same organization.

Conflicts of interest are insidious; one can slip into them without realizing it. Sometimes, there is a fine line between acceptable and unacceptable behavior, a pragmatic view recognizing that the relationships of normal business often create a duality of interests, which may result in actual conflicts of interest.

Relationships among staff members can cause dualities of interest that result in an actual conflict of interest, or certainly the appearance of a conflict.

Sometimes More than Friends

Mary and John work in the medical imaging department of a large community hospital. Mary is a radiographic technologist who earned an MBA online. She was appointed the administrative head of the department 2 years ago. She supervises 14 techs, 5 clerical staff, and 4 transporters. About 2 years ago, Mary hired John to be a transporter. John had a strong recommendation from a radiologist in the department, who is a family friend. Mary and John developed a good relationship and sometimes had lunch together or took breaks at the same time. Their friendship did not seem to interfere with their jobs; they always acted professionally at the hospital.

About a year after John was hired, there were rumors that Mary and he were dating. A few months later, Mary told her staff that she and John had eloped and were married. Now, they spent even more time together. They arrived at work together, joined each other for meals and breaks, and left together. The staff began to pay close attention to how Mary treated John and if there was any favoritism. Sometimes, the other transporters grumbled that John got more attention from Mary when he had problems and that he was getting physically less demanding transport assignments.

One of the senior techs spoke to the human resources (HR) director about what she thought was a developing problem in the department. The director told her that there were no hospital guidelines on nepotism. The HR director told the tech that she could file a grievance if she felt that John was receiving preferential treatment, or if she thought their marriage was interfering with good management in the department.

The Latin root of nepotism is *nepoti*, defined as child, grandchild, or nephew. Niccolò Machiavelli touted the value of *nepoti*—especially nephews—in government as the best means of maintaining control and wielding power effectively. He argued that great benefits resulted from keeping control and power within the family. The contemporary view of nepotism in organizations is that it should be avoided or, if allowed, minimized and controlled. Nepotism has the potential to decrease objectivity, cause behavioral problems to be ignored, result in favoritism, produce an unhealthy work environment, cause poor workplace decision making, diminish morale among non-*nepoti*, and not stand up to public scrutiny. Well-managed organizations have guidelines on nepotism. Commonly, relatives are not allowed to report to one another, or even to work in the same department. As important as the actual presence of problems is the perception of unequal or inequitable treatment. The halo effect (perceived positive qualities as to one attribute cause a perception of similar qualities in related things) and stereotyping (conceptions of an individual based on prior assumptions) are two examples of problems when there is nepotism. Generally, policies—such as those on nepotism—help managers make decisions that further the interests of the organization and its patients. In addition, they can be used by those who may not want to supervise or work in the same department with a relative as a reason to avoid doing so. HR should take the lead in developing a policy on nepotism. Managers need guidance in such matters, and the certainty of policies furthers the organization's effectiveness.

Managers' relationships with the organization and interactions with the health system and other organizations in it can cause conflicts of interest. In addition to potentially affecting managers' relationship with the organization, conflicts of interest can affect managers' relationships with the profession and their personal development.

Conflicts of interest are often subtle and can affect all managerial activities. Has the manager who uses a position of influence and authority to gain titles, stature, and income at the expense of the organization or patient care acted ethically? Is the manager who is lax in developing and implementing an effective patient-consent policy and process acting ethically? Is it ethical for a manager to review and cleanse negative information from reports to the governing body? Is it ethical for a manager who has reason to believe that quality of care problems may exist in a clinical department to do nothing to prove or disprove their presence? Is it ethical for managers who have serious concerns about their abilities to continue managing? To the complexity of such questions from an ethical perspective must be added the legal implications. Regardless, managers must first be concerned about their independent, positive duty to the patient.

There is significant evidence that many conflicts of interest are not consciously understood by persons making decisions—they honestly believe that what they are doing is in the best interest of the organization or individuals involved. Compensation program incentives may subconsciously drive decision making that leads to conflicts of interest.[1] Yet, managers must avoid any hint of wrongdoing, especially the suggestion of divided loyalties. A bad odor emanates when a hospital's chief executive officer (CEO) owns stock in a corporation that contracts for the hospital's data processing business, and in which the principal stockholder and CEO is the hospital's comptroller. The odor lingers regardless of discounted price or other advantages the hospital may gain. Outside observers will certainly think that the relationships have hidden aspects that are detrimental to the organization or its patients, and that managers are reaping a personal advantage. Attempts to convince the public otherwise probably reinforce the perception of wrongdoing. The only course of action is to avoid arrangements or entanglements that contain any hint of duality of interests that could lead to conflicts of interests. The problem is well put by Harlan Cleveland in *The Future Executive*: "If this action is held up to public scrutiny, will I still feel that it is what I should have done, and how I should have done it?"[2] Cleveland's criterion of public scrutiny can be called the "light of day" test; its simplicity is compelling.

FIDUCIARY DUTY

Fiduciary is an ethical and legal concept arising from Roman jurisprudence. A fiduciary relationship exists whenever confidence and trust on one side result in superior position and influence on the other. Superior position and influence result in duties of loyalty and responsibility. This definition suggests that numerous fiduciary relationships exist in health services. Governing body members, for example, are fiduciaries. Their duty of loyalty prevents them from using their position for personal gain, and they must act only in the organization's best interests. This definition has been interpreted to mean that no secret profits can be made in dealings with the organization and that the governing body member may not accept bribes or compete with the organization. The duty of responsibility requires governing body members to exercise reasonable care, skill, and diligence, as demanded by the circumstances.[3] Members of governing bodies have a duty to avoid both errors of omission and errors of commission. Breaching these duties could result in personal liability, whether or not the corporation is organized for profit.

Trusts are common in the health services field. Many not-for-profit health services organizations engaging in charitable activities were founded because of a gift or bequest that established a trust; trustees manage the assets of the trust. Examples are trusts to defray the costs of a patient unit or specific clinical activity in a hospital. Other uses include funding schools of nursing or providing scholarships to educate health services personnel.

The term *trustee* is commonly used to describe governing body members of not-for-profit corporations in the health services field, even though there is no trust and they are not true trustees. Technically, the legally correct term is *director* or *corporate director*. The title *trustee* is preferred in the not-for-profit sector, however, perhaps because governing body members want to be distinguished from governing body members in for-profit organizations, in which *director* is used.

The legal standard for true trustees is much more stringent than that applied to directors of corporations or to individuals responsible for monies or properties not held in trust. True trustees actually hold title to property or the corpus of the trust, and manage it for the beneficiary. True trustees must act in good faith and practice undivided loyalty in administering the trust. All situations and relations that interfere with discharging these duties must be avoided. Breaching these standards results in personal liability.

In many jurisdictions, the standard of care required of directors of not-for-profit corporations who are not true trustees is higher than that required of other corporate directors. The usual standard for directors who are not true trustees is that they are liable for ordinary negligence (e.g., errors in judgment). The minority rule is that to be legally liable, directors must have committed an act of gross negligence, usually defined as an intentional failure to perform a manifest duty, with reckless disregard of the consequences.

Sibley Memorial Hospital

An important court case involving governing body members of a health services organization is *Stern et al. v. Lucy Webb Hayes National Training School of Deaconesses and Missionaries et al.* (1974).[4] The members of the governing body of Sibley Memorial Hospital, a not-for-profit hospital in Washington, D.C., were called "trustees" even though they were not true trustees. David M. Stern brought a class action suit against the hospital on behalf of his minor son and other patients, alleging that patients had overpaid for care because several governing body members had engaged in mismanagement, nonmanagement, and self-dealing (succumbing to self-interest). The suit alleged that the acts of omission and commission resulted from a conspiracy between those "trustees" and various financial institutions with which several "trustees" were affiliated. The court found no evidence of a conspiracy. In considering the other allegations, however, it determined that

> The charitable corporation is a relatively new legal entity which does not fit neatly into the established common law categories of corporation and trust. . . . The modern trend is to apply corporate rather than trust principles in determining the liability of the directors of a charitable corporation, because their functions are virtually indistinguishable from those of their "pure" corporate counterparts.[5]

This ruling meant that defendant "trustees" were held to a less stringent standard of care.

The court found that the "trustees" had violated their duties as fiduciaries, even when held to the lesser, corporate standard. Mismanagement occurred because the "trustees" ignored the investment sections of yearly audits, failed to acquire enough information to vote intelligently on opening new bank accounts, and generally failed to exercise even cursory supervision over hospital funds. Nonmanagement was evidenced by the same failure to exercise supervision. In the starkest example, although certain "trustees" were repeatedly elected to the investment committee, they did not object when the committee did not meet in more than 10 years. The allegation of self-dealing was substantiated by the following: A number of "trustees" were officers of banks in which Sibley kept hundreds of thousands of dollars in noninterest-bearing checking accounts and in which interest-bearing accounts paid less than market conditions would have permitted, and one "trustee" advised approval of and voted to approve a contract for investment services with a corporation of which he was president.

The court did not find evidence of personal gain by the "trustees," although in several instances they had been associated with organizations that had benefited from transactions with the hospital. That there was no evidence of a conspiracy seems significant to the ruling.

The court did not order any "trustees" removed from the governing body, and no personal liability attached to their wrongdoing. To prevent similar problems in the future, the court ordered the governing body to adopt a written investment policy, review relevant committees to determine if hospital assets conformed to the policy, and establish a regular process of disclosure of governing body members' business affiliations. Before the case was decided, the governing body adopted the then-current guidelines on conflicts of interest published by the American Hospital Association (AHA). That action occurred long after the fact but demonstrated the governing body's good faith. The AHA's conflict of interest statement (which is now out of print) reflected the less stringent corporate director standard.

The decision in Sibley was handed down by a federal trial court and has limited legal significance as a precedent. Nevertheless, it is one of the few cases that considers the standard of care for governing body members (directors) of not-for-profit organizations. Fiduciary duty requires that governing body members exercise reasonable care, skill, and diligence; under a negligence theory, they are liable for acts of commission or omission that violate this standard. *Reasonable care* is the care an ordinary, prudent director would exercise under the same or similar circumstances. The rule enunciated in Sibley is that governing body members (directors) of a not-for-profit corporation who are not true trustees may be liable for ordinary negligence as well as gross negligence or willful misconduct. This standard is usually imposed on the board of directors of a business enterprise.

CEOs and other managers are not fiduciaries in the same sense as directors, but they are held to a similar standard: a duty to exercise reasonable care, skill, and diligence, or the care that an ordinary, prudent manager would exercise in the same or similar circumstances. Many states' laws provide immunity from liability for governing body members of not-for-profit organizations. Often, however, the statutes contain limitations and exclusions from immunity, loopholes, and vague language, thus providing little real protection for directors and officers against liability.[6]

An infrequently discussed aspect of fiduciary duty is the politicization of healthcare. In addition to fiduciary duty, politicization may cause conflicts of interest, which were discussed earlier in this chapter. The risk of politicization is high when programs owe their existence to public funding sources; it can also occur in any organization with a defined constituency, especially if that constituency is also a major source of funding. Public health managers and their organizations and activities are at greater risk because they have a unique relationship with government and the political process. They are heavily dependent on the goodwill of government officials and politicians for their funding. This puts them at risk of adopting prevailing political viewpoints to the exclusion of objective, scientific-based decision making. Politicization arises most often in the macroallocation of resources. If public health organizations and practitioners lose, or appear to lose, their objectivity because they are too closely tied to one point of view, the public may no longer have confidence in them—they will be seen as but an extension of only that viewpoint. Once lost, trust is regained only with difficulty and over time. It will take courage and the ability to persuade through use of science and objective data to protect the public's health without diminishing its autonomy or violating the precepts of beneficence, nonmaleficence, and justice for the public. Successful managers will have a well-developed, clearly identifiable personal ethic that will help them avoid or minimize the problems of politicization.

ETHICAL OBLIGATIONS OF TRUSTEES AND DIRECTORS

Legal standards stand as the minimum required level of performance. What are the ethical obligations of trustees and directors? Policies on conflicts of interest emphasize disclosure—putting other governing body members on notice about potential or actual conflicts. In the Sibley case, it is uncertain that disclosure would have made a difference. The "trustees" almost certainly knew about their colleagues' outside affiliations and activities. Adopting the AHA guidelines and knowing their content might have alerted them to the ethical problems of self-dealing and mismanagement. A conflict of interest statement probably would have made no difference as to nonmanagement because the "trustees" did not take seriously their fiduciary duty to invest hospital funds prudently.

Health services managers have the characteristics of fiduciaries. They are also moral agents, and an important part of their work is assisting the organization, through the governing body, to meet its ethical and legal obligations. Concomitant with this effort, managers have a duty to help the governing body avoid conflicts of interest and problems of nonmanagement. Managers are the conscience of the organization; they recognize potential administrative and biomedical ethical problems and act to avoid them or minimize their effect.

Hermann Hospital

A scandal uncovered in early 1985 involved activities of both administrators and trustees of the Hermann Hospital, an 800-bed facility, and the Hermann Hospital Estate, a trust established in 1914 to provide charity care to the poor of Houston, Texas. An investigation of the two entities showed evidence of theft, kickbacks, insider stock deals, lavish perquisites and expenditures, and costly trips taken by trust and hospital executives and employees at the trust's expense. Among the allegations were that the former executive director of Hermann Hospital paid money to his mistress for work that was never done and that he received kickbacks from overcharges paid by Hermann Hospital to a company of which he was president. The trust sued the former hospital executive director, asking that he repay $100,000 in kickbacks, $500,000 that he allegedly paid his pregnant mistress, and other funds he allegedly laundered. The suit also alleged that he took improper trips that, with related expenses, cost the hospital $250,000. In addition, it alleged that he used Hermann Hospital's name, credit, and money to create an interior decorating firm for his mistress, most or all of whose business came from the hospital.

The Hermann Hospital Estate's former executive director was alleged to have stolen more than $300,000. Allegations against a trust employee stated that a luxury automobile was traded in at less than 20% of its market value for a new automobile paid for by the trust. The employee then purchased the undervalued automobile at a grossly understated price. In addition, there was evidence that trustees and employees had entertained lavishly at trust expense. Newspaper accounts stated that the Hermann Hospital Estate actually spent less than 3% of its funds on financially disadvantaged patients.

As a result of the investigation, two trustees and eight high-ranking trust and hospital executives resigned. Three individuals connected with the estate, including a trustee, were indicted on criminal charges.[7]

Many of the activities at Hermann Hospital and the Hermann Hospital Estate were unethical because they violated the law. The misconduct involved in this case goes well beyond a breach of that minimum standard. By squandering funds that should have benefited patients, the trustees violated their fiduciary duty to protect trust assets. True trustees and directors alike must avoid anything that could be considered a conflict of interest and/or an improper benefit from their association with an organization. Similarly, hospital managers must be above reproach in all that they do. They act unethically when there is self-dealing or when organization assets are diverted, whether or not these are criminal offenses.

Cedars of Lebanon Hospital

Unlike Sibley Memorial Hospital but like Hermann Hospital, circumstances at the Cedars of Lebanon Hospital in Miami involved a hospital CEO whose behavior was both unethical and criminal. The latter resulted in a prison term for the CEO. As noted, criminal behavior is in itself unethical. In addition to conflict of interest, the case contains instances of self-dealing, bribery, and violations of federal laws:

- The CEO owned a consulting firm in the Caribbean with which the hospital contracted for architectural consulting services that were never performed.
- The CEO falsified governing body minutes to cover the fraudulent contract with his own consulting firm.
- The CEO received more than 2,500 shares of stock with a market value of $75,000 in a computer company from which the hospital had purchased a $1.8 million diagnostic computer to be used for multiphasic screening; later underutilization of the equipment caused a loss of more than $2,000 per day.
- The CEO bribed public officials to obtain approval for construction and loans for an unnecessary addition to the hospital.
- The CEO attempted to ease the hospital's desperate cash flow situation by not paying federal withholding on employees' salaries.[8]

Other violations of ethical principles occurred, but these five are illustrative. The CEO's activities forced the hospital into receivership; he was later convicted and sent to prison. Important in the Cedars of Lebanon case is that governing body members were negligent in monitoring the CEO and failed to meet their duties as fiduciaries.

Clinical Conflicts of Interest

The preceding discussion focused on conflicts of interest involving governing bodies and administrators. Conflicts of interest arise in clinical decision making, too. For example, is an orthopedic surgeon obliged to disclose to his patients that he will use an artificial joint that he has developed and on which he receives a royalty? Similarly, should physicians who helped develop a new drug and on which they receive a royalty have to disclose that information to patients for whom the drug is prescribed? Or, is the physician who refers a patient to an imaging center in which he has an ownership interest (that meets federal guidelines) obliged to disclose this information? Each of these examples describes a duality of interests that rises to an actual conflict of interests. The facts of each situation will determine the seriousness of the conflict. To minimize the potential for a conflict of interest, the health services organization should provide guidance to clinicians about a duality of interests that could lead to a conflict of interests. Failure to provide guidance increases the likelihood that physicians will fall into the trap of conflicts of interest, with the embarrassment and negative publicity that invariably result.[9]

CODES OF ETHICS AND CONFLICTS OF INTEREST

As noted, conflict of interest may be only a matter of degree—certain behavior, if limited, is unlikely to cause, or is presumed not to cause, a problem. Exaggerated, the same behavior will have the appearance of a conflict of interest, though there may not be an actual conflict. Gratuities are an example in applying this criterion. Few would say that a conflict of interest arises when a sales representative treats a manager to lunch in the organization's cafeteria. A 2-week, all-expenses-paid vacation suggests something very different. Extravagant gratuities, benefits, kickbacks, and gifts that are intended to be a quid pro quo are reasonably assumed to encourage or reward certain behavior. Nevertheless, the appearance of a conflict of interest results by accepting *any* gratuity from those with whom business is done—even to the extent of a small gift or inexpensive lunch.

Even gratuities of insignificant value have a cumulative effect—they bind the giver and recipient in a way that diminishes the recipient's objectivity. Keeping such relationships at arm's length is key in business transactions.

Healthcare executives are expected to conduct themselves personally and professionally so that all decisions are in the best interests of the organization and those it serves. They are expected to disclose to the appropriate authority direct or indirect personal or financial interests that pose potential or actual conflicts of interests, as well as to inform the appropriate authority of appointments or elections to governing bodies or committees inside or outside the executive's organization that result in a duality of interests that may lead to a conflict of interest. Gifts or benefits are not to be accepted if offered with the express or implied expectation of inappropriately influencing management decision making. Regardless of intention, the perception raised by the fact of the gift or benefit will suggest impropriety.

These guidelines rely on the judgment of managers. Only they possess the knowledge about personal activities and those of the organization that will permit them to determine when there are potential or actual conflicts, when a solution is required, or when certain facts should be disclosed or brought to the attention of the appropriate authority. As noted, conflicts of interest are often subtle and insidious—avoiding them or minimizing their effect once they occur requires constant vigilance.

The Code of Ethics of the American College of Health Care Administrators (ACHCA) assists managers in preventing and solving conflicts of interest. It states that the healthcare administrator shall

> Disclose to the governing body or other authority as may be appropriate, any actual or potential circumstance concerning him or her that might reasonably be thought to create a conflict of interest or have a substantial adverse impact on the facility or its residents. [Furthermore, he or she shall not] participate in activities that reasonably may be thought to create a conflict of interest or have the potential to have a substantial adverse impact on the facility or its residents.[10]

ACCEPTING GRATUITIES AND BENEFITS

Health services organizations must help staff avoid conflicts of interest by adopting policies to guide their decision making in the acceptance (or nonacceptance) of gratuities and benefits. Failing to receive guidance, staff and managers will act in ways that they believe are consistent with reasonable practice and the organization's culture.

Bits and Pieces

John Henry Williams liked his new job in the radiology department of Affiliated Nursing Homes and Rehabilitation Center. He had been appointed acting head when his predecessor, Mary Beth Jacobson, asked for a 6-month maternity leave. John Henry would be responsible for two and one-half technicians, an appointments clerk, and $350,000 in equipment. He would have the authority to purchase radiographic supplies, the annual value of which was approximately $110,000. Most supplies were obtained from three vendors, companies from which the Center had bought for years.

As Mary Beth oriented John Henry, she emphasized how much she liked the meetings with sales representatives from the three vendors. Over the years, one had become a close friend. She told John Henry that most meetings were held at the nice restaurant near the Center. Some were held in her office, and, if so, the reps always brought along "a little something." When John Henry asked what she meant, Mary Beth gave some examples: perfume, a bottle of brandy, and a pen set in a leather case. John Henry remembered thinking that his wife would like the perfume, but he was more interested in the lunches. It would be a chance to get away from the dreary cafeteria as well as his boring sandwich from home. Mary Beth said the lunches were nothing fancy. She estimated the cost to the sales rep to be similar to that of the small gifts—in the $40–$50 range.

John Henry asked Mary Beth whether there was a policy about accepting gifts from vendors. Mary Beth was upset by the question, which implied something might be wrong with what she was doing. She responded curtly that the Center trusted its managers and allowed them discretion in such matters. John Henry then asked if accepting gratuities might suggest to other staff that her decisions were influenced by the pecuniary relationship with the sales reps. Mary Beth's anger flashed: "I know you think that what I'm doing doesn't look right. That's not fair! I work long hours as a manager and get paid very little extra. It takes effort and time to order and maintain proper inventory. If things go wrong, it's my neck in a noose. The lunches and small gifts make me feel better about my efforts. My work has been exemplary. I'd be happy to talk to anyone who thinks otherwise!"

This case illustrates a problem common to health services organizations. Several facts support Mary Beth's position: Taking clients to lunch and providing small gratuities is common in business relationships. The organization incurs no direct cost because everything is paid for by the sales representatives, who use their expense accounts. At least one sales representative has become a personal friend. Taken individually, it seems unlikely that Mary Beth's judgment could be influenced by the modest value of the lunches and gratuities, but a long-term pattern could result in a different interpretation. It must be asked, however, whether other potential vendors are being ignored because of what have become "cozy" relationships with vendors.

Apparently there is no organizational policy to guide John Henry. Neither the American College of Healthcare Executives (ACHE) code nor that of the ACHCA addresses the more subtle aspects of conflicts of interest. Although it is impossible to judge the giver's true intentions, vendors try to develop good relationships with buyers, and gifts are one way this is done. External evidence, including what is offered and accepted, must be used to infer that a conflict of interest exists.

Decision makers may gain from conflicts of interest in many ways. Often ignored are situations in which the parties understand that the decision maker will be considered favorably for employment or other benefits in the future. A promise or suggestion of future benefit necessarily creates a duality of interests that can lead to actual conflicts of interest and should be prohibited in professional codes of ethics. Nonhealth-sector examples of these circumstances are common. Active-duty military personnel interact with contractors and suppliers; upon retirement, they accept employment with those same organizations. Former members of Congress and staff of federal agencies find lucrative employment as lobbyists or employees of organizations they formerly affected. Federal law limits how soon such contacts can occur, but advising those who actually make contact is permitted—a very large loophole. Former health services executives are employed by consulting firms with which their organizations have done business. Such problems in the health services field are more than theoretical, and their likelihood increases as healthcare becomes more politicized and as large aggregations of health services organizations become more common.

Anyone who takes something of value, knowing the giver intends to influence the recipient, acts unethically. Bribery is obvious: The recipient knows what is being done and what (or who) is being bought. Typically, however, the relationship of giver and recipient is subtler. What does the hospital pharmacy director do about the proffered lunch from the drug detailer? Does the CEO stop a dietitian from accepting holiday chocolates from a wholesaler? What about a modest gift from the equipment salesperson who was the successful bidder during the renovation program completed 3 years ago? Or 10 years ago? Such transactions suggest potential conflicts of interest. The gift might be given to receive special consideration in the future, or it might be payment for past decisions.

Such situations become even more complex because it is difficult to distinguish the conflict-fraught activities of managers and staff from normal interactions. People develop relationships and friendships, whether as buyer and seller or as professional colleagues. As friends or professional colleagues, however, one should expect the buyer to be equally generous in buying meals or making gifts to the seller. The street should go in both directions.

Health services organizations must establish a policy on gratuities and benefits. There are three basic options. The least complicated is to prohibit staff from accepting any gratuity or benefit offered in the course of business. Such a policy is simple—there is no need to try to judge the giver's intent. This clear, unequivocal rule can be used by staff to refuse gratuities and benefits that may make them feel uncomfortable, thus adding to its usefulness. Declining gratuities of trivial value may make some staff feel awkward, but this is not a significant negative aspect. Most important, such a policy eliminates the need to judge whether there is an expectation of influencing management decision making. The first option is the position of the Association for Healthcare Resource & Materials Management, whose code of personal ethics states, "Never enter into any transactions that would result in personal benefit or a conflict of interest."[11]

The second option is pragmatic but more complex because judgment and difficult decisions are occasionally required. A criterion of reasonableness is applied to the first option. This allows for various circumstances and recognizes that staff members have friends and relationships. What must be assiduously avoided, however, is any hint of wrongdoing or suggestion that a decision creates a conflict of interest. As noted, such balancing is achieved only with difficulty. The test should be what the reasonable person objectively viewing the situation would conclude about the intent of the giver and the effect of the gratuity or benefit on the decision maker.

A third option is a hybrid of the first two and is a compromise for organizations that prefer not to enforce an absolute prohibition, but want to minimize conflicts of interest and provide staff with a reference point. This policy considers all gratuities and benefits as coming to and belonging to the organization. They are made available for its use by sending them to the director of supply chain, either for redistribution to staff or for other corporate uses. If given to the organization or widely shared with staff, the potential for a personal conflict of interest ceases to exist, even though a conflict between the organization and patient care may continue.

This option is similar to a health services organization that receives gratuities and benefits from businesses. Suppliers of goods and services commonly make cash or in-kind contributions to not-for-profit organizations. Accepting them is not a conflict of interest. The contribution benefits the organization directly and as a whole, just as would a price cut or a discount. This option makes it difficult to accept consumable gratuities or benefits such as meals and paid travel, but even here accommodations can be made. Free travel, for example, can be raffled to staff or used to reward someone for a significant success. The gratuity or benefit does not accrue to one person, even though the reflected glory of such contributions may enhance the reputations of those who manage the organization. In addition to enhancing management's reputation, it raises the question of future favorable treatment for vendors because of gifts made previously. The practice of accepting in-kind or cash gifts from vendors is widespread and unlikely to change even though it raises ethical concerns.

Only a Matter of Degree

Stimson received four Super Bowl tickets in the mail. Attached was a note from the local sales representative for a major equipment manufacturing company, which read, "Thought you might be able to use these." The nursing facility of which Stimson is CEO recently decided to build an addition for a rehabilitation unit. The sales representative's company manufactures equipment that could be used in the unit. Stimson had called the manufacturer several months earlier to discuss equipment that might be available in order to make the specifications for the bidding process more precise.

Stimson is in a difficult situation. Super Bowl tickets are expensive, difficult to obtain, and highly prized in many circles. However, their intrinsic value is subjective; some recipients would place little value on them. Absent a personal relationship, such as a long-standing friendship, the proffered tickets seem intended to influence the CEO's decision. Important to discussing this conflict is whether Stimson is the sole owner of the organization. If so, Stimson's interests and the organization's are one—there is no economic conflict of interest. Nevertheless, the owner's financial interests may conflict with the interests of facility residents, which is a different type of conflict.

APPROVAL OF SELF-DIRECTED EXPENDITURES

More subtle questions of conflict of interest can be self-induced. It seems a safe assumption that health services managers usually identify a personal obligation to put patient interests before their own. How much, then, should be spent to refurbish the CEO's office? What types of automobiles should be leased for senior management? Answers to such questions vary by type of organization and ownership.

Patient or Self?

Anderson is the CEO of Community Hospital, a not-for-profit organization, for which he has assembled an effective administrative staff. Because Anderson's results have been good year after year, the governing body pays little attention to internal operations and focuses on fund-raising and community relations. Anderson has a large discretionary fund available. In the past, it has been used for entertainment, gifts, and staff education.

At the urging of several governing body members and managers, Anderson redecorated the administrative suite. Rosewood and leather sofas were ordered, elegant carpet and drapes were installed, a burled oak desk was delivered, and several original oil paintings were purchased through the interior decorator. The project's cost totaled $50,000.

When the cost was criticized, even by the more financially successful members of the medical staff, Anderson reacted defensively. Anderson's primary argument to justify the expenditure was that the CEO of a multimillion-dollar enterprise needed the accouterments of his office in order to be effective. Few critics were placated.

Whether such expenditures are appropriate varies by context and setting. A big private hospital with a large endowment, in which the CEO's office is expected to reflect success and sophistication, will view this case differently from a public hospital, in which each nickel is spent reluctantly. Organizations at either extreme, however, could fund worthwhile administrative and clinical projects with $50,000. No one expects a CEO to sit on a lawn chair or use brick and board bookshelves, but the criterion should be good judgment tempered by reason. Again, it is useful to view such actions as would an informed, objective outsider. The "light of day" test enunciated by Cleveland has application here.

CONFLICT OF INTEREST WITH NO DIRECT PERSONAL GAIN

The case of Miriam Hospital is similar to that of Hermann Hospital.[12] Both lie between Sibley Memorial Hospital and Cedars of Lebanon Hospital. This case has an element of conflict of interest, though other aspects make it unique.

Miriam Hospital

Before 1980, routine blood tests at Miriam Hospital in Providence, Rhode Island, were performed by a 6-channel analyzer. In 1980, the hospital purchased and put into operation a 12-channel analyzer. Because of a computer programming error, patients continued to be charged for both sets of tests, even though only the 12-channel machine was used.

A year later, Blue Cross raised questions about the unusually high laboratory charges at Miriam as compared with other hospitals. The explanation was that doctors at Miriam simply ordered more laboratory tests. In 1982, a professional standards review organization audit clerk uncovered the double billing. The manager of information systems was ordered by his immediate superior to eliminate the programming error. Shortly thereafter, however, he was told by top officials at Miriam to reinstate the programming error.

Later in 1982, a Blue Cross auditor uncovered the same problem and asked for a copy of the program. The manager of data processing was told to erase any evidence in the program that showed that the original error had been reintroduced. Blue Cross received the sanitized program.

A short time later, two data processing personnel were accused of allowing an outside company to use Miriam's computer in contravention of hospital policy. Each was offered the opportunity to resign. Fearing he would be made a scapegoat, one data processor told his story to Blue Cross, who went to the state's attorney general. Six months later, a grand jury handed up indictments against the hospital and several senior managers. The charges included obtaining money under false pretenses, conspiracy, and filing false documents. The alleged overbilling totaled almost $2.8 million.

The hospital's and managers' defense was based on their interpretation of the rules under which reimbursement was made. They argued that the rules required hospitals to continue using the same accounting methods for the entire fiscal year, even though there were errors such as those found here. An end-of-fiscal-year audit would determine what financial adjustments were needed.

Unlike Cedars of Lebanon Hospital and Hermann Hospital, there is no evidence that managers at Miriam gained personally from their decisions. Miriam Hospital was the only direct beneficiary of the double billing. This explanation does not excuse the action, ethically or legally, but does put it in a different light. Unlike Sibley, these executives did not benefit other organizations to the hospital's detriment. Regardless, to the extent that double billing improved Miriam's financial situation, the managers enhanced their positions. Thus, they benefited through continued employment, better status and reputation, and, perhaps, proffered financial rewards from the organization. Miriam's financial position was unclear; some sources stated that it could not afford to refund the overcharges, even though management stated that doing so posed no problem. If true here, saving a financially troubled organization at personal risk is altruistic, self-sacrificing, and reflects virtue ethics. Such efforts also benefit managers, however. Nevertheless, selfless or self-sacrificing activities cannot take precedence over other virtues and moral values. The end cannot be used to justify the means. These managers ignored the virtues of honesty, integrity, and trustworthiness, which are ethically more demanding.

SYSTEMS CONFLICTS

Health services managers typically serve on governing bodies of health-related organizations. Examples of such organizations include health planning agencies, charities, insurance companies, Blue Cross plans, managed care organizations, and hospital associations. Increasingly, the duality of interests caused by such service has great potential for conflicts of interest. Conflicts of interest can be prevented by proactive disclosures to the governing body (and other parties) of service on governing bodies or committees outside the manager's organization. Such information puts the organization on notice and allows it to judge the extent of the potential conflict of interest. If an actual conflict occurs, the manager must withdraw. However, changes in the health services environment may have rendered these precautions inadequate.

The dilemma begins with the manager's civic obligation and professional responsibility based on a general duty of beneficence to assist the community in meeting its health needs. These efforts are reinforced by codes of ethics and the stimulus of governing bodies. Health services managers should be encouraged to apply their professional expertise to improving community health services, but the potential for conflicts of interest is apparent and can be present even if other health services providers are not discussed. If a health services manager is a governing body member of an insurer, for example, there are potential conflicts of interest as to rates, programs, and covered services. Furthermore, some insurers are becoming competitors of traditional health services organizations by developing service delivery capability. Even if managers abstain from debating or voting on matters directly affecting their organizations, it is impossible to avoid becoming privy to corporate thinking and strategies for other activities that in general and specific ways affect the managers' health services organizations. Once obtained, this knowledge cannot be ignored.

Increased competitiveness in the field of health services makes all information about one's competitors important in order to meet threats to market share or to blunt unfriendly initiatives. In fact, the virtues of loyalty and conscientiousness require a manager to preserve or expand the organization's market share. If managers minimize the problem of conflict through disclosure and withdrawal when necessary, they both diminish their effectiveness as a governing body member of the external organization and potentially violate their fiduciary duty. Furthermore, they risk charges of impropriety simply by participating in outside organizations.

How is this problem solved? How does a health services organization obtain important expertise without exposing itself and manager-directors to charges of impropriety and conflicts of interest? One option is to permit service only by individuals from noncompeting organizations. This solution has the disadvantage of potentially excluding individuals with operational experience in the relevant geographic or service area. However, over time, out-of-area directors will develop expertise. This solution is complicated by the growing number of integrated delivery systems, which replace traditional, local organizations with those that are regional or national.

A second option is that health services organizations use full-time governing body members—persons who are governing body members of noncompeting organizations and who are not employed elsewhere. Full-time directors are common in business enterprise but rare in health services, especially the not-for-profit sector. These individuals are usually paid, an expenditure that should pose no problem for health services organizations, especially the larger ones. Organizations unable to bear the cost should consider the following course of action.

The third option uses professionally prepared and experienced individuals not actively managing health services organizations. Examples include retired health services managers and health services administration educators. Physicians and well-informed members of the public could also serve effectively. This option possesses most of the advantages of the second option. Here, some payment is desirable because it will produce higher levels of commitment and higher-quality involvement.

Managers working to improve community health services through cooperative efforts face an increasingly competitive environment. This challenge makes some types of cooperation difficult or impossible. Other types, such as sharing services and participating in joint ventures, are stimulated. Survival is a primary corporate goal for health services organizations, and new ethical guidelines are needed to address these problems.

CONCLUSION

Avoiding conflicts of interest requires constant vigilance. Managers of government-owned facilities risk fines and criminal charges for conflicts of interest. The likelihood of legal penalties is less pronounced in the private sector. This does not obviate the ethical problem, however. The ACHCA stresses disclosure in order to eliminate or minimize the problem. Disclosure presumes that one recognizes duality of interests that could lead to conflicts of interest. Failure to recognize conflicts means that managers may be well into a conflict situation before they realize it. Conflicts of interest can be subtle, and continual questioning and self-analysis are needed to identify them. Their potential and actual effect will increase as competition intensifies.

In addition to disclosure, conflicts of interest may be avoided or eliminated in other ways, including divesting a potentially conflicting outside interest, seeking guidance from the governing body, and not participating in or attempting to influence matters in which conflicts may exist. Such steps eliminate the conflict or put the governing body on notice. Both are important, but managers must remember their moral agency and must prevent conflicts of interest or work to minimize their negative effects once they are present.

Systems conflicts will cause unique problems as well as opportunities in competitive environments. To avoid conflicts of interest, managers must be alert and may need to withdraw from all governing and advising involvement with competing or potentially competing health services organizations. Nontraditional means will be required to maximize the assistance that individuals experienced in health services can offer while minimizing the potential for systems conflicts.

NOTES

1. Mahzarin R. Banaji, Max H. Bazermand, & Dolly Chugh. (2003, December). How (un)ethical are you? *Harvard Business Review 81*(7), p. 61.
2. Harlan Cleveland. (1972). *The future executive* (p. 104). New York: Harper & Row.
3. Arthur E. Southwick. (1988). *The law of hospital and health care administration* (2nd ed., pp. 123–126). Chicago: Health Administration Press.

4. Stern et al. v. Lucy Webb Hayes National Training School of Deaconesses and Missionaries et al., 381 F. Supp. 1003 (1974).

5. *Ibid.*, p. 1013.

6. James E. Orlikoff. (1990, January). What every trustee should know about D & O liability. *Trustee 43*, pp. 8–9.

7. *Houston Post*, articles dated March 5, 9, 10, 12, 13, 16, and 19, 1985, and *Washington Post*, article dated March 21, 1985.

8. Summarized from a case study written by the late Milton C. Devolites, Professor Emeritus, Department of Health Services Administration, George Washington University, Washington, D.C. The case was prepared from various issues of the *Miami Herald* and the *Miami News* published in 1974.

9. Cheryl Clark. (2010, July 1). 99% of teaching hospitals lack clinical care conflict of interest policies. *HealthLeaders Media*. Retrieved October 24, 2010, from http://www.healthleadersmedia.com/content/QUA-253272/99-Of-Teaching-Hospitals-Lack-Clinical-Care-Conflict-Of-Interest-Policies.html.

10. American College of Health Care Administrators. (2003). *Advocacy: Code*. Alexandria, VA: Author.

11. Association for Healthcare Resources & Materials Management. (2003, August 27). *Code of ethics and professional conduct*. Chicago: Author.

12. *Providence Journal-Bulletin*, articles dated September 22, 1983; October 2, 5, and 6, 1983; and May 16, 1984.

CHAPTER 7

ETHICAL ISSUES REGARDING ORGANIZATION AND STAFF

A wide variety of administrative ethical issues arise as health services managers do their jobs. Issues linked to employee performance appraisal, for example, are a function of formal relationships. Other issues, such as working with independent practitioners of the medical staff, often result from less formal organizational relationships. Managers have an ethical and legal fiduciary relationship with the organization as represented by the governing body. In an ethical sense, managers are fiduciaries for all staff in the organization, and this relationship raises special obligations. Self-dealing was examined briefly in Chapter 6 but is addressed further in this chapter.

In carrying out their duties, health services managers are privy to copious confidential and insider information. Much is sensitive; almost all is proprietary. Administrative information is distinguished from that collected, used, and maintained for patient care. Using and safeguarding both types of confidential information is a major ethical concern in health services organizations.

ORGANIZATIONAL CONTEXT OF RELATIONSHIPS

Managers are employed to carry out the organization's mission in the context of its philosophy. As one of its most important responsibilities, the governing body selects and evaluates the chief executive officer (CEO). In turn, the CEO selects and evaluates subordinate managers, perhaps down to middle management. Regardless of organizational level, managers are moral agents who are ethically accountable for the effects of nonfeasance, misfeasance, and malfeasance affecting patients, staff, and organization. Managers' decisions are not excused because they are employees or because they were only "following orders." The law may hold individuals who are not prime actors or decision makers to a different standard, but managers remain morally accountable.

As an employee, the manager has a duty of loyalty to the organization and its staff. In terms of the organization, this duty means that the manager supports the employer's goals and activities and keeps confidential what is learned. Disagreements about policy and its implementation are neither broadcast nor otherwise shared with individuals who have no "need to know." The duty of loyalty has special importance in light of a common malady, backbiting the employer. Backbiting is not the grumbling or complaining usually considered normal, perhaps even healthy behavior. Although employees may have a legitimate reason to complain about their treatment (even the best employer does not get it right every time), rabid, negative comments are problematic. Employees who persistently speak ill of their employer act in an unacceptable fashion and should find new employment, voluntarily or involuntarily.

Managers must achieve the difficult balance between loyalty to the organization and fidelity to their personal ethic and professional integrity. Where does the manager draw the line? How far should a manager go in following the crowd or in standing alone? A clear and well-considered personal ethic is needed to answer questions such as these. Professional codes of ethics play a role but provide only general guidance and are unlikely to be useful in helping a manager decide what to do in specific cases. At the extreme, the limits of loyalty are part of whistle-blowing, which is examined in Chapter 8.

As posited previously, the manager has an independent duty and responsibility to the patient; at minimum, this means that managers protect patients from unnecessary risk and work to further their interests. What follows from that duty is the need for integrity and the courage to speak out and act to make that responsibility a reality. What happens, however, when the duty to protect the interests of patients conflicts with the duty of loyalty in achieving part of the organization's mission?

She Only Had to Ask

Richard Weidner experienced angina during mild exercise. His internist referred him to a cardiologist at University Hospital for a cardiac catheterization. After the cardiologist examined Weidner, she explained the procedure and obtained his consent. As the cardiologist turned to leave, Weidner asked her, "You'll be taking care of me, won't you, Doc?" The doctor replied, "I'll see you in the cardiac cath room." Weidner was reassured and especially pleased that he had had such a long, friendly visit with his cardiologist.

That afternoon, Weidner was lying on the table waiting for the catheterization to begin. He had a clear view of the television monitor, and as the procedure began he saw the catheter moving from his groin toward his heart. At one point he asked a question and was startled when his cardiologist appeared near his head and described what was happening. When Weidner asked who was threading the catheter, she told him it was a resident in cardiology.

Later, Weidner was in the recovery area waiting to be discharged. He was quite agitated that a resident had performed the procedure, especially because he thought he had an understanding with his cardiologist. He described what had happened to the nurse and demanded an explanation. The nurse tried to calm him. "You know," she said, "this is a teaching hospital—we train residents so they can perform these procedures to help other people." Weidner was not placated. He said, "Had I been asked, I probably would have agreed to have the resident participate. But they didn't ask me, and I'm damned angry about it. Please tell a manager to see me immediately. I want some answers!"

Weidner was not harmed physically, but he was emotionally distraught. He believed that he was misled and that a promise was broken. Weidner was concerned about who would perform the procedure and sought reassurance from the cardiologist, whom he trusted. Her answer was, at best, evasive. She purposefully or negligently misled him and thus breached her obligation to tell the truth. In sum, Weidner was deceived and treated disrespectfully. What happened does not seem to be the result of maliciousness; all involved would likely be distressed to learn of Weidner's anger about his treatment. Weidner's understanding was unmet, however.

What should the manager of cardiology do when Weidner relates his story? Except to reassure and placate, little can be done for Weidner. Perhaps a promise to Weidner that it will not happen again (to him or to other patients) will be helpful. More important is what should be done to prevent similar problems. The manager of cardiology should be the force for staff education and necessary process changes. The personal ethic of this manager's peers and the organizational philosophy should demand this level of attention to the principle of respect for persons and the virtues of trustworthiness and integrity.

To become fully qualified, physicians in residencies need specialized training, which can only be gained by treating patients. Far less acceptable, of course, is the assumption that all patients are willing to participate in medical education. Being used as a means to an end is a crude summary of utilitarianism and one incompatible with the principle of respect for persons; specifically, the elements of autonomy and truth telling were violated in this case.

The forms used to admit patients to teaching hospitals disclose their involvement in medical education. Few patients, however, read or understand the implications of that disclosure. Judged by legal standards of informed consent, the act of signing such a form has questionable validity. More important than the law, however, is the organization's ethical obligation to inform patients of what being a teaching institution means in terms of their care. Even if the form has been read and understood, minimum ethical conduct demands that patients are actively informed when teaching activities occur and that permission is again obtained. Medical education and consent are covered more fully in Chapter 9.

ORGANIZATIONAL INFORMATION

In addition to some types of clinical information, the manager is privy to confidential information about the organization. As with patient information, a basic criterion for other confidential information is "need to know." Examples of confidential organizational information include decisions about capital equipment, medical staff recruitment and development, business and marketing strategies, and financial and human resources programs. Equally important, but less commonly included, is general information concerning the staff and organization and specific information such as the strengths, weaknesses, and peculiarities of individual managers or governing body members.

In a competitive environment, "loose lips" will result in significant adverse consequences. It is unethical to make confidential information available, deliberately or negligently, to unauthorized organizations or individuals. This is true regardless of whether the manager's organization is put at risk or actually experiences a loss, or whether the manager disclosing the proprietary information gains personally.

The 2007 American College of Healthcare Executives (ACHE) code directs healthcare executives to "respect professional confidences." This wording provides little guidance about use of confidential information in the organization. Managers, governing body members, and staff must ensure that confidential information, which is usually proprietary, is safeguarded. Physicians who are independent contractors—a typical arrangement in hospitals—have limited loyalty to the organization; this makes sharing proprietary information with them problematic. In a competitive environment, which likely includes competition from physicians on their own medical staff, health services organizations increasingly provide confidential information to physicians only on a "need to know" basis.

Self-Dealing

Narrowly defined, self-dealing occurs only when a person with access to confidential information uses it for advantages such as monetary gain, unfair personal advantage, or self-aggrandizement. Misuse of confidential information that does not involve self-dealing is simply a breach of confidentiality. Examples of misusing insider information include the following: a manager, knowing that the organization will establish a surgicenter in a specific location, purchases the property through a straw man (an agent), who then resells it to the organization at a profit that the two share; a manager discloses information about organizational decision making that gives acquaintances an advantage in doing business with it (misuse of confidential information); and a manager seeking revenge for perceived insult discloses market strategies to competitors, with no resulting personal gain. Strictly speaking, only the first scenario illustrates self-dealing. If the manager in this example is the decision maker for both the sale and the purchase, there is also a conflict of interest.

What's a Manager to Do?

S.L. Rine joined the management staff of a large health services provider after working at a similar organization for several years. Rine is a member of ACHE and wants to build the best set of credentials in the shortest time. His goal is to become a CEO.

Rine is responsible for several support departments as well as the administrative aspects of some clinical areas. Shortly after beginning employment, Rine realized that the organization is very political. Much of what happens at the senior level is the result of personal relationships and obligations.

Maintenance is one of Rine's departments; it is responsible for all the grounds. Rine learned that grounds crews were being sent to the homes of senior members of the governing body to maintain their lawns, shrubs, and trees. Rine asked the maintenance director to explain and was told that the practice had a long history and should be left alone. When Rine asked the director for a cost estimate of the grounds work being done at the private homes, the director refused, saying that he feared the wrath of the governing body members who were benefiting. Rine pondered what to do.

Soon after talking to the maintenance director, Rine had lunch with the laboratory director. Without discussing specifics, Rine described the problem in maintenance. The laboratory director exclaimed, "That's nothing!" and went on to describe how two governing body members were selling reagents and supplies to the laboratory at higher-than-market prices. Rine asked the laboratory director why she had not done anything about the situation. She replied that her predecessor had tried to stop the practice and was fired. Again, Rine pondered what to do.

This case has two dimensions, one involving governing body members, the other involving managers. Governing body members whose yards are maintained by the organization or who sell to the laboratory at inflated prices are implicitly or explicitly using their authority for personal benefit. Selling overpriced reagents and supplies to the laboratory seems more unethical than receiving free grounds maintenance; morally, however, the two acts are indistinguishable. Both improperly divert (steal) organizational resources. Most destructive for the organization's moral health is that governing body members are setting a bad example, which, at best, makes the staff cynical; at worst, staff is encouraged to use their authority improperly as well.

The second dimension of "What's a Manager to Do?" is the role of managers. Knowing about improper (i.e., unethical or illegal) behavior, but not acting to affect it (nonfeasance), is no better than committing an unethical act (malfeasance). Codes of administrative ethics are of limited help. Rine and the laboratory manager agree that the behavior is unacceptable. Their ethical obligations are clear; they should act on them.

By confronting those involved, Rine will achieve little more than embarrassing them, and he may be fired. Managers can and should take any available steps, however. One is to question generic unethical activities at every opportunity and to encourage colleagues to speak out. If several managers agree that certain behavior is unethical, they draw strength from one another. They can implement (or at least try to implement) a policy of competitive bidding for all purchases, including those for the laboratory. They can develop and propose an organization-wide policy on self-dealing and abuse of authority. In short, they must take whatever steps they can to end unethical practices. As moral agents, they cannot close their eyes to such problems. Nonfeasance is not an option.

Misuse of Insider Information

Persons in an organization with access to information not available to the public are known as insiders. Ethical problems arise when managers use such information in a manner that is inconsistent with their fiduciary duty, the obligation to be trustworthy. Benefiting oneself or one's associates are examples. Some misuse of confidential information has a salutary effect and must be distinguished. An example is whistle-blowing that occurs when internal efforts at reform fail and the manager's moral agency demands external disclosure of information about practices that may affect the safety of patients or the public. The protection of such groups takes precedence over a duty of loyalty (fidelity) to the organization, even if the manager becomes subject to civil or criminal sanctions.

A common misuse of confidential (nonpublic) information occurs when employees (insiders) use it to make advantageous stock market transactions. Historically, health services organizations were largely unaffected because few were publicly traded, for-profit stock corporations. This status has changed dramatically since the late 1960s. Regulation by the Securities and Exchange Commission or state counterparts does not diminish the seriousness of the unethical conduct inherent in misusing insider information. Again, the law is a minimum that does not necessarily set an appropriate level of ethical behavior.

Just Part Owner

Jane Abernathy is the CEO of a large urban not-for-profit nursing facility. She is a voting member of all governing body committees. Following a retreat, the governing body's planning committee recommended that rehabilitation become a significant new initiative. For the past several months, the capital expenditures committee has considered the purchase of equipment to increase the nursing facility's capacity in rehabilitation. The part-time physician-director of rehabilitation wants to become a full-time employee.

Following an uncle's death 2 years ago, Abernathy inherited 1,000 shares of INCO, Inc., stock. She submits an annual statement of her investments and holdings as part of the governing body's conflict of interest disclosure requirement. The next report is due in 8 months. INCO's last annual report stated that 10 million shares of common stock are publicly held. INCO manufactures rehabilitation equipment similar to that which Abernathy's facility may buy.

The capital expenditures committee's draft report includes the purchase of INCO equipment. Abernathy dislikes making private information available to the governing body and is distressed about this apparent need for special disclosure.

In theory, Abernathy faces a duality of interests that could lead to a conflict of interest. Also, there is a potential to misuse confidential information to engage in self-dealing if Abernathy recommends purchasing equipment from a manufacturer in which she owns stock. Abernathy's ownership interest is remote, however—a mere .01% of the company's stock. Thus, the personal gain is so small that it is unlikely Abernathy's decision could be influenced by her stock ownership or, if it were, that she would enjoy any measurable benefit. Abernathy's objectivity becomes more suspect as her ownership interest increases. Nevertheless, Abernathy should disclose her holdings in INCO, even though it is distasteful to her.

RELATIONSHIPS WITH THE GOVERNING BODY

The CEO is the governing body's agent in achieving the organization's mission. In turn, the CEO selects, hires, evaluates, and retains subordinate managers. The CEO and other managers and staff are moral agents, not just the organization's morally neutral arms and legs.

As previously noted, some sectarian health services organizations require that mid- and senior-level managers are adherents of the religion of the sponsoring organization. This requirement is too restrictive; coreligionists often hold different views about various doctrines and the rigor of their application. An effective corporate culture is built on managers (and other staff) who understand and accept the organization's philosophy. Nonsectarian philosophies and secular humanism commonly have values like those of organized religion. Culling for values occurs in recruiting and selecting staff, and it is here that ethical compatibility should be determined. Applicants, too, should assess their fit with the organization's culture during the interview.[1] Focusing on congruence of values widens the field from which to recruit competent managers; such diversity inevitably benefits the organization.

The governing body and the CEO and senior management (shown in Figure 6 as "Administration") must define the scope of their respective functions. Figure 6 also suggests the need to distinguish senior and middle management. Governance, administration, and management must understand their respective activities or they will interfere in one another's spheres, with resulting inefficiency and frustration of organizational goals. The diagram is not intended to depict relationships and spheres as isolated. It must include permeability of ideas and communications, but separateness as well as unity must be clear.

Early leaders in hospital administration asserted that the risk of conflicts of interest when the CEO or members of the medical staff are members of the governing body far outweighs any benefit.[2] The environment has changed dramatically, however. Current thinking is that disclosing

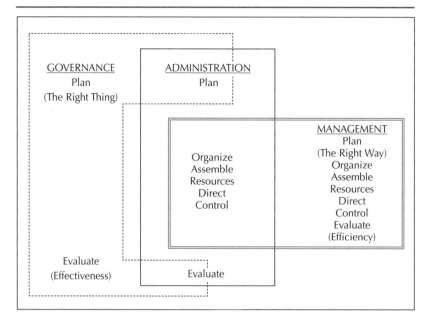

Figure 6. A model of hospital governance, administration, and management. (Reprinted from *Trustee,* 34, p. 6, by permission, June 1981. Copyright © 1981, American Hospital Publishing, Inc.)

duality of interests or potential conflicts of interests prevents or minimizes their occurrence. In 1989, 42% of hospital CEOs were full voting members of the governing body, an increase from 38% in 1985.[3] That study found that, on average, two physicians with medical privileges at a hospital were members of its governing body.[4] The trend toward membership of senior managers and medical staff members on the governing body has continued; as of 2011, it is considered essential that they participate in governance.

Anecdotal evidence suggests a trend toward a greater proportion of internal governing body members (senior managers employed by the organization) relative to external members. Internal members are desirable because of their general and organization-specific expertise. This duality of interests necessarily increases the potential for conflicts of interest, however. Governance has a specific and important role. The board reviews, evaluates, and directs senior management and its performance. It is a buffer, as well as a connection, between the organization and the ownership— stockholders in the case of for-profit corporations, or the community (service area) in the case of not-for-profit organizations. The governance and management functions are combined to the potential detriment of the organization, but especially to those served by it.

Regardless of governing body membership, the CEO and senior managers link governance to the operating components of the organization. As the governing body's agents, they provide it with the information and recommendations upon which macro-decisions are made. This enables senior managers to filter or sanitize data and make themselves look good or to mislead, as occurred in the Cedars of Lebanon case (see Chapter 6). A key issue is how much and what types of information the governing body should receive. The governing body must make this determination. The CEO and senior managers should make recommendations, but governing body members must be sufficiently informed to know which data it needs and how to interpret them. Level of involvement and expertise are special problems in organizations that have voluntary governing body members. A partial answer to improving performance of governance is to identify the qualities, skills, and education that board members of healthcare organizations should have. To stimulate such efforts, several states have adopted voluntary certification for hospital trustees; some have mandatory requirements.[5]

It is natural that managers want their performance to be viewed in a good light. Pressures in the external environment may tempt managers to engage in "creative reporting" about their performance. However, managers are obliged to be truthful in governing body interactions, an ethical duty arising from virtues such as courage, trustworthiness, veracity, and candor. Deception is antithetical to these virtues. This does not mean staff must emphasize unfavorable information; a balanced picture is prudent and desirable. It does mean that the governing body must be informed of problems honestly and in a timely manner. Managers must be alert to understated or misrepresented problems from their subordinates as well. Truthfulness is linked to whistle-blowing, which is discussed in Chapter 8. Standardized and routinized reporting minimizes the potential to manipulate the system or the data.

I Wonder If They Even Care?

Stu White had just returned to his office from a monthly governing body meeting. His assistant, Barbara Jones, noticed that he was agitated and asked, "How was it?" White responded by describing the governing body's chronic problem, something Jones had heard before. He said, "I think I could tell them that the moon is made of green cheese and they would believe it! They don't seem to know, or care, what happens in this nursing home!" White described how he did all the thinking for the governing body. He also described how there was no reporting system until he had established one. He emphasized that the organization had been lucky to have honest managers because, as he put it, "anybody else could have been hauling it [money] out of here by the carload."

The information-flow problem White faces results from governing body members' lack of awareness or their unwillingness to be fully involved and accountable for the organization, duties that are unquestionably theirs. White is in a powerful position. He works with a governing body that takes little interest in understanding the organization's affairs, and he determines what information it receives. This problem is not uncommon, even if not as extreme as described here. CEOs and other senior managers possess knowledge superior to the governing body's in at least two respects. They are expert about health services generally and they intimately understand the organization's activities and functions. Managers' fiduciary relationship requires them to be certain that they provide information the governing body needs. They act ethically when they present and interpret information that accurately portrays the organization. White must educate the governing body as to its responsibilities, including legal requirements. Next, he must help them identify the data and reports they need to meet those responsibilities. Failing to change the governing body's culture sets a scenario with potential for significant harm to the organization. Someone less scrupulous than White would be in a position to delay or withhold negative information, thus preventing timely action and increasing the probability of damage.[6]

RELATIONSHIPS WITH THE MEDICAL STAFF

Relations among physicians and the organization and its managers raise several ethical issues that are present whether it is a matrix organization or one organized as a traditional functional hierarchy. Schulz and Johnson[7] suggested that the CEO's role has evolved from business manager to coordinator to corporate chief to management team leader, the predominant role at this writing. As a management team leader, the CEO is a partner with physicians in their joint efforts to efficiently provide the best possible care. This evolution causes the green-eyeshade mentality of health services managers to become no more than a historical curiosity. In collegial relationships, peers identify and solve problems of mutual concern.

Regardless of the role and degree of collegiality, the CEO has duties and responsibilities that inevitably cause disagreements with physicians.

But He's Already Dead!

Dr. Reddy is an interventional radiologist who practices at Community Hospital. She has been an active and respected member of the medical staff for a dozen years. Dr. Reddy was on call the second weekend of March and was paged by the supervisor of the emergency department at Community.

When they spoke, Dr. Reddy was told that she would have to come to the hospital as quickly as possible. A 25-year-old gunshot-wound patient had been declared brain-dead and his family had given permission to harvest his organs. Dr. Reddy was needed to prepare the deceased for transport by beginning perfusion of his body, which would allow the organ-harvest team to obtain the highest quality organs. The organs would be harvested at University Hospital, which is one hour away by helicopter. Transport could not begin until perfusion was started.

Dr. Reddy was silent for a few moments, as though she were mulling over her options. The pause was somewhat startling to the supervisor, but not nearly as much as the response from Dr. Reddy: "It will be at least two hours before I can get there. I don't think that there's any rush—he's already dead, isn't he?"

The response stunned the supervisor. She was quick to remind Dr. Ready that the optimal time to begin perfusion is within one hour. Brusquely, she added, "As you know, the organs will suffer significant damage if perfusion is started beyond the critical one-hour window." Dr. Reddy did not reply. The next sound heard by the supervisor was the phone being disconnected. The supervisor called and paged Dr. Reddy repeatedly; there was no response. Frantically, the supervisor placed a call to the vice president for medical affairs.

Managers are ethically (and legally) expected to be aware of the quality of clinical practice and to intervene, as necessary. This expectation reflects their ethical obligations to protect and further the interests of patients. Dr. Reddy's refusal to come to the hospital has no element of clinical judgment. She simply failed to meet on-call obligations. This significant lapse should result in disciplinary action as required by the medical staff bylaws and rules and regulations. Dr. Reddy failed her duty of promise keeping and virtues such as trustworthiness. In addition, the principles of beneficence and nonmaleficence have been violated for those who might benefit from the transplantable organs.

Although not competent to judge the quality of clinical practice, managers act through experts who are. This situation is similar to that of a manager responsible for pharmacy or dietetics. Here, too, the manager relies on technical expertise to assess performance and make decisions. Some physicians react negatively to the slightest hint of such involvement, which they see as interference in clinical decision making. In fact, managerial involvement also serves the physician's best interests because it helps to ensure that high-quality medicine is practiced. Anecdotal evidence suggests that more competent physicians are less likely to object to review of their work. It must be stressed that the manager is not judging quality of care directly, but only in cooperation with those clinically competent to do so. Differing interests, perhaps even conflicts of interest, arise because managers must maintain harmonious relationships with physicians while ensuring patient safety. As moral agents, physicians are expected to meet the principles of respect for persons, beneficence, and nonmaleficence, as well as the virtues of courage, compassion, and caring. Lapses do occur, however.

The manager must be attentive to the needs and activities of physicians because they are essential to patient care. Their clinical service to and relationships with patients are the reason the organization exists. Conflicts with the medical staff result from enforcing medical staff bylaws, resource allocation decisions, and relationships between physicians and staff. Other important responsibilities of senior management are to help the medical staff keep its bylaws and rules and regulations current and to assist in enforcing their administrative provisions. A typical example of the latter responsibility occurs when a hospital CEO or medical director applies the medical staff bylaws and its rules and regulations to suspend a physician's admitting privileges. This action occurs most often because of tardy completion of medical records. Absent dire circumstances in which summarily suspending a physician's privileges is warranted, disciplinary actions use established procedures and are not undertaken single-handedly. Because of the independent duty owed to patients, even exclusively clinical problems cannot be ignored by managers. Clinical and nonclinical managers must act as the need arises. Sometimes mistakes occur.

Oops!

Dr. M is a graduate of a foreign medical school who has been a successful cardiologist on the staff of a large Midwestern hospital for more than 20 years. Occasionally, there have been rumors of Dr. M's alcohol abuse and disruptive behavior. Until a month ago, however, the only formal report nursing administration had received was from a registered nurse, who stated that Dr. M had been verbally abusive and had embarrassed her in front of a patient and his family. Recently, nursing administration received two incident reports: one oral, the other written. Both stated that Dr. M smelled of alcohol and seemed mentally and physically impaired. The information was forwarded to the medical director, Dr. G, a hospital employee and a member of the administration.

Dr. G called an emergency meeting of the medical staff executive committee, which the chief operating officer (COO) could not attend because of a professional meeting out of town. After discussing the information but without a formal investigation, the committee agreed to immediate termination of Dr. M's medical staff privileges. A registered letter was sent to Dr. M describing the action and the reasons for it. Another cardiologist was asked to treat Dr. M's hospitalized patients. Upon her return a week later, the COO was aghast to see the letter terminating Dr. M. She realized immediately that Dr. M's privileges should have been suspended, not terminated, pending an investigation.

Dr. M was enraged and retained legal counsel. The hospital withdrew the termination letter 2 weeks after it was sent and reinstated Dr. M's staff privileges pending a full investigation. Dr. M was not placated, however, and filed suit against the members of the executive committee and the hospital, alleging antitrust violations, defamation, and tortious interference with his business relationships.

Dr. G erred in terminating Dr. M's privileges; suspension pending an investigation was the appropriate disciplinary action. Dr. G acted to protect patients; secondarily, he wanted to protect staff. Both actions are ethically correct. However, he mistakenly chose too punitive a disciplinary action. This error was costly for the hospital in terms of public controversy and embarrassment, legal bills, medical staff disruption, and probable lingering ill will.

The hospital failed to adequately prepare Dr. G for his duties; furthermore, the medical staff bylaws and rules and regulations should require an expedited review process for such actions when patient harm is not imminent. The future holds a greater risk for this hospital, however. Managers and members of the medical staff may be reluctant to act in such cases, even when the facts are more egregious, because they fear doing the wrong thing. Had there been no action and a patient had been harmed because of Dr. M's impairment, the public outcry would have been greater. The lesson for the hospital is that all those in managerial positions must be prepared for the demands of their jobs.

Dr. M's right to due process was violated. His anger was justified, but it is not clear that he suffered significant professional or economic injuries. The termination was rescinded soon after imposition. Even if the executive committee had taken the correct disciplinary action, he would have been suspended from admitting patients pending an investigation. Regardless, Dr. M was not treated fairly. He gained sympathy (perhaps unwarranted) from physician colleagues and other staff members. This will make future disciplinary actions against him all the more difficult, should they be needed.

RELATIONS WITH NONPHYSICIAN STAFF

Like staff in other types of organizations, health services professionals seek various goals, objectives, and interests. Their work in the organization is a primary focus of their lives, but the congruence between personal goals and objectives and those of the organization is likely to be less than total. Chapter 3 noted that employees must understand that they and the organization possess the same core principles of working in the patient's best interests. This attitude must be reflected in action, not just in written organizational philosophy and policies. If employees and physicians perceive that the organization places greater value on performance other than that which reflects ethical interaction with patients (e.g., increasing hospital revenues), the principles of respect for persons, beneficence, and nonmaleficence cannot be satisfied. Because the organization can act only through its staff, this lapse is serious. If staff members fear that intervening on the patient's behalf jeopardizes their relationship with their colleagues and the organization, they will be discouraged from acting as they should.

The "Uncooperative" RN

Sally Hansen, a registered nurse with 10 years experience, works nights. At the start of her shift she noted that a urinary catheter had been ordered for a post-surgical male patient with acute urinary retention. Following established procedure, she paged the resident on duty. A first-year resident appeared and told her that he would insert the catheter. Hansen accompanied him to the patient's bedside and watched him remove the catheter from its package. He looked at the package, apparently for instructions, but found none. The resident began to insert the catheter into the patient's penis, but faltered. It was clear that he did not know what he was doing and that the patient was in great pain.

The resident turned and asked for assistance, but Hansen refused, saying that inserting a catheter was the job of a properly trained resident. "Really, you shouldn't attempt something you don't know how to do," she said. She also reminded the resident of hospital policy that prohibits a female nurse from performing certain intimate procedures on male patients. The resident yelled at

Hansen and stormed off. Hansen paged the chief resident, who catheterized the patient, but offered no explanation when she described the incident with the inexperienced resident.

The next day, Hansen was awakened at home by a call from the vice president for nursing. She told Hansen that the inexperienced resident had filed a formal statement accusing her of insubordination. The resident was adamant about pressing the issue with nursing administration and the chief of his service. The vice president for nursing said she could not be sure of the outcome.

What was Hansen's proper role in this matter? Where did her duties lie? Clearly, her duties lay with the patient and she acted properly. Even had she known how to insert the catheter, she was constrained by hospital policy from doing so. Stopping the resident protected the patient from pain and potential injury. A reprimand from nursing administration will greatly diminish Hansen's willingness to intervene to protect a patient in the future. The hospital must encourage appropriate action by all staff as it seeks to deliver high-quality care and protect the patient. Teaching is not an issue in this case; the resident was not competent to undertake the procedure—a failure of instruction, not of nursing—a failure that should be addressed with the hospital's director of medical education.

Other issues are present. One is the traditional subservient role of nurses, partly due to sexism. Poor relations between doctors and nurses do not result only from sexism, however. Anecdotal evidence suggests that the problem exists even where sexism is not a factor (e.g., male doctors–male nurses, female doctors–female nurses). A second issue is that a resident attempted a procedure beyond his training. He should have asked for help from the senior resident. Here, too, bravado, ego, and the culture of medical education may have caused an unwillingness to seek help. The third issue is that the limits of residents' clinical activities are unclear. In this regard, the procedures and safeguards in the medical education program may need review. The American Nurses Association Code for Nurses requires Hansen's action: "As an advocate for the patient, the nurse must be alert to and take appropriate action regarding any instances of incompetent, unethical, illegal, or impaired practice by any member of the health care team or the health care system."[8] Implicit in this statement is accountability for one's actions as a nurse—a professional ethic—not merely accountability through the organizational hierarchy.

The organization must support its staff with an unequivocal commitment that encourages them to intervene when a patient is at risk. This policy should be communicated and enforced. Action in such situations may cause some individuals to accuse caregivers of spying on one another. This charge is unfounded. Spying is a negative process and has no place in health services. The focus here is on an organization-wide effort—an ethic—to protect and serve the patient. If caregivers are able to minimize their ego involvement in the care process and keep their eyes on these goals, this problem will lessen or disappear.

Ignoring problems will not solve them. This maxim is especially true if patients are at risk. As the Watergate (1970s) and Clinton-Lewinsky (1990s) political scandals showed, problems can be ignored or covered up for a time but will come to light eventually. The public reacts to such revelations by assuming that others in the organization knew, yet did nothing. The public wonders how such situations could occur or be allowed to continue. In addition to the moral guidelines of respect for persons and the virtue to be honest in all interactions, the likelihood of discovery is a utilitarian reason for recognizing and solving such problems early.

Deadly communicable diseases and other high-risk situations raise special issues in the relationship between organization and staff. Both parties are ethically bound to protect patients and further their interests. It is ethically unjustifiable for an organization, through its managers, to put clinical staff at risk by failing to properly train or equip them, for example. All potentially dangerous situations should cause managers to consider the need to protect staff from unnecessary risk; failing that, the organization cannot meet its ethical obligations to them. In turn, staff will be unable to meet their ethical obligations to patients. The paradigmatic examples of human immunodeficiency virus/acquired immunodeficiency syndrome (HIV/AIDS) and other deadly infectious diseases are discussed below. They receive further attention in Chapter 8.

HIV/AIDS and Other Severe Infectious Diseases

Since it was first identified in the early 1980s, HIV, which leads to AIDS, has proved an elusive foe. Its spread continues, though more slowly since the late 1980s. Both the pessimistic prediction of a major outbreak in the general population and the optimistic prediction that it would be eliminated have proved wrong. There have been scientific breakthroughs in understanding HIV and treating AIDS. Unlike the vaccines for hepatitis A (HAV) and hepatitis B (HBV), however, HIV has neither a vaccine to prevent infection nor a cure once infected. A second strain of HIV was isolated in the late 1980s, and a new strain entered the United States from Africa in summer 1996; it is probable there will be others. Work on a vaccine is tempered by knowledge that HIV's rapid mutation makes developing a vaccine with long-term effectiveness difficult, if not impossible. Even if a successful vaccine were developed, several years of testing and clinical trials would be required before it could become generally available. Meanwhile, the attention to prevention and education is unprecedented in modern public health.

In 2008, the World Health Organization estimated that 33.4 million people worldwide were living with HIV.[9] The number of individuals living with HIV in the United States in 2006 was 1.1 million.[10] By comparison, there are approximately 3.2 million persons infected with hepatitis C (HCV), the most common chronic blood-borne infection in the United States.[11] People with AIDS are living longer as a result of more effective medical management using combinations of drugs and healthier lifestyles, including better nutrition and preventive measures that reduce risk of re-infection. The result may be that AIDS will become a chronic rather than an acute disease, a development with significant implications for health services organizations.

Legal Aspects of HIV/AIDS

Legally, HIV/AIDS is daunting to health services organizations. Already by 1990, the number of AIDS-related lawsuits was the largest attributable to any disease in U.S. legal history.[12]

One major legal issue with HIV/AIDS is confidentiality. Dimensions include confidentiality of patient names and records, reporting HIV infection, and a duty to warn third parties. Legal protections against breaching medical confidentiality are well established. The AIDS epidemic caused states to pass laws safeguarding the confidentiality and privacy of people infected or thought to be infected with HIV.[13] Like other serious communicable diseases, all states have made AIDS a reportable disease. Contact tracing, a historically important role for health departments, is belatedly being applied to HIV infection as an effective measure to diminish its spread. The American Medical Association (AMA) supports HIV testing of physicians and healthcare workers in appropriate situations. It opposes mandatory testing for medical staff privileges but urges physicians to voluntarily determine their HIV status and/or act as if their serostatus is positive.[14]

A second legal dimension and area of litigation results from special risks present when staff members work with AIDS patients. The Occupational Safety and Health Act of 1970 (OSHA) requires employers to provide a place of employment free from recognized hazards that cause, or are likely to cause, death or serious physical harm. OSHA requires universal blood and body substance precautions.

Third are the legal concerns of the risk to staff and other patients from patients infected with HIV and the opportunistic diseases that develop as HIV progresses to frank AIDS. In protecting patients and staff, health services organizations must avoid discriminating against people with HIV/AIDS, whom the law defines as having a disability. The ADA (Americans with Disabilities Act of 1990, PL 101-336) strengthened the right to full public accommodations for people with disabilities.[15] The ADA protects people with HIV or AIDS from discrimination in places of public accommodation, which include professional offices. Physicians or dentists can only refuse to treat a patient with HIV or AIDS under limited circumstances, such as when needed care is beyond the provider's expertise.[16]

Risk to staff and patients from staff infected with HIV is a fourth legal dimension. Health services organizations are subject to Section 504 of the Rehabilitation Act of 1973 (PL 93-112), which prohibits discrimination against qualified employees with disabilities. Those protections were strengthened by the ADA, which requires that employers make reasonable accommodations for employees with disabilities. To establish a violation of either of these statutes (Section 504 of the Rehabilitation Act and Title II of the ADA), a plaintiff must prove: 1) that he or she has a disability; 2) that he or she is otherwise qualified for the employment or benefit in question; and 3) that he or she was excluded from the employment or benefit due to discrimination *solely* on the basis of the disability. As to the second requirement, individuals are not "otherwise qualified" if they pose a significant risk to the health or safety of others because of a disability that cannot be eliminated by reasonable accommodation.[17]

In 1987, the United States Supreme Court considered a case analogous to that of an HIV-positive employee. In *School Board of Nassau County, Florida v. Arline*,[18] a teacher with recurring tuberculosis was discharged because of the health risk to students. The Court determined that tuberculosis was a disability protected by Section 504 of the Rehabilitation Act of 1973 and developed a four-part test: 1) nature of the risk (how the disease is transmitted); 2) duration of the risk (how long the carrier is infectious); 3) severity of the risk (potential harm to third parties); and 4) probability that the disease will be transmitted. No HIV/AIDS case has been considered by the Supreme Court.

Cases litigating whether HIV-positive health services staff are "otherwise qualified" under the ADA turn on the potential risk of harm to patients, even when harm is remote. An HIV-positive cook in a nursing facility was found otherwise qualified. Medical evidence showed that HIV is not transmitted by preparing and serving food and beverages and that his HIV status did not restrict him from performing his job.[19] Conversely, a surgical technician with HIV who assisted in exposure-prone invasive procedures was not protected by the ADA and the Rehabilitation Act of 1973. The court determined that his HIV status disqualified him from working as a surgical technician and that he was not otherwise qualified to perform his job. Evidence showed that his duties occasionally required him to place his hands on and in surgical incisions and that this put him at risk for needle sticks and minor lacerations. Expert testimony showed the risk of transmitting HIV to a patient to be very small. Nonetheless, the trial court applied the four-part test enunciated by the Supreme Court in *Arline* and agreed with the defendant hospital that there was a real possibility of transmitting HIV, and that because the consequence of infection is death, the nature, duration, and severity of the risk outweighed the fact that the chance of transmission was slight.[20]

The legal theory of a duty to warn suggests the extent to which caregivers (and, likely, organizations) may be legally obligated to protect third parties in immediate danger. *Tarasoff v. Regents of the State of California*[21] held that a psychotherapist who reasonably believes that a patient poses a direct threat to a third party must warn the person in danger. The state supreme courts that have adopted *Tarasoff* limit the duty to warn to identifiable third parties at risk of real and probable harm.[22]

Protecting Staff from HBV, HCV, and HIV

The underlying ethical premise is that health services organizations must respond to life-threatening infectious diseases by doing all they can to protect staff. This is supported by the virtue of fidelity (faithfulness, loyalty) and by the principle of nonmaleficence. Through its managers, the organization has a duty to provide a safe work place. Rawls's difference principle (special benefits may be given to small groups if doing so is in the interests of the least advantaged) supports this duty, as does the theory of utility (the greatest good for the greatest number). An effective workforce is sustainable only if there are safe working conditions. Having identified that there is an ethical priority not to put staff at unnecessary risk, the health services organization must create and maintain an environment compatible with the obligation to provide services to the community and treat individuals with infectious diseases such as HBV, HCV, and HIV.

Although present in all body substances of those who are HIV positive, the virus apparently can be spread only by sexual intercourse or intimate contact with body substances, especially blood. Though the risk to healthcare workers is low, the consequences of severe infectious diseases such as hepatitis and AIDS make infection a major concern for them and the organization. The Centers for Disease Control and Prevention and the Occupational Safety and Health Administration guidelines for universal precautions must be used in all health services organizations.

Some physicians and staff are reluctant or unwilling to treat people with AIDS. In 1987, the AMA Council on Ethical and Judicial Affairs issued a statement that physicians behave unethically if they refuse to treat people with AIDS whose medical conditions are within their competence, and this continues to be its position.[23] In mid-1987, the American Hospital Association (AHA) issued recommendations about clinical management of AIDS patients.[24] These recommendations have not changed.[25] They are consistent with CDC guidelines and state that universal blood and body substance precautions are the best protection for caregivers. They require that all patients' blood and body substances be considered hazardous and that all patients be subject to the infection-control guidelines originally established for hepatitis and HIV. This means that isolation and biohazard precautions should be used for all patients, regardless of infectious status, and that healthcare workers should protect themselves against blood and body substances and patient contact. Under CDC guidelines in effect since 1987, hospitals should judge whether their patients' characteristics are such that all admissions should be tested for HIV.

Staff compliance with the requirements for universal precautions has been and continues to be a problem and a challenge for the health services manager.[26,27] In addition to consistent use of universal precautions, the proper disposal of contaminated materials, including needles, is a problem.[28] Enhanced education can be only a small part of the answer. No caregiver can be ignorant of the risk of HCV and HIV and the importance of universal precautions. Management must identify and correct structure and process inhibitors that reduce staff willingness or ability to comply with universal precautions.

In 1987, the CDC confirmed that three hospital staff had become HIV positive after occupational exposure to contaminated blood. The risk to healthcare workers who work with patients who are HIV positive is now well documented, and there have been 57 confirmed cases of transmission of HIV, almost all the result of percutaneous (puncture/cut injury) exposure to HIV-infected blood.[29] Three large studies in the late 1980s estimated the risk of contracting HIV after being stuck accidentally with a contaminated needle at approximately 1 in 250.[30] Recent estimates are lower, with a finding that the average risk of HIV transmission after percutaneous exposure to HIV-infected blood is approximately 0.3% (1 in 300). The risk of infection after percutaneous exposure to hepatitis B (6%–30%) and hepatitis C (1.8%) is significantly greater.[31]

CDC estimated that approximately 800,000 healthcare workers in the United States would be injured by patient needles in 1998. Combined estimates from the CDC and EPINet—a computer-based standardized injury tracking system used by approximately 1,500 U.S. hospitals—suggested that more than 2,000 of those workers would test positive for new infections of HCV. Another 400 would get HBV, and 35 would contract HIV. HIV is the most feared, but HBV, for which there is a vaccine, and HCV, for which there is no vaccine, are life threatening because they can lead to liver damage, cirrhosis, and cancer.[32] The risk of infection by HBV, HCV, or HIV after occupational injuries from sharps when the source is noninfectious or unknown appears to be relatively small.[33] Prudence in all sharps injuries is the best course, regardless.[34] Attention should be paid, as well, to the psychological aspects of blood and body fluid exposure.[35]

The CDC reports that almost 25,000 adults with AIDS have a history of employment in healthcare.[36] Of concern, too, are the opportunistic diseases that accompany progression to frank AIDS. These include tuberculosis and *Pneumocystis carinii* pneumonia (PCP). At special risk in healthcare settings are older adults and persons with compromised immune systems.

Increasing numbers of infectious diseases in health services organizations pose special problems for managers and caregivers. As they seek to comply with legal requirements, the ethical obligations owed to staff and patients cannot be put at risk. Meeting the expectations of beneficence and nonmaleficence should always be foremost in the minds of all who deliver and manage services.

NEW RELATIONSHIPS WITH MEDICAL STAFF

Beginning in the late 1980s, significant changes occurred in relationships between physicians and health services organizations, a movement led by acute care hospitals. These arrangements are designed to add an economic dimension to relationships that emphasizes clinical activities. The *MeSH (medical staff–hospital)* concept was introduced in the 1980s but gained only limited acceptance; then, the *joint venture*, which included undertakings such as medical office buildings and the lease or purchase and operation of high-technology equipment, became the focus of economic relationships between organizations and practitioners. In the 1990s, both concepts were replaced by the *PHO (physician–hospital organization)* and integrated health networks, both of which focus on primary care but seek to deliver a continuum of services to a defined population. The economics of clinical practice must be tied to the organization so that each may assist the other to survive.

Such arrangements are fraught with potential ethical problems. A mildly adversarial relationship between medical staff and managers is useful because it provides checks and balances in maintaining high-quality patient care. This relationship requires that each party remember that its reason for being is to serve and protect the patient. When management and clinical practice are economically bound together, patient interests may suffer. The potential for conflicts of interest increases if the physicians involved in these arrangements are also part of the governing body. Evidence of actual conflicts of interest and fear of their potential have led to the passage of federal and state laws regulating certain clinical referrals.

APPRAISAL OF MANAGERIAL PERFORMANCE

A principal role of the governing body is appraising the CEO's performance, even as the CEO appraises subordinate managers. W. Edwards Deming rejected management by objectives (MBO) for general use in organizations. He argued that MBO pits managers against one another and leads to internal competition and suboptimization of the affected systems; ultimately, the entire organization is suboptimized. Despite Deming's concerns, MBO continues to be common in organizations.[37] In its pure form, MBO, as first conceptualized by Peter Drucker, is consistent with Deming's theory. Its use, however, has deviated from the original intent.[38]

Despite the controversy over MBO, formal appraisal of CEOs using specific criteria is appropriate. Their responsibility for the organization carries broad authority. Their interests are consistent with its optimization, and appraising them should reflect this consistency. Harvey used MBO to evaluate hospital CEOs.[39] His list of competencies necessary for managerial effectiveness included planning and organizing, achieving hospital objectives, maintaining the quality of medical services, allocating resources fairly and efficiently, resolving crises, complying with regulations, and promoting the hospital. These criteria are generalizable to any health services organization in which performance is compared against predetermined measures and standards. Current theory applies similar criteria in an MBO format.[40] One study of CEOs found that 1 in 10 had *never* had a performance appraisal, despite the Joint Commission on Accreditation of Healthcare Organizations requirement and an appraisal being an indicator of good governance.[41] Another study found that 76% of governing bodies in responding hospitals formally evaluated their CEO.[42] Ongoing informal evaluation and annual formal evaluation of CEO performance are considered essential to organizational effectiveness. Anecdotal evidence suggests, however, that relatively few CEOs are evaluated against specific criteria, especially with the specificity recommended by Harvey.

To avoid conflicts of interest when they are evaluated, CEOs must limit their role to explaining organizational performance. The CEO's performance should be reviewed without the CEO present but with feedback provided later. Like all staff, the CEO is owed fairness in the review process, especially if negative outcomes that might result in termination are possible. Problems are minimized if the governing body employs a formal process to evaluate the CEO's performance, one based on predetermined objectives that are to be attained during the period under evaluation.

CEOs evaluate the work of subordinate managers directly or in coordination with other senior managers. This includes evaluating administrative dimensions of clinical managers' work. Personal and professional relationships may interfere with objective appraisal, or, in some cases, even day-to-day management.

A Little Too Close

Sue Rosen has been a successful health services executive for more than 20 years. She is currently the CEO of an addiction treatment center that provides a full range of in- and outpatient services. Approximately 4 years ago, she experienced significant job-related stress. In addition, she had had emotional problems in her personal life, which became more complex after her divorce and difficulties with her only child.

She recognized her need for professional help and sought the services of Dr. Eisenbard, a clinical psychologist. In addition to his private practice, Eisenbard consulted for several addiction treatment centers. Rosen received 32 sessions of therapy over 2 years. Eisenbard was of great assistance and their final session occurred 2 years ago.

Recently, Rosen's clinical director, a clinical psychologist, resigned. Eisenbard responded to a blind advertisement and sent his resume to a post office box. The director of human resources brought the resume to Rosen, who was surprised to receive it. Rosen has high regard for Eisenbard but is concerned about the implications of his application.

A previous therapeutic relationship will make it impossible for Rosen to interact effectively with Eisenbard, either as colleagues or as superior–subordinate. Rosen will not feel at ease, and, if needed, disciplinary actions against Eisenbard will be difficult, perhaps impossible. Eisenbard may not wish to enter into a managerial relationship with Rosen, but at this point he is unaware that she is his potential employer. Regardless of Rosen's high estimate of Eisenbard's professional abilities, this employment relationship should not be undertaken, as it is fraught with problems.

Governing bodies should be evaluated, and properly applied MBO is also appropriate at this level. Objectivity and comprehensiveness will be enhanced if an external expert assists in the evaluation. Important in evaluating governing body members is input from the CEO and other managers who interact with them.

PROFESSIONAL CREDENTIALS

The process of verifying credentials begins when a physician first applies for medical staff membership and clinical privileges. All aspects of the candidate's education and training, licensure, and clinical preparation are reviewed. Regular periodic reviews ensure that physicians continue to be qualified. Renewal of privileges depends on demonstrated current competence. All clinical staff with independent access to patients receive a similar review, whether or not they are members of the medical staff. Preventing legal actions and bad publicity are important, but the primary reasons to be concerned about competence are the principles of respect for persons, beneficence, and nonmaleficence, as well as various of the virtues.

Occasionally, there are reports of persons claiming to be physicians but whose credentials are partly or wholly false. The problem of over-stated, misrepresented, or false credentials is extensive in the business world, and there is reason to believe health services management is infected with the same virus. Examples of misrepresented credentials include inflated job titles, responsibilities, and duties; exaggerated or falsified academic preparation and credentials; and falsified or misleading information about professional achievement and activities.[43] Some ruses are elaborate and very effective at misleading others.[44] Recent studies have found significant levels of plagiarism in original essays (known as personal statements) among applicants to medical residencies.[45] Such actions are dishonest and unethical.

Even a cursory check by a potential employer will usually uncover nonexistent formal credentials, such as licenses and academic degrees. More subtle and pervasive is the problem of "creative" resume writing. One need only look at resumes produced by some employment and executive search firms to realize that it is possible to make trivial management positions appear significant. Uncovering exaggerated or overstated credentials can be difficult because specific details of employment must be verified. Even job descriptions may not adequately reflect what the incumbent actually did in a particular position. For this reason, marginal cases may slip through.

Managers who encounter a management applicant who has presented dishonest credentials have one course of action—exposure and disciplinary action through the professional society. Appropriate action is less clear when it is discovered that current employees have falsified or misrepresented their credentials. Nevertheless, action must be taken. Counseling is a first step, whether or not the employee is to be retained. Beyond counseling, the action taken should be proportionate to the seriousness of the problem. Current job performance and the reasons for the falsified credentials should be considered. Serious falsifications and misrepresentations must be reported to the professional society and to the authorities if there is criminal behavior.

What action should be taken if one has personally overstated, misrepresented, or falsified qualifications? Managers with such problems should inform their superiors and offer the strongest possible rationale for the action. This is a sound course of action even when the claimed credential does not exist but was material to the hiring decision. The employer may not take drastic action, especially if the reasons for what was done are compelling. The employer is likely to consider current job performance. The manager must be prepared for termination, however. Continued concealment is unacceptable: As one rises to a more senior level, the stakes are higher and the potential for devastating damage to one's career increases. Misrepresented or falsified credentials are a burden to the individual because they will eventually be uncovered, and because of the chronic, nagging fear of being caught. It is better that corrections be made when there is less to lose. This is a compelling utilitarian argument. The Kantian and virtue ethicist, however, would quickly add that it should be done because it is right and honest to do so.

Slovenly verification by potential employers greatly eases the use of false or exaggerated credentials. Inadequate verification is a problem for any position in the organization. Managers breach their moral obligation if they fail to perform effective credentials checks because patients are at risk, for example, if an incompetent administrative or clinical practitioner is hired. The employer is responsible for adequately checking credentials and acting when dishonesty is uncovered. Discovery of significantly misrepresented or falsified credentials should be reported. It should cause the professional association to take disciplinary action up to and including expulsion. Representation of a fictitious academic degree or position is significant to both employer and professional organization.

Employers are morally obligated to accurately and comprehensively report the performance of former employees. In the case of serious problems such as drug addiction or other criminal behavior, specific information should be reported, whether or not it was requested. The legal concept of a duty to warn reinforces managers' ethical obligation to provide information about a former staff member's significant problems. Less serious problems should be communicated as part of a balanced appraisal of strengths and weaknesses.

A Massachusetts case raised questions about ethical behavior when physicians writing references neglected to include information about the character and criminal behavior of former residents in anesthesiology.

But Is It Relevant?

The Massachusetts Medical Society investigated three physicians at a leading Boston hospital who wrote highly laudatory letters recommending a colleague only a few days after he was sentenced to jail for raping a nurse.

The convicted physician was able to use the letters to get a new job as an anesthesiologist at the Children's Hospital in Buffalo, where officials said they were unaware of his legal troubles. He was charged later in another Boston rape case, dating back to 1978, involving patients.

Medical officials said the case, involving physicians at the Brigham and Women's Hospital, was the most striking example they have encountered of how letters of recommendation for hospital jobs have lost their value in recent years, as physicians become cautious about writing anything critical about colleagues for fear of being sued.

Other physicians on the staff of the hospital said they believed the letters were written after consulting the attorney for the Brigham and Women's Hospital. Because the rape did not occur within the hospital, they suggested that the attorney had advised the physicians that they had no basis for being critical of the physician's medical performance.

In commenting on the case, B.J. Anderson, associate general counsel for the American Medical Association, said that the association advised directors of departments in hospitals to be candid when writing letters of recommendations despite the threat of lawsuits: "Too frequently hospitals that have had a problem with a physician will write a glowing letter because it is easier to export your problems across a state line than to resolve them yourself."[46]

After an investigation by the Massachusetts Medical Society, the three physicians who wrote the letters of recommendation were censured and placed on probation for a year. The controversy over the letters prompted appointment of a panel to suggest guidelines for preparing letters of recommendation. Its report advised physicians to follow a Golden Rule of letter writing: "A letter should contain the information known to the writer that he would like to have were he to receive the letter." The report also stated that "information regarding personal character is of great importance in the case of physicians."[47]

Whether or not the physicians who wrote recommendations violated the letter of the law, they certainly failed to honor its spirit. All health services organizations hiring this physician or appointing him to its medical staff would find it relevant that he had been convicted of a felony. This is especially true of the crime of rape, which is so inimical to the intimacy of the patient–physician relationship. As with nonphysician staff and employees, the organization, through its managers, is morally obliged to report relevant information about physicians (and all staff) honestly and objectively. Reluctance to communicate information about former staff to potential new employers facilitates movement of incompetent and even dangerous clinical staff from job to job, despite spotty employment records and investigations.[48] Even state statutes that protect references if they are truthful have given limited reassurance to former employers because references tend to be subjective.[49]

CONCLUSION

This chapter identified and analyzed the ethical problems managers experience in their relationships with the organization and staff. These relationships are analyzed within the context of the manager's ethical obligations to patients. Managers have access to patient and proprietary information, most of which is confidential. This accessibility suggests the potential for inappropriate disclosure, self-dealing, and misuse of insider information.

The unique relationships that senior managers, especially CEOs, enjoy with governing bodies and staff were examined within the context of various ethical duties. Managers must act to protect patients when questions of clinical competence arise. Taking this action includes having the policies, procedures, and resources needed to minimize the risk of inadequate practice and to eliminate it should it occur. Managers must establish a culture that emphasizes patient care and safety, and they must support all staff in their efforts to maintain this focus.

New relationships among organizations and with physicians raise ethical issues, most of which result from the potential for conflicts of interest.

Emphasizing financial aspects makes it easy to forget that the patient is the primary reason for the existence of health services organizations.

The chapter concluded with an examination of falsified or overstated personal qualifications and the obligation of managers to act when these problems come to their attention. Thorough background checks and the provision of honest recommendations assist organizations in their work, protect patients, and maintain the integrity of the profession.

NOTES

1. Diane M. Barowsky. (2003, September/October). Assessing cultural fit during the interview. *Healthcare Executive 18*(5), pp. 62–63.
2. See, for example, Charles U. Letourneau. (1959). *Hospital trusteeship* (pp. 90–91). Chicago: Starling Publications; Charles U. Letourneau. (1969). *The hospital administrator* (p. 45). Chicago: Starling Publications; and Malcolm T. MacEachern. (1962). *Hospital organization and management* (pp. 87, 97). Berwyn, IL: Physicians' Record Co. T. MacEachern. (1962). *Hospital organization and management* (pp. 87, 97). Berwyn, IL: Physicians' Record Co.
3. Jeffrey Alexander. (1990). *The changing character of hospital governance* (p. 13). Chicago: Hospital Research and Educational Trust.
4. *Ibid.*, p. 18.
5. Melanie Evans. (2009, March 2). Raising the bar for boards. *Modern Healthcare 39*(9). Retrieved November 12, 2010, from http://www.modernhealthcare.com/article20090302/reg/902279962.
6. Paul B. Hofmann. (2003, September/October). Revealing inconvenient truths. *Healthcare Executive 18*(5), pp. 56–57.
7. Rockwell Schulz & Alton C. Johnson. (1990). *Management of hospitals and health services* (3rd ed., pp. 87–95). St. Louis: Mosby.
8. American Nurses Association. (2011). *Code of ethics for nurses with interpretive statements.* Retrieved January 4, 2011, from http://www.nursingworld.org/MainMenu Categories/EthicsStandards/CodeofEthicsforNurses/Code-of-Ethics.aspx.
9. AIDS epidemic update (report). (2008, December). UNAIDS, World Health Organization.
10. HIV prevalence estimates—United States, 2006. (2006, October 3). *Morbidity and Mortality Weekly Report 75*(39), p. 1073.
11. Andine Davenport & Frank Myers. (2009, May). How to protect yourself after body fluid exposure. *Nursing2009 39*(5), p. 23.
12. AIDS-related lawsuits will continue to rise, report shows. (1990, April 16). *AHA News 26*, p. 3.
13. Ronald Bayer & Larry Gostin. (1990). Legal and ethical issues relating to AIDS. *Bulletin of the Pan American Health Organization 24*, p. 457.
14. American Medical Association. (2003, November 25). *Report 4 of the Council on Scientific Affairs* (p. 4). Chicago: Author.
15. Robert E. Stein. (1991, June). The Americans with Disabilities Act of 1990. *Arbitration Journal 46*, pp. 6–7.

16. Kenneth E. Labowitz. (1992, March). Refusal to treat HIV-AIDS patients: What are the legal obligations? *Trial 28*(3), p. 58.
17. Barry R. Furrow, Thomas L. Greaney, Sandra H. Johnson, Timothy S. Jost, & Robert L. Schwartz. (1997). *Health law: Cases, materials and problems* (3rd ed., pp. 487–488). St. Paul, MN: West Publishing Co.
18. School Board of Nassau County, Florida v. Arline, 480 U.S. 273 (1987).
19. Raintree Health Care Center v. Human Rights Commission, 655 N.E. 2d 944 (1995).
20. Mauro v. Borgess Medical Center, 886 F. Supp. 1349 (1995). The trial court decision was affirmed on appeal at 137 F. 3d 398 (6th Cir. Feb. 25, 1998). In Scoles v. Mercy Health Corporation of Southeastern Pennsylvania (887 F. Supp. 765 [1994]), a federal court held that an HIV-positive surgeon was not "otherwise qualified" under Section 504 and the ADA and could be prohibited from performing exposure-prone procedures, despite the virtually nonexistent risk of infection. A federal court upheld the suspension of a neurosurgical resident from his residency in Doe v. University of Maryland Medical System Corporation (50 F. 3d 1261 [1995]) because he posed a significant risk to his patients' health and safety that could not be eliminated by reasonable accommodation.
21. Tarasoff v. Regents of the State of California, 17 Cal. 3d 425 (1976).
22. Ronald Bayer & Larry Gostin. (1990). Legal and ethical issues relating to AIDS. *Bulletin of the Pan American Health Organization 24*, pp. 461, 462 (notes).
23. American Medical Association. (Updated June 1996 and June 1998). *Opinion 9.131: HIV-infected patients and physicians.* Retrieved January 3, 2011, from http://www.ama-assn.org/ama/pub/physician-resources/medical-ethics/code-medical-ethics/opinions9131.shtml: "A physician who knows that he or she is seropositive should not engage in any activity that creates a significant risk of transmission of the disease to others. A physician who has HIV disease or who is seropositive should consult colleagues as to which activities the physician can pursue without creating a risk to patients."
24. American Hospital Association. (1987–1988). *AIDS/HIV infection: Recommendations for health care practices and public policy.* Chicago: Author.
25. Diana Culbertson, AHA Resource Center, American Hospital Association, personal communication, January 12, 2011.
26. Mary Koska. (1989, September 5). AIDS precautions: Compliance difficult to enforce. *Hospitals*, p. 58.
27. Cynthia Carter Haddock, Gail W. McGee, Hala Fawal, & Michael S. Saag. (1994, Fall). Knowledge and self-reported use of universal precautions in a university teaching hospital. *Hospital & Health Services Administration 39*(3), pp. 295–307.
28. Shelley A. Harris & Laura Ann Nicolai. (2010, March). Occupational exposures in emergency medical service providers and knowledge of and compliance with universal precautions. *American Journal of Infection Control 38*(2), pp. 86–94.
29. Centers for Disease Control and Prevention. (2011). *Preventing occupational HIV transmission to healthcare personnel.* Retrieved January 7, 2011, from http://www.cdc.gov/hiv/resources/factsheets/hcwprev.htm.

30. Susan Okie. (1990, January 16). HIV-infected workers undercounted. *Washington Post*, p. A5.

31. Centers for Disease Control. (2003, July). *Exposure to blood: What health care personnel need to know.* Retrieved November 12, 2010, from http://www.cdc .gov/ncidod/dhqp/pdf/bbp/Exp_to_Blood.pdf.

32. Kathleen F. Phalen. (1998, August 11). Needle stick risk. *Washington Post*, p. 11.

33. Ziya Kuruuzum, Nur Yapar, Vildan Avkan-Oguz, Halil Asian, Ozgen Alpay Ozbek, Nedim Cakir, & Ayse Yuce. (2008, December). Risk of infection health care workers following occupational exposure to a noninfectious or unknown source. *American Journal of Infection Control 36*(10), pp. 27–31.

34. Davenport & Myers.

35. Jaye Wald. (2009). The psychological consequences of blood and body fluid exposure injuries. *Disability and Rehabilitation 31*(23), pp. 1963–1969.

36. Centers for Disease Control and Prevention, Division of Healthcare Quality Promotion. (2003, December 11). *Surveillance of healthcare personnel with HIV/ AIDS*, as of December 2002. Retrieved January 2, 2004, from http://www.cdc .gov/ncidod/hip/BLOOD/hivpersonnel.htm.

37. Edward Marlow & Richard Schilhavy. (1991, January/February). Expectation issues in management by objectives programs. *IM*, pp. 29–32.

38. Philip E. Quigley. (1993, July). Can management by objectives be compatible with quality? *Industrial Engineering 14*, p. 64.

39. James D. Harvey. (1978, Spring). Evaluating the performance of the chief executive officer. *Hospital & Health Services Administration 23*, pp. 5–21.

40. Beaufort B. Longest, Jr., & Kurt Darr. (2008). *Managing health services organizations and systems* (5th ed., pp. 548–549). Baltimore: Health Professions Press.

41. Daniel R. Longo, Jeffrey Alexander, Paul Earle, & Marni Pahl. (1990, May). Profile of hospital governance: A report from the nation's hospitals. *Trustee 43*(5), 7.

42. J. Larry Tyler & Errol L. Briggs. (2001, May). Practical governance: CEO performance appraisal. *Trustee 54*(5), 18.

43. Physicians are not immune. A study by Gail Sekas and William R. Hutson of applicants to a gastroenterology fellowship found that nearly one-third of the 53 applicants who said they had published articles in scientific journals misrepresented themselves. Misrepresentations included citations of nonexistent articles in actual journals, articles in nonexistent journals, or articles noted as being in press. Review of applicants to an infectious disease fellowship suggested that the problem of misrepresentation is not confined to gastroenterology. The authors of the study posit but do not answer the question of what those discovering the deception should do. They urge that guidelines be developed. See Gail Sekas & William R. Hutson. (1995). Misrepresentation of academic accomplishments by applicants for gastroenterology fellowships. *Annals of Internal Medicine 123*, pp. 38–41.

44. Marilynn Marchione. (2010, December 12). Fake doctor: Pilot duped AMA with fake M.D. claim. *Huffington Post.* Retrieved February 28, 2011, from http:// www.huffingtonpost.com/2010/12/12/fake-doctor-pilot-duped-a_n_795548 .html.

45. Scott Segal, Brian J. Gelfand, Shelley Hurwitz, Lori Berkowitz, Stanley W. Ashley, Eric S. Nadel, & Joel T. Katz. (2010, July 20). Plagiarism in residency application essays. *Annals of Internal Medicine 153*(2), pp. 112–120.
46. Fox Butterfield. (1981, September 24). Doctors' praise assailed for peer in rape case. *New York Times*, p. A16.
47. Doctors censured in Massachusetts. (1982, February 4). *New York Times*, p. D27.
48. Michelle Garcia. (2003, December 26). Nurse investigation expands: Five counties, 2 states to cooperate in probe of patients' deaths. *Washington Post*, p. A4.
49. Amy Joyce. (2003, January 4). Who cares about references? Employers should though it may be difficult to get thorough answers. *Washington Post*, p. F5.

CHAPTER 8

ETHICAL ISSUES REGARDING
PATIENTS AND COMMUNITY

This chapter identifies the special relationships between managers (and their organizations) and patients and the community. The personal duties and obligations of managers, as well as the responsibilities to their profession, were noted in Chapter 4 in the context of the moral philosophies and the ethical principles of respect for persons, beneficence, nonmaleficence, and justice, in addition to various of the virtues. That chapter highlighted the need for managers to have a well-defined personal ethic to guide their decision making on administrative and biomedical ethical problems within the context of the organizational philosophy.

This chapter reinforces the book's underlying premise that the manager is a moral agent with independent duties to the patient. Managers must juxtapose their relationship with and duty of loyalty to the organization with their patient relationships. The reciprocal duties of colleagues are a part of belonging to a professional group that has expectations and demands certain behavior. In many ways, organization and manager are one. Managers must keep this in mind because their actions and decisions are judged in that context—they personify the organization. However, there are ethical limits to what the organization can expect of those working for or affiliated with it. Managers must know the limits of their personal ethic and must speak out when the organization infringes on those limits.

MAINTAINING CONFIDENTIAL INFORMATION

Patient Records

Through their managers, health services organizations are charged with duties regarding patient information. Medical records are essential for good patient care and they must be legible, current, complete, and authenticated. The legal duty to maintain their confidentiality and security is met by providing adequate and effective personnel, systems, and procedures in medical records activities, and by ensuring that medical staff bylaws, rules, and regulations are enforced. Much can be done to prevent or minimize unauthorized access to paper medical records. The increasing use of electronic records raises significant new confidentiality issues.

The federal Health Insurance Portability and Accountability Act (HIPAA) passed in 1996 and became effective for medical privacy in 2003. It places substantial restrictions on how health information is obtained, managed, stored, transferred, and used. Much attention is paid to the need for patients to consent for any use of their health information, including among various types of personal and institutional providers.

State legal requirements vary, but individuals working in health services organizations have an ethical duty to ensure the confidentiality and appropriate use of patient information. A common breach of this ethic occurs when patients are discussed with or in the presence of persons with no need to know. Hospital-based research has found significant breaches of patient confidentiality and other types of inappropriate comments, such as concerns about a staff member's ability or desire to provide high-quality patient care, concerns about poor-quality care in the hospital, or derogatory remarks made about patients or their families.[1] Idle chatter or gossip may be titillating, but it is ethically unacceptable inside and outside the organization. Breaches of patient confidentiality can also occur through improper disposal of electronic patient records (e.g., those stored on computer hard drives).[2] In addition, conflicts may arise between maintaining confidential information about patients and furthering organizational interests.

Mailing Lists

University Hospital has a very active cardiac medicine section in its department of medicine. Across several decades, it has treated thousands of people with heart problems ranging from angina to congestive heart failure. Its patients have been included in several research protocols, many of them funded by the National Institutes of Health or various national heart associations.

Periodic questionnaire surveys are conducted as part of long-term patient follow-up. To complete these surveys, an extensive database and mailing lists are maintained by the cardiac medicine section. On one occasion, the development office of University Hospital used the mailing lists to solicit general contributions. On another occasion, it undertook a special fund-raising effort to assist in converting and equipping a cardiac intensive care unit. Contributions by the cardiac program's current and former patients have been excellent, primarily because the program maintains superior rapport with its patients.

The physician-director of the program and her administrative assistant have been approached by a prominent and respected national insurance company impressed by the results of the program. It wants to use the mailing lists to market life insurance to the program's participants. The proposal is attractive because the opportunity to obtain life insurance will benefit present and former patients, many of whom are insurable only with very high premiums. The proposal is also attractive because any data obtained by the insurance company will be available to the hospital at cost if the mailing lists are provided to the insurance company.

The physician-director and administrative assistant are enthusiastic about the clinical possibilities in addition to the opportunity to help patients. The director of development views the sale of mailing lists as a way to raise money for the cardiac program's activities. Both he and the physician-director spent an hour trying to convince the chief executive officer (CEO) that it is appropriate to release the mailing lists for this worthy purpose.

As stated, the proposal violates the privacy rule of the HIPAA because medical information from a covered entity—in this case, a hospital—is being used to market a product or service without the patient's written authorization.[3] Because breaking the law is unethical per se, University Hospital must obtain consent before it can use the mailing lists as proposed.

An ethical analysis produces virtually the same result as that obtained by applying HIPAA. This case suggests the legitimate but opposing and competing considerations that are a part of patient care, research, fundraising, and a limited duty of general beneficence to help patients solve problems indirectly linked to medical treatment. The case highlights the ethical problems of safeguarding the confidentiality of patient information. Using the information in the way requested violates the confidentiality of patient treatment and diagnosis. Some direct benefits may inure to patients (e.g., opportunity to obtain life insurance) and some indirect benefits may inure to the organization (e.g., improved data for epidemiological studies). Nevertheless, using the mailing lists as suggested serves no valid research purpose, nor does it directly further patients' medical treatment. Data that do not identify patients serve the same epidemiological purposes. The promise of mortality data on insurance purchasers is incidental to the research effort, and the money earned selling the mailing lists is likely to be modest. Regardless, these utilitarian arguments are irrelevant because such uses are incompatible with the principle of respect for persons, which includes confidentiality. Previous use of the lists to solicit contributions was questionable and cannot be used to support making the lists available now.

A weightier ethical argument for using mailing lists could be made if all University Hospital patients were included, rather than only those identified by diagnoses. Mailing to all former patients identifies only that they were patients at University Hospital, but even this activity may raise concerns over confidentiality for some former patients. The problem of mailing lists can be minimized by determining upon admission whether patients are willing to be on mailing lists used for hospital purposes, such as fund-raising.

University Hospital's use of mailing lists must be distinguished from selling or renting them. Patients must be informed if the hospital intends to use a mailing list commercially. Chapter 9 discusses several of the issues incident to obtaining consent in similar situations. Confidentiality concerns change, and patients should know that they can ask that their names be removed from a mailing list at any time. Rental or sale of mailing lists in health services settings is fraught with ethical problems and is best avoided.

MONITORING CLINICAL ACTIVITIES

Managers are agents of the organization, but as decision makers whose actions have moral implications and as members of a profession, they are never simply instruments of the organization. Managers have duties to patients independent of those the organization has to the patient, or those the physician has to the patient. Managers' concerns and duties are not limited to problems with the business office or the quality of food but extend to clinical activities. In terms of the patient, the manager is the organization's conscience.

Nonphysician managers do not judge clinical activities as would physicians. Just as they use technical experts to develop a new computer system or prepare a loss prevention management program, managers rely on experts in nursing and medicine to assist in understanding these activities and their outcomes. Experienced managers have considerable knowledge about clinical medicine; in a gross fashion, this knowledge enables them to determine when problems may be present. Regardless of their clinical sophistication, their purpose is not to be junior physicians but to understand what physicians do and what they need and want. The primary reason to understand clinical activities is to help the organization serve patients safely and effectively.

The health services organization benefits most when involvement is bidirectional—managers should expect and seek physician participation in administrative decision making. Hospitals in which physicians participate in management decision making achieve superior results.

An important role of managers in clinical settings is to link the formal and informal organizations. Anecdotal evidence suggests that informal communications are helpful, perhaps critical, in identifying clinical problems, and that they are an important supplement to formal systems. Nursing is especially important as an informal link. Deficient performance by physicians is often initially identified by nurses. Information from them can alert the formal system and be a starting point for further inquiry. Disciplinary actions cannot be based on rumor, however; managers must ensure adequate follow-up and investigation in conjunction with normal monitoring of clinical outcome data. As necessary, the manager must take action to protect the patient. As a moral agent, the prudent, ethical manager cannot ignore situations that jeopardize the patient or the organization. Sometimes, however, the tables are turned.

A Different Kind of Risk

Dr. Sagatius has just returned to his office after seeing the risk manager. He was very upset and slammed the door behind him before slumping into his chair. He would not stand for it, not again, he said to himself. This was the final straw. Administration was not going to push him around!

He thought back to the two previous incidents in the pediatrics unit and considered their similarity. Now there was a third incident, this time involving a different nurse. Another one of his patients had been medicated incorrectly—actually overdosed. Luckily, Sagatius had been able to intervene once again before serious consequences occurred. The child would have to stay in the hospital several days longer to be sure that the child was stable. He had reported the first two instances to the nurse supervisor. Now he would have to take other action.

The day following the third incident, Sagatius was asked by the risk manager to stop by her office. While there, he saw the child's medical record lying on her desk. Sagatius noticed that the risk manager had changed the medication record, which he knew had previously shown the overdose. When he asked the risk manager about it, she said that it did not matter because no apparent harm had come to the child. "Why needlessly upset the parents?," she asked. When Sagatius protested that this was dishonest, the risk manager became hostile and reminded Sagatius that a malpractice suit would hurt all those affiliated with the hospital, including the doctors, who were almost certain to be sued should the error come to light. She warned him not to discuss what happened with anyone, especially not with the parents.

Sagatius planned to tell the parents about the overdose, believing that they were owed an explanation for the extra days in the hospital. In addition, they had to watch for signs of long-term effects of the overdose and seek medical treatment for the child should they occur.

Sagatius weighed his options. He knew he had to tell the parents to watch the child closely, even if he did not discuss the overdose. He retrieved the parents' telephone number from his computer.

Dr. Sagatius faces two ethical problems. The first concerns the risk manager. Ethically, Sagatius's primary duty is to protect the interests of his patient, which means that he must provide the parents with the information they need to monitor their child; doing so meets the principles of beneficence and nonmaleficence. How can he carry out this duty given the position of the risk manager? The risk manager has violated the principle of respect for persons, specifically truth telling. In addition, by covering up clinical failures, the risk manager is enabling a system that violates the principle of nonmaleficence, as well as the virtues of honesty and trustworthiness. The dishonesty is inconsistent with the typical organizational philosophy. Furthermore, it will thwart the investigation to find the root cause of a type of problem that appears systemic.

The second ethical problem involves the nursing supervisor, who has not acted to prevent a serious, recurrent problem in the pediatrics unit. Such inaction is inconsistent with the principles of beneficence and nonmaleficence and the ethical obligations under the Code of Ethics for Nurses. Sagatius is ethically obligated to report the persistent quality problem to more senior leaders through the nursing and medical staff hierarchy or other appropriate means.

Medical record falsification is rare, even though it is human nature to want to hide problems. The manager's ethical obligations commonly become submerged in the legal dimensions of a problem, despite the fact that in this case, the risk manager's action was illegal. As a result, the patient becomes the enemy, and those in the organization move into a defensive posture. Patients and family sense this and are spurred even more to press for an explanation, a kind word, or perhaps even an apology. Patients and their families understand that errors and mistakes can occur, and it is increasingly clear that they are less likely to take legal action if they believe that they have been treated fairly and everything was done to ease the effects of the error. What they cannot understand and often will not accept are deceit and coldness. Hiding the truth and lying to patients and families angers them; angry patients and their families are much more likely to file a lawsuit. This utilitarian argument also supports the unpleasant but ethically preferred course of forthrightness and honesty with injured patients or their families, as appropriate. Doing so has been shown to be successful in some settings.[4]

Organizations that acknowledge their mistakes and strive to make things right are better served ethically—and, apparently (with limited evidence), legally—than those who fight to the end. In this regard, it is important to note that admitting an error, accepting responsibility for an error, or even admitting negligence are not the same as admitting liability. A finding of liability requires negligence (departure from the standard of care), injury (harm to the patient), and proximate cause (the harm must have been caused by the departure from the standard of care). The plaintiff has the burden of proving *all* these elements; it is the causal relationship that remains to be proved even when negligence has been admitted.

Since the early to mid-1990s, a small number of organizations determined that their ethical duty to disclose treatment errors was greater than the potential risk of legal action against them. After acting to minimize the error's clinical consequences, they informed patients (and family, as appropriate) about what happened and why, apologized, and sought a fair solution to the medical and economic effects of the error. Money may or may not have changed hands.

Being honest with patients gained momentum in 2001 when the Joint Commission on Accreditation of Healthcare Organizations (The Joint Commission) amended its patient safety and medical and healthcare error reduction standards. The changes require that patients and families, as appropriate, be informed of unanticipated outcomes, including medical error. Medical error was defined as "an unintended act, either of omission or commission, or an act that does not achieve its intended outcome." The Joint Commission addresses medical error by requiring that "patients and, when appropriate, their families are informed about the outcomes of care, treatment, and services, including unanticipated outcomes." The responsible licensed independent practitioner or designee provides this information.[5] Honestly admitting mistakes carries potential harms as well as benefits to patient and practitioner.[6]

All members of the organization have a shared responsibility to scrutinize the services delivered and take action as necessary. If this is seen as "ratting someone out" or being a "stool pigeon," the organization's culture is in desperate need of change. Identifying problems should be an important part of the culture and everyone should be committed to correcting them once identified.

This type of culture will make whistle-blowing unnecessary. Such a negative interpretation is possible only if one ignores the reason for being of the organization and those who work there. Both exist to further the interests of patients. When problems occur in the delivery of services, the organization and its managers must act to minimize loss and injury and do whatever is possible to make the patient whole. The manager must be involved, as necessary, to eliminate or reduce the recurrence of problems.

WHISTLE-BLOWING

Whistle-blowing occurs when an employee reveals information about illegal, inefficient, or wasteful action that endangers the health, safety, or freedom of the public.[7] This definition is broad enough to include revelations of mismanagement, including nonfeasance, misfeasance, and malfeasance. Many contemporary discussions of whistle-blowing focus only on fraud and abuse or other illegal activities under state and federal law. Here, however, the broad definition is used.

Whistle-blowing affects the private and public sectors and includes disclosing information both internal and external to the organization. Generally, internal whistle-blowing is much more likely to be seen as positive because the organization has the opportunity to correct the problem. External whistle-blowing usually occurs after internal reporting has proved fruitless; it may have significant negative effects on the organization. Negative reaction from managers is likely to be a function of the perceived or real level of embarrassment and threat to them and the organization. Whistle-blowing results from the activities of both individuals and the organization.

An example many health services managers will recognize is an organization that harbors a clinical or management staff member whose incompetence or incapacitation is known, except, of course, to those outside the organization. Despite this knowledge, nothing is done. The organization's culture discourages acting against those "in the club," or the lack of support in remedying the problem and the fear of retribution make the price too high. Thus, the problem continues until a catastrophe occurs or the situation becomes intolerable to a critical mass of managers and staff and action is forced. Much of the stimulus is fear of public exposure and the embarrassment or disciplinary action that is likely to result. Such motivation is not the stuff of moral agents, who act because it is right to do so.

Three types of activities result in whistle-blowing: clear illegality, potential illegality or danger, and the organization's social policy.[8]

Clear illegality occurs when the law is knowingly violated. Examples include falsifying information reported to the government, bribing inspectors, making illegal campaign contributions, falsifying audits, deliberately violating labor laws, discriminating in employment because of race or gender, and improperly disposing of hazardous wastes.[9]

The second type of activity affected by whistle-blowing involves *potential illegality or danger*. A growing body of regulations and case law protects employee health, patient safety, public health, and the environment. In addition, managers and employees are moral agents who are obligated to take action when there is reason to believe that patients are at risk, regardless of other requirements. In most situations in which whistle-blowing occurs or should occur, the whistle-blower acts in the belief that a given practice, process, or result is either not in compliance with accepted standards or that it places the patient at risk unnecessarily. "In any well-run enterprise, management should be seriously concerned about such violations and should welcome warnings by its own employees."[10]

The third type of activity affected by whistle-blowing involves the *organization's social policy*. An employee may become concerned about the morality of a management policy and its effect on patients or society. For example, an employee may believe that the net revenue of a not-for-profit health services organization is excessive or spent inappropriately and that too little is used for indigent care. Speaking out or refusing to participate is likely to be protected by conscience clauses in state or federal statutes or by the U.S. Constitution, if state action is involved. Assuming the policy is legal, employee protest raises two issues: the employee's right to free speech and the employee's responsibility as a moral agent. Employees are entitled to the same constitutionally protected right of free speech as are other individuals. Furthermore, as moral agents, they have an ethical duty to speak out when policies and actions could or do adversely affect patients or society. The controversy usually arises when an employee exercises the right of free speech or the duty of moral agency by speaking publicly against an organization's lawful policy, thereby harming its reputation and market advantage.[11]

Health services organizations create a paradox when they encourage managers and staff to act responsibly in all situations without causing unnecessary disruption. When the organization or individuals in it act illegally, inefficiently, or wastefully, staff is expected to be loyal and not speak out. This paradox is less easily resolved as organizations become more competitive because employees are asked to deal aggressively with external competitors but to be complacent internally.

An important dimension of whistle-blowing is found in federal law. In 1986, Congress amended the False Claims Act, which was originally passed during the Civil War to reduce fraud in federal contracting. The amendments added important protections and rewards for individuals who blow the whistle. These whistle-blowers are known as relators. The lawsuits they can bring are known as *qui tam* actions (an abbreviation of the Latin phrase *qui tam pro domino rege quam pro se ipso in hac parte sequitur,* meaning "he who sues in this matter for the king as well as for himself"). The law protects relators against wrongful dismissal, and they are allowed reinstatement with seniority, double back pay, and compensation for discriminatory treatment.[12] After relators file suit, the case is sealed for 60 days while the U.S. Department of Justice (DOJ) decides whether it will intervene. If the DOJ does not intervene, the whistle-blower may proceed independently. Assuming a successful outcome (and a significant role on the part of the relator), the whistle-blower may receive 15%–30% of any double or triple damages and fines imposed.[13] The vast amounts spent for Medicare and Medicaid, as well as other federal healthcare and healthcare-related programs, offer great potential for fraud; for that reason, many *qui tam* suits are brought in the health services sector. Since 1986, more than $27 billion has been recovered. In fiscal year 2010, $2.5 of $3 billion was recovered from healthcare fraud.[14] Federal false claims law is supplemented by state laws.

Examples of Whistle-Blowing

When considering these cases, it is important to bear in mind that employees and managers are moral agents with an ethical duty to speak out when policies and actions could or do affect patients or society adversely. This is true regardless of other requirements, such as the law.

How Sweet It Is!

Dr. A. Grace Pierce joined the research staff of Ortho Pharmaceutical Corporation in 1971. In 1975, she was part of a team developing a prescription drug known generically as loperamide. The drug was used to treat acute and chronic diarrhea in infants, children, and older adults. Saccharin was used to make it palatable by masking its bitter taste.

The research team agreed that the formula was unsuitable because it substantially exceeded U.S. Food and Drug Administration (FDA) saccharin limits. Management was informed of this fact but decided nevertheless to file a new drug application with the FDA. Other members of the research team continued development, but Dr. Pierce refused. Although she was offered work in other projects at no decrease in pay, she resigned her position, apparently believing her refusal had irrevocably damaged her career at Ortho.

Later, she sought relief in the courts, alleging wrongful discharge. The New Jersey Supreme Court ruled that Ortho had not acted illegally and that there were no grounds for a cause of action.[15]

The court placed substantial weight on the fact that there was no imminent harm to the public. The court ruled that the ethic of the Hippocratic oath did not contain a clear mandate of public policy that would have prevented Dr. Pierce from continuing her research. Similar cases have occurred in organizations that deliver health services.

It's Really Only an X-ray

Frances O'Sullivan was an x-ray technician employed by several radiologists and a hospital. She sued for breach of an employment contract after she was fired. She alleged she was fired for refusal to perform catheterizations, a procedure she had not been trained to perform. O'Sullivan could not legally perform catheterizations in New Jersey, where only licensed nurses and physicians may do so. The issue involved was unique because the plaintiff had been asked to perform an illegal act. The superior court denied the defendant physicians' and hospital's motion to dismiss.[16]

Denying the motion to dismiss meant that O'Sullivan was entitled to a trial on the merits of the case. No report exists that this occurred, and it may be assumed that the case was settled before trial. In light of the illegality of what O'Sullivan was asked to do, she acted properly.

Don't Speak Now and Forever Hold Your Peace

Linda Rafferty was a psychiatric nurse at a state institution in which the conditions were appalling. The abuses Rafferty claimed to have observed included the staff failing to protect patients from sexual abuse by other patients and from sexual exploitation by outside employees, providing improper nonpsychiatric medical care, allowing patients to keep medications in their rooms, locking up fire extinguishers, leaving blank prescription forms that were signed in advance by physicians in unlocked drawers for nurses to fill out on weekends, and hospital medical staff being chronically absent from work. Rafferty repeatedly complained to her superiors but resigned when her protests brought no change.

She was hired at another institution, Community Mental Health Center, as supervisor of nurses. Before she began work, she gave an interview to a Philadelphia newspaper in which she was sharply critical of treatment at the state institution. The morning after the story appeared, she was fired from her new position because "staff members were upset about the article." No other reasons were given until trial, when the Community Mental Health Center alleged inadequate job performance in addition to the previous reason.

Rafferty brought suit alleging she had been deprived of her constitutional rights. The court ruled that she be reinstated and be awarded more than $3,000 in back pay.[17]

These whistle-blowing cases resulted in court decisions, which makes them a matter of public record. The types and number of whistle-blowing cases are legion. Senior administrators at the University of California–Irvine Medical Center were fired for allegedly retaliating against employees who had reported physician misconduct at the center's fertility clinic. Whistle-blowers said that physicians were implanting eggs and embryos into patients without donor consent. An internal investigation supported the whistle-blowers' allegations and showed that after they reported the wrongdoing, they were treated badly by medical center management and clinic physicians and were subsequently fired.[18] Another whistle-blower case alleged that 132 research center hospitals conspired to deliberately miscode procedures and manipulate patient records so as to obtain $1 billion in federal reimbursement for the use of investigational devices, which are not covered under Medicare and Medicaid guidelines. The hospitals argued that diagnosis-related groups pay by diagnosis rather than by products used, and thus payment was due regardless of treatment. The facts suggest that this was a *qui tam* case brought under the federal False Claims Act.[19]

An example of *qui tam* occurred at a community hospital in Pineville, Kentucky, at which a new physician found that several physician colleagues were not performing some patient histories, physical examinations, and other services listed in patient records. Hospital medical records clerks wrote histories and physicals based on information in the medical records or, sometimes, by interviewing patients. The document created by the clerk was used to bill Medicare. At discharge, clerks used the medical record to prepare a discharge summary, which was stamped with the physician's signature and used by the physician's office to bill Medicare for a discharge examination and treatment plan. After repeated efforts to change the practice, the new physician brought a *qui tam* suit. The hospital settled the case for $2.3 million; each physician paid $100,000. Had they been imposed, maximum damages and penalties could have totaled $31 million. Allegedly, hospital administration hindered efforts to end the fraudulent practices. Not unexpectedly, many at the hospital and in the community saw the whistle blower as the problem.[20]

Qui tam cases cover a gamut: TAP Pharmaceuticals agreed to pay nearly $600 million over allegations of kickbacks to physicians and false Medicare claims regarding treatment of their patients. Beverly Medical Care paid $175 million to settle allegations that employees of its nursing homes were exaggerating claims of time spent attending Medicare patients.[21] McAllen (Texas) Hospitals agreed to pay the United States $27.5 million to settle claims that it violated the False Claims Act, the anti-kickback statute, and the Stark law (which regulates physician self-referrals for Medicare and Medicaid patients) between 1999 and 2006 by paying illegal compensation to physicians in order to induce them to refer patients to its hospitals.[22] St. Joseph Medical Center in Towson, Maryland, paid $22 million to settle federal claims that it had engaged in a decade-long kickback scheme involving cardiologists who allegedly performed unnecessary procedures.[23]

Cases such as these highlight the three significant issues relating to whistle-blowing as an ethical problem in health services organizations. The first is staff responsibility and accountability, something that applies to all employees, whether or not they are managers. The second is fair practices. To encourage responsibility and accountability, due process procedures are necessary to protect employees—whether or not these are *qui tam* cases—who consider themselves moral agents and are courageous enough to speak out. Due process regarding employee disciplinary actions (both in terms of procedure and substance) is necessary, whether the organization is one to which federal or state constitutional protections apply. Being bound by such requirements will also encourage others to act when they should. Methods must be developed to balance the individual's duty to the employer against the duty to the public. This can be difficult because "many of the rights and privileges . . . so important to a free society that they are constitutionally protected . . . are vulnerable to abuse through an employer's power."[24] The third issue is how to encourage employees to speak out in appropriate ways in order to meet their independent duty to the patient, without causing unnecessary damage to the indispensable cooperative and trust relationships that exist within the organization as well as between them and their communities.

Negative Aspects of Whistle-Blowing

Several negative aspects temper what is positive about whistle-blowing: Determining the accuracy of whistle-blowing charges is not always easy. Whistle-blowers may be incorrect in what they allege to be the facts of management's misconduct. The danger exists that incompetent or inadequate employees may become whistle-blowers to avoid facing justifiable disciplinary actions. Employees can blow the whistle in unacceptably disruptive ways, regardless of the merits of their protest. Some whistle-blowers are not protesting unlawful or unsafe practices, but rather social policies by management that the employee considers unwise or unethical. The legal definitions of a safe product, danger to health, or improper treatment of employees are often not clear. The efficiency and flexibility of human resources management could be threatened by the creation of legal rights to dissent and legalized review systems. Risks to the desirable autonomy of the private sector are possible because a review of allegations by whistle-blowers will expand government's role too deeply into internal business policies.[25]

Courses of Action

Managers with the authority to remedy a problem are morally bound to do so. If persons in authority will not act, there are alternatives consistent with the duty of loyalty that managers and staff have to the organization, even if these alternatives ultimately involve public disclosure. It is ethically appropriate to act early, even at the risk of embarrassing an organization, than to await further corruption, with its attendant greater risk of harm to others as well as the organization. The alternatives involve whistle-blowing of various types. Regrettably, whistle-blowing has a bad connotation for many. It suggests disloyalty to the group, if not to the organization—the person who blows the whistle is considered an informer, a betrayer. This attitude is perverse. How, for example, could one be considered disloyal by informing senior management of illegal or incompetent actions that risk the health of patients or staff? Establishing a culture that makes whistle-blowing unnecessary is a major challenge for management. Making the environment risk-free in terms of retribution against those who are willing to speak out (i.e., internal whistle-blowers) is an essential first step.

One type of whistle-blowing involves stimulating action by approaching those in authority directly. Working with persons of like mind—finding allies and gaining strength in numbers—can reinforce and stimulate the need to act. In an environment of fear, anonymous communication with those who are able to remedy the problem may be necessary to try to produce the desired result.

It is crucial that there is a change in the atmosphere typically found in an organization—the "I win, you lose" (*zero-sum*) approach to whistle-blowing. Responsible reporting will benefit employees, employers, and, most important, patients. As Bowman, Elliston, and Lockhart[26] point out, "Directing corrective efforts to [whistle-blowers] instead of the policy or practice they protest will not alter the conditions that make whistle-blow-ing necessary." As noted above, this attitude was pervasive at Pineville.

Place of Whistle-Blowing

Leading commercial companies have created ombudsman programs in which one person receives, investigates, and responds to employee com-plaints. Such programs are important for employees who believe illegal or improper conduct is occurring. The problem is that the ombudsman may lack the authority to solve problems in line departments. The ombudsman may not be empowered to deal with senior managers who actively promote illegal or improper conduct as an organizational imperative.[27]

Even where employees are protected by law, as in federal employ-ment, they fear reprisals. The U.S. Merit Systems Protection Board found that 50% of employees who said they knew firsthand of illegal acts or waste in federal government failed to report it. Only 13% of whistle-blowers were given credit by management for doing the right thing; 71% said their supervisors or upper management became unhappy with them. Of whistle-blowers, 37% said they had experienced or had been threatened with re-taliation, which included poor performance appraisals, being shunned by coworkers and managers, and verbal harassment or intimidation.[28] These findings were confirmed by a later survey showing that 25% of employees believed their government agency would not protect them from retaliation for whistle-blowing.[29] Research on whistle-blowing in the private sector has similar findings. For example, half of management accountants who observed wrongdoing did not report it.[30]

Doorway Consultations

A consulting ethicist for a large nursing facility was asked by a nurse to discuss a problem concerning a physician, several of whose patients are residents in the facility. The nurse said she had an ethical quandary and was not sure what to do. She continued by describing how the physician routinely looked into his patients' rooms from the doorway and then made chart entries indicating he had had a professional visit with them. The nurse said that she had heard of physicians who would "survey" the dining room at mealtime and then make chart entries indicat-ing a professional visit. She said that behavior was only slightly worse than what she had seen. In fact, she said, one of her patients asked if her doctor was coming in because she had questions for him. "What should I do?," asked the nurse.

Quality of care questions aside, the physician is acting unethically. If he bills for these "visits" he is committing fraud; this makes him subject to criminal prosecution and other sanctions. The nursing code of ethics and the expressed personal ethic of this nurse require that she report her concerns within the nursing administration hierarchy—that she become an internal whistle-blower. Failing action, the nurse should consider external whistle-blowing or a *qui tam* action if federal or state programs are involved.

Organizational Culture

The word *whistle-blowing* is unfortunate terminology. In historical context, it suggests a police officer who used a whistle to stop criminal activity and summon assistance. It would be far better to make the concept one of highlighting the compliant culture that emphasizes quality—one in which calling attention to a problem is considered positive, not negative. An open culture that stresses honesty, integrity, quality of care, fairness, and concern for patients and staff—an environment with shared values—will result in proper treatment of patients and staff, safe surroundings, and honest billing practices. This makes a compliance officer and compliance program largely redundant. Even if both are necessary because of legal or regulatory requirements, their roles will be to communicate information, educate staff, and assist in establishing policies and procedures that enable compliance. Assigning "ethics" to an individual or a program is foolhardy and will never create a culture of shared values. It bears repeating that meeting the law's demands (compliance) is only the base expectation for an organization. An ethical organization, through its managers, holds itself to a higher standard of performance. Larson noted this:

> Take the example of a homeless person who repeatedly comes into the ER for care. Compliance dictates only that the patient be stabilized, then released or transferred. Ethics ask us: What can we do for this patient? . . . Do we pass the buck or is it our turn? Should we do more? Compliance is the minimum, but ethics mean addressing all that is necessary.[31]

Managers must work to establish and nurture a largely risk-free culture in which problems of nonfeasance, malfeasance, or misfeasance are easily communicated and action taken. Such a culture is the ounce of prevention that is worth a pound of cure. The acculturation begins in the recruitment and selection processes and continues with new employee orientation. Later, it must be reinforced by the example of formal and informal leaders. The importance of example setting from the governing body down through the management ranks cannot be overstated.

This culture of responsibility, openness, and commitment on the part of management is essential to developing a meaningful internal policy on whistle-blowing. Also essential is drafting the principles and policy statements that apply management's intention throughout the organization and communicating these statements to employees. The importance of middle and line managers must be stressed. Not only must they be knowledgeable about the principles and policy statements, but their evaluations must encourage widespread adherence.

Identifying, communicating, and solving problems are made easier if fear and fault finding are removed from the equation, an approach consistent with the philosophy of W. Edwards Deming. Even Deming recognized that the employee causes a small percentage of problems, but that the greatest gain in quality will occur by improving the process.[32] In the case of impairment because of substance abuse or other willful acts with negative effect, however, focusing on the individual is a necessary first step.

Summary

The concept of moral agency and the willingness to speak and act as necessary remain central, recurring themes for managers and caregivers alike. Professional dissent is critical to the field of health services administration and the delivery of health services. No morality exists without action; ethics will survive only if people speak out when it matters. Professionals are distinguished by the ability to recognize ethical problems and to act as moral custodians of the organization in which they work.

ASSESSING AND IMPROVING QUALITY OF CARE

Through their organizations, health services managers are charged with the weighty responsibility of assessing and improving the quality of patient care. Managers cannot directly assess clinical quality, but they are ethically bound to support and encourage the efforts of experts who can. Sometimes, managers must stimulate quality assessment and corrective action. More important, managers are key in leading the organization to adopt the philosophy and concepts of quality improvement and to apply its methods.

Consistent with the manager's duties of beneficence and nonmaleficence—as well as virtues such as courage, compassion, discernment, and conscientiousness—is to discourage or actively oppose establishing or continuing clinical services that expose patients to unnecessary clinical risk.

One source of risk occurs when health services organizations perform low volumes of a surgical procedure or treat few patients with a specific medical condition. Early studies suggested that successful cardiac surgery was correlated positively with the number of procedures and that hospitals performing few procedures had poorer outcomes than hospitals performing many. Explanatory factors may have included patient acuity and a willingness to accept higher risk patients, but their contributions were not examined. Absent explanation of the differences, the studies recommended closure of low-volume/high-risk programs.[33]

Data published in the mid-1990s supported these recommendations and included physician and geographic area volumes, as well as improved outcomes and lower costs.[34] Research published in 2000, 2002, and 2003 provides further support for the proposition that there is a positive relationship, albeit variable, between higher volume providers and better outcomes, including better results for high-risk patients. These studies analyzed a broad range of surgical procedures; one also showed similar benefits for high-volume site treatment of HIV.[35]

Thus, evidence of the link between volume and quality of clinical outcome continues to mount. There is a clear ethical imperative for managers whose organizations either have a low-volume service or are considering undertaking a service whose volume is likely to remain low.

Higher-Risk Procedures

Teaching Hospital was established in 1907 with a grant from a wealthy local industrialist. The star of its long history of educating nurses and physicians is a surgical residency program, a key element of which is cardiac surgery. Two years ago, the cardiac surgery program was set back substantially by the death of the chief of cardiac surgery and the departure of a member of the team. Referrals declined markedly, and the volume of open-heart procedures dropped to five per month. This occurred despite significant efforts to build referral volume.

The quality department performs special studies for various clinical services. Recently, it reviewed mortality data from cardiac surgery and found that mortality rates were more than double the rates found in the literature. The director of quality expressed concern as she discussed the report with the CEO. She noted that the literature reported an inverse relationship between mortality rates and the number of procedures performed. It seemed that technical competence could be only gained and retained by performing a high volume of procedures.

Soon after, the CEO saw the medical director at lunch. During their conversation, the CEO asked whether he had any reason to believe that the cardiac surgery program was of lower quality than it had been in the past. The medical director replied, "As far as I know, things are fine." When she inquired as to the reason for the concern, the CEO replied that the frequency of performing cardiac procedures had declined and the literature suggested that this had implications for quality of care. In fact, the hospital's review had been confirmatory. The medical director said she would look into it. The discussion moved to other matters.

The ethical issue for Teaching Hospital and its patients is apparent. An ethical problem exists because patients undergoing cardiac surgery there are at higher risk than they would be in a high-volume hospital, and this violates the principle of nonmaleficence. The CEO may not ignore what is happening; to do so is inconsistent with the manager's role as a moral agent, as well as that of a professional with an independent duty to protect patients. What is the next step? Discontinuing the program immediately may be politically and economically impossible, but steps must be taken now to gain the support of the medical staff and to apprize the governing body of the problem. Whether or not the medical staff lends its support, the CEO must urge the governing body to suspend the program.

What happens if working internally proves fruitless? What if the problem is acknowledged but those in authority will not act? This situation is a significant test of the manager's ethic because it poses a true ethical dilemma: The manager is confronted with conflicting moral duties. On the one hand, information about the cardiac surgery program is confidential and the manager has a duty of loyalty to the organization. On the other hand, organization inaction places patients at special risk. Weighing these conflicting moral duties should lead the manager to conclude that the higher duty is that of protecting patients. The manager must press and pursue, even to the point of releasing information outside the organization if corrective action is not taken. Going public with such damaging information (whistle-blowing) is a last resort and an act of great moral courage. External whistle-blowing will make the manager a pariah who is likely to be terminated for what will be seen an act of betrayal.

The CEO might consider two other options that are more pragmatic but ethically less desirable. One option is to ignore the short-term implications of the decline in quality of care and find ways to build on program strengths to increase volume and quality. Another option is to determine the types of procedures with better results and focus on performing them. Both approaches may place patients at unnecessary risk, although special attention could reduce the risk to acceptable levels. This option seems unconscionable in terms of the virtues of caring, trustworthiness, and integrity, and the principles of beneficence and nonmaleficence. Absent an emergency or triage situation, one cannot justify the harm to some (patients) because of benefit to others (e.g., surgeons and residents;

hospital income and status). Using patients as a means to an end is morally wrong.

Other clinical quality issues go beyond reviewing and ensuring a clinician's competence. These include ensuring the adequacy of support staff and equipment, evaluating the patient's clinical appropriateness for a procedure, and acting when a clinician's abilities decline. Often, the problem is apparent only in retrospect. Some processes allow concurrent control of quality, however, and these should be used.

Operating Beyond His Skill?

Jim Hudson picked up the form that had been delivered by the operating room (OR) scheduling clerk and began to review the procedures scheduled for 2 days hence. Hudson's job is to ensure that surgical packs, equipment, time, and personnel are adequate to meet the demands of scheduled surgery. The list included a procedure that Hudson had never seen scheduled before. Looking at the column that showed whether special equipment or supplies were needed, Hudson saw a note that the attending surgeon would provide the items. This notation puzzled him because it was the responsibility of the OR supervisor or the purchasing department to provide everything needed for a surgical procedure. Hudson called the chief of surgery, to whom OR staff reported clinically. He was unavailable, but his secretary promised he would return the call.

When the chief of surgery called, he was noncommittal. "If the procedure is scheduled," he said, "it's probably okay for it to be done." The clear implication was that the surgeon would not perform a procedure with inadequate preparation.

Hudson was unsure what to do. Not being a physician, further action by him would be seen as inappropriate meddling in clinical matters. Nevertheless, further checking seemed necessary.

This case focuses on a problem of clinical quality. Hudson must do more than ponder what the facts suggest. Hudson should query the attending surgeon, and if that does not produce satisfactory information, the problem should be taken higher up the administrative hierarchy. Additional information may clear up the questions; it may also cause the procedure to be canceled.

To obtain routine information on quality of services, health services organizations establish systems to review the content of clinical and administrative activities. The two have many parallels. It should be stressed, however, that these are primarily objective functions and measures. The judgments and conclusions of individuals reviewing the data are also required. It is these conclusions that trigger action. Table 2 shows examples of quality measures.

Table 2.   Some measures of hospital quality

Feature	Measures of patient care quality	Measures of administrative quality
Structure	Accreditation	Accreditation
	Medical staff qualifications	Administrative staff qualifications
	Professional staff qualifications	Employee development programs
	Professional staff training	Staff per occupied bed
	Special care unit availability/ utilization	Services provided
Process	Medical staff peer review	Use of management studies
	Average length of stay	Occupancy rate
	Autopsy rate	Management planning activities
	Community involvement	Community involvement
Outcome	Patient outcome	Cost per unit of output
	Surgical procedures assessment	Staff hours per patient-day
	Adjusted death rate	Financial stability
	Hospital-acquired infections: reported/treated	Compliance
	Malpractice suits	
Attitude	Expert evaluation of patient care	Expert evaluation of administrative performance
	Patient satisfaction (dissatisfaction)	Employee satisfaction (dissatisfaction)

From Grimes, R., & Moseley, S. (1976, Fall). An approach to an index of hospital performance. *Health Services Research, 2,* 289; adapted by permission.

543 943   Mondrian Art 2019 !

MAINTAINING RELATIONS WITH THE COMMUNITY

Health services organizations are considered quasi-public, regardless of ownership. They have a service orientation and a moral obligation to meet community health needs. This relationship necessitates building and retaining community confidence, and it means taking steps to act in the interests of people in the community who are as yet only potential patients. If potential patients risk acquiring an infection or are in danger because the facility is operating with safety code deficiencies, the organization has special obligations to these individuals.

Protecting Patients and Community from Staff with Severe Infectious Diseases

Chapter 7 provided background on HIV/AIDS, hepatitis B (HBV), and hepatitis C (HBC) and issues related to protecting staff. Legal dimensions and the obligations of health services organizations to staff and physicians were discussed. Medical advances in the last two decades allow health services organizations to treat patients with AIDS more effectively and increase their longevity. The result will be more episodes of hospitalization, as well as treatment at organizations such as nursing facilities and hospice. Protecting patients and staff from infected staff and maintaining confidentiality will be a major challenge for providers.

Of the infectious disease, HIV has unique aspects in terms of its spread. A critical context for analysis is that for reasons unknown, the probability that caregivers will become infected when exposed to blood and body substances from patients who are HIV positive is several magnitudes greater than that patients will become infected from caregivers who are HIV positive. With two *possible* exceptions, there are no known cases in which a caregiver with HIV has infected a patient. There have been numerous instances of surgeons and other physicians with frank AIDS performing exposure-prone and invasive procedures. However, screening their patients found no transmission of HIV after exposure. This suggests unique aspects of HIV and the likelihood of cofactors in transmissibility as well as infectivity and progression to frank AIDS, cofactors that are not present in the general population. The Centers for Disease Control and Prevention (CDC) defines an invasive procedure as "surgical entry into tissues, cavities, or organs, or repair of major traumatic injuries," and identifies treatment locations and types of procedures.[36]

> Characteristics of exposure-prone procedures include digital palpation of a needle tip in a body cavity or the simultaneous presence of the healthcare worker's fingers and a needle or other sharp instrument or object in a poorly visualized or highly confined anatomic site.[37]

These definitions should guide health services organizations in assigning staff members.

Currently, the AMA advises physicians and other healthcare workers with HIV to disclose their serostatus to a state public health official or to a local review committee to establish practice limitations. The review committee will determine which activities can be continued without risk of infecting patients. The current policy recommends that physicians *should* refrain from conducting exposure-prone invasive procedures or "perform such procedures with permission of the local review committee and the informed consent of the patient. HIV-infected physicians . . . must err on the side of protecting patients."[38] The American Dental Association's approach is similar:

A dentist who becomes ill from any disease or impaired in any way shall, with consultation and advice from a qualified physician or other authority, limit the activities of practice to those areas that do not endanger the patients or members of the dental staff.[39]

Most states require patient notification for exposure-prone invasive procedures when the physician is HIV positive; many also require notification for invasive procedures that are not exposure prone.[40]

In meeting their ethical duties, clinical staff should want to know whether they pose a risk to patients and other staff. Because of the opportunistic diseases they contract as HIV progresses to frank AIDS, infected staff may pose a risk to patients, many of whom are immunocompromised or physically weakened. Staff members with AIDS may also pose risks to other employees and to visitors. These risks should cause managers to err in favor of caution in assigning staff. As staff who are HIV positive become increasingly immunocompromised, infectious diseases common in health services organizations will pose risks to them. If the organization is to discharge its ethical obligations to staff, it must be able to consider such information in job assignment. Given how much is *not* known about transmissibility of the virus, staff who are HIV positive or who have other significant infectious disease should be encouraged to accept nonpatient care assignments. Physicians who wish to continue performing exposure-prone invasive procedures pose a special problem, but as noted in Chapter 7, the law is generally well settled. Given the unknown but possible risk to patients, it is prudent to prohibit physicians and other staff who are HIV positive from performing exposure-prone invasive procedures, as reasonably defined. Protecting confidentiality to the greatest extent possible is crucial to the success of any such effort.

Despite some legal uncertainty, health services organizations should know the significant infectious disease status of staff who engage in exposure-prone invasive procedures. It is ethically appropriate (and legally prudent) to prohibit them from performing exposure-prone invasive procedures. Such a rule meets the ethical principle of nonmaleficence, which is that the caregiver's first duty is "do no harm." That there have been only two cases of HIV transmission from caregiver to patient—one is "confirmed" but challenged and the other is "not entirely conclusive"— suggests that the risk of being infected by a healthcare worker with HIV is infinitesimally small. Notably, the risk of transmitting other significant infectious diseases is much higher.

In early 1999, a French study provided strong evidence that an infected orthopedic surgeon transmitted HIV to a patient during surgery. Of the almost 1,000 patients on whom the orthopedist had performed surgery who were tested, only one had contracted HIV. "The evidence . . . is not entirely conclusive, but provider-to-patient transmission during orthopedic surgery is the most plausible explanation for the . . . infection."[41]

The CDC has estimated that the risk that an infected surgeon will transmit HIV during an exposure-prone invasive procedure is between 1 in 40,000 and 1 in 400,000, and that the risk of transmission from an infected dentist is between 1 in 200,000 and 1 in 2,000,000.[42] By way of context, HBV is a greater threat to patients than HIV. In 1996, a thoracic surgeon was found to have transmitted HBV to 19 patients during surgery despite evidence that he used adequate infection control procedures.[43] This incident, plus that of a Spanish cardiac surgeon who infected five of his patients with HCV, supports mandatory testing for HBV, HCV, and HIV among caregivers who perform exposure-prone invasive procedures.[44]

Something Must Be Done, But What?

Stunned, Carolyn Aubrey, the CEO of Metropolitan Hospital, sank into her chair and stared out the window for a very long time. She realized that something was afoot when Dr. Midmore's wife had angrily insisted on seeing the CEO. Even in her worst nightmare, Aubrey could have never imagined that Mrs. Midmore would tell Aubrey that she was suing her husband, an orthopedic surgeon, for divorce because he had given her AIDS. As Mrs. Midmore left Aubrey's office, she had turned back and said, "I was sure you'd want to know. Surely you'll have to do something."

Aubrey thought Mrs. Midmore's statements might be nothing more than the ravings of an angry, vindictive wife, but that was not likely. As she considered what she had just learned, she recalled an incident several years ago involving Dr. Midmore and a male orderly. In retrospect, it suggested that Dr. Midmore might be bisexual. Aubrey also thought about the department of surgery meeting last year when there had been a long discussion about the desirability of knowing the HIV status of all surgical patients. The special risks to surgeons of torn gloves and cuts during orthopedic surgery had been described in detail.

Now it seemed that Dr. Midmore's patients might be at risk. Aubrey called operating room scheduling and learned that Dr. Midmore was maintaining a full surgical load. Aubrey asked her secretary to call the hospital attorney and the medical director and set up an emergency meeting for 7:00 the following morning. Mrs. Midmore had been right, thought Aubrey. We'll have to do something, but what?

This case suggests several ethical (and legal) issues. Protecting patients is key, and Midmore's surgical privileges must be suspended immediately.

Once Midmore no longer poses a risk to patients, further action can follow in an orderly and deliberate manner. Meeting the principle of justice requires that the investigation is fair to Midmore in terms of process and substance. If Midmore is HIV positive, the hospital may choose from two courses of action: 1) allow Midmore to continue performing surgery if he follows CDC guidelines that physicians who are HIV positive notify their patients before performing exposure-prone invasive procedures; or 2) terminate Midmore's surgical privileges. The first choice maximizes patient autonomy, but the hospital must ensure that Midmore actually informs patients that he is HIV positive and that patients understand the implications of this information. As a practical matter, few patients are likely to allow him to perform their surgery after learning his HIV status. The second choice meets the principle of nonmaleficence by preventing potential harm to patients, but it is paternalistic by not allowing Midmore's patients to make their own choice. Prudence, however, demands terminating his surgical privileges. All actions must be consistent with protecting patients and meeting the requirements of the medical staff bylaws and rules and regulations, as well as state and federal law.

Confidentiality regarding Dr. Midmore's HIV status must be safeguarded. Such efforts can never compromise patient safety, however. The issue of confidentiality takes on further complexity if Midmore leaves the staff and applies for surgical privileges elsewhere. The hospital is ethically bound to communicate what it has learned in the course of its investigation. Applying the legal principles in the Tarasoff case discussed in Chapter 7, the hospital has a legal duty to warn.

Health services organizations must be alert to the special problems of confidentiality when they treat patients with HIV/AIDS or other significant infectious diseases. Within the constraints of state law, however, the first obligation must be to safeguard staff and other patients. An added benefit is that identifying these patients will be an important additional stimulus that encourages staff to comply with universal precautions.

Protecting staff confidentiality to the greatest extent possible is crucial to the success of any such effort. Consistent with the ethical principle of respect for persons, health services organizations must be alert to the special problems of confidentiality when treating patients with infectious diseases. Within legal constraints, however, the organization's first obligation is to safeguard other patients and staff.

HIV/AIDS is only one infectious disease that raises ethical (and legal) problems for health services organizations and their managers. Events at University Hospital suggest yet another.

Protecting the Community

University Hospital plays a unique role in the community. It is a tertiary referral hospital for the region and a major source of healthcare to the community.

In 1977, it experienced an outbreak of legionella (Legionnaires' disease). A number of patients contracted the disease; several died.

Legionella is a bacterial infection of the respiratory tract and lungs that may result in death if not diagnosed and treated early. It is especially dangerous for older adults and people with medical problems that weaken their general resistance. A factor requiring even greater caution on the part of hospital management is that at the time of the outbreaks, the process for identifying the organism in the laboratory took several days. Thus, patients were at greater risk until a confirmatory diagnosis was obtained.

Epidemiological studies showed a relationship between the fine aerosol mist that the hospital's air conditioning cooling tower gave off and the spread of the disease. Employees exposed directly to the aerosol contracted severe cases of legionella. Chlorinating the water in the cooling towers eliminates the organism. Although the cooling tower was suspected in the 1977 outbreak at University Hospital, the relationship was never confirmed. The hospital's infection control committee did not develop any standing orders or policies after the first outbreak.

In May 1982, there was evidence of another outbreak of legionella. The cooling tower water was immediately chlorinated and the number of new cases dropped dramatically. However, an undetected failure in the chlorination system brought a second outbreak in early June.

When the first cases were detected in May 1982, the hospital administrator was notified. He met with various staff members, including physicians. It was decided that information about the outbreak should be kept from the community, lest a panic and sudden drop in patient census occur, as well as loss of public confidence. A confidential letter was sent to staff physicians advising them of the problem and asking that they keep in mind the potential for infection when making admissions decisions. Admissions were not limited to emergencies, however, and there was neither a prospective review of elective admissions to determine whether patients at risk for pulmonary infections such as legionella should be sent elsewhere, nor a review of indications for and necessity of admission. The medical staff developed a protocol stating that unexplained, acute-onset pneumonias were to be treated immediately with a potent antibiotic known to be effective against legionella. However, no provision was made for effective review to determine that the protocol was actually followed.

The administrator at University Hospital faced several problems, all with ethical dimensions:

1.   The medical staff wanted to continue elective admissions.

2.   The community could lose confidence in the hospital if it learned that there was an epidemic of a potentially fatal disease.
3.   The administrator and management staff could lose face, and even their jobs, should the infection become common knowledge.
4.   There was potential legal liability.

Solving this ethical problem is difficult but not impossible. Similar situations arise in nursing facilities that are threatened with closure because their physical plants violate fire safety requirements and in hospitals in which outbreaks of meningitis or salmonella occur in the newborn nursery. How does the organization protect current as well as potential patients in such situations? More important, what is the manager's role?

One feature that distinguishes this legionella outbreak from other, similar cases is the difference in duty owed to potential rather than actual patients. The law recognizes a difference. Generally, unless there is a special relationship with potential patients, one has no duty to act on their behalf. In this case, however, there would be a duty to warn elective admissions who are at risk from legionella.

The legal distinction is useful in ethical analysis. The duty toward actual patients is immediate and more compelling than the duty owed potential patients. Potential patients should be put at risk of legionella only if their medical condition puts them at greater risk outside the hospital. Inpatients who might benefit from a continued stay but who are at greater risk by remaining in the hospital should be discharged. It is incumbent on the managerial and clinical staff to convince caregivers of their obligation to protect the patient.

The argument that the administrator must protect the reputation of the organization in the community has merit. First, healthcare has a significant psychological component and potential patients will benefit from having confidence in their providers. Second, those needing hospitalization should not fear receiving it, because deferring care may exacerbate their condition. Finally, individuals may be at greater risk by not obtaining treatment than from potentially contracting legionella.

On admission, potential risk becomes actual risk. Emergency admissions pose no ethical problem if an alternative source of care is unavailable and the risk of no care is greater than that of harm from contracting legionella.

Elective admissions are quite different, however. At the very least, the organization, led and prompted by its managers, should have developed and applied policies and procedures separating high- from low-risk elective admissions and made special provision either to send the former group elsewhere or to take special precautions regarding them. Ethically, it could not rely only on the discretion of the admitting physician. As with any quality assessment activity, management has a responsibility to review decision making about care and do so in a fashion consistent with the level of risk. Here, concurrent review is required.

Obvious potential conflicts of interest exist. It is natural for managers to protect their positions and reputations. They do so out of loyalty to the organization but also from selfish motives. A typical response is to cover up. Concealment seems an easy way to reduce the risk of personal and professional damage. Experience suggests, however, that from both an ethical and pragmatic standpoint honesty is the best policy. Rumors will be carried into the community by staff and patients, and the potential tarnish to the organization's reputation may last much longer than if the community is informed that there is a problem and that steps are being taken to protect patients. This tactic may raise questions about the cause of and responsibility for the problem, but the community will not distrust the organization. Furthermore, in terms of guiding ethical principles, the organization must treat individuals in the community with respect and dignity by being truthful, and managers must live by the virtues of trustworthiness and conscientiousness.

CONCLUSION

Just as they rely on computer programmers or wage and salary experts for reports, advice, and counsel, health services managers rely on technical expertise and assistance to monitor, review, and maintain the quality of clinical services. Managers provide clinical staff with the systems, procedures, and resources needed to be effective in delivering and monitoring clinical care. Beneficence and nonmaleficence—as well as the virtues of compassion, caring, and courage—demand that managers are sufficiently aware of what is expected and how that expectation is measured to determine that the goal of delivering quality health services is being met. Managers are remiss in meeting their ethical (and legal) duties if they occupy themselves exclusively with nonclinical activities and claim that clinical matters lie outside their ken and range of responsibilities. The manager is accountable to the governing body for all activities, and this requires active involvement and effective partnerships between managers and clinicians.

This chapter identified and examined several generic ethical problems arising from the duties owed by managers to patients and community. The duties are not always clear and may be further obscured by accompanying problems, such as bureaucratic inertia and medical staff relations. They become clear if managers focus on the primary reasons for the organization's existence—serving and protecting the patient and community.

NOTES

1. Peter A. Ubel, Margaret M. Zell, David J. Miller, Gary S. Fischer, Darien Peters-Stefani, & Robert M. Arnold. (1995, August). Elevator talk: Observational study of inappropriate comments in a public space. *American Journal of Medicine 99*, pp. 190–194; Simone N. Vigod, Chaim M. Bell, & John M.A. Bohnen. (2003, November 1). Privacy of patients' information in hospital lifts: Observational study. *British Medical Journal 327*, pp. 1024–1025.
2. Richard Perez Pena. (2011, March 9). New Jersey nearly sold secret data. *New York Times*. Retrieved March 17, 2011, from http://www.nytimes.com/2011/03/10/nyregion/10computers.html.
3. Horty, Springer & Mattern. (2003, July 10). *Question of the week*. Retrieved July 2003 from http://www.hortyspringer.com/.
4. Steve S. Kraman & Ginny Hamm. (1999, December 21). Risk management: Extreme honesty may be the best policy. *Annals of Internal Medicine 131*(12), pp. 963–967.
5. Joint Commission on Accreditation of Healthcare Organizations. (2004). Ethics, rights, and responsibilities. In *Hospital Accreditation Standards* (p. 110). Oakbrook Terrace, IL: Author.
6. Albert W. Wu, Thomas A. Cavanaugh, Stephen J. McPhee, Bernard Lo, & Guy P. Micco. (1997, December). To tell the truth: Ethical and practical issues in disclosing medical mistakes to patients. *Journal of General Internal Medicine 12*, pp. 770–775.
7. James S. Bowman, Frederick A. Elliston, & Paula Lockhart (Eds.). (1984). *Professional dissent: An annotated bibliography and research guide: Vol. 2* (p. 3). New York: Garland Publishing.
8. Alan E Westin. (1981). *Whistleblowing! Loyalty and dissent in the corporation* (p. 140). New York: McGraw-Hill.
9. *Ibid.*, p. 139.
10. *Ibid.*, p. 140.
11. *Ibid.*
12. Whistle-blowing. (2001). *The Columbia Encyclopedia* (6th ed.), as cited on Bartleby.com. Retrieved November 7, 2003, from http://www.bartleby.com/65/wh/whistlebl.html.
13. U.S. Department of Justice. (2010, November 22). *Department of justice recovers $3 billion in false claims cases in fiscal year 2010*. Retrieved November 28, 2010, from http://www.justice.gov/opa/pr/2010/November/10-civ-1335.html.
14. Ibid.
15. Pierce v. Ortho Pharmaceuticals, 84 NJ. 58, 417 A.2d 505 (1980).
16. O'Sullivan v. Mallon et al., 160 NJ. Super. 416, 390 A.2d 149 (1978).

17. Commonwealth of Pennsylvania ex rel. Rafferty et al. v. Philadelphia Psychiatric Center, 356 F. Supp. 500 (E.D. Pa. 1973).
18. Louise Kertesz. (1995, July 3). Execs fired in whistleblower case. *Modern Healthcare*, p. 11.
19. Lisa Scott. (1995, August 21). Whistle-blower suit alleges patient records doctored. *Modern Healthcare*, p. 34. Another example of a *qui tam* suit occurred in United States ex rel. Brandimarte v. Wurtzel, Civ. Action No. 94-2398 (E.D. Pa. Nov. 3, 1995), in which defendants settled allegations of making false and fraudulent claims for psychotherapy services under the Medicare and Medicaid programs by paying $500,000 to the U.S. government and $50,000 toward the whistle-blower's legal fees and costs.
20. Berkeley Rice. (1995, August 7). When a doctor accuses colleagues of health fraud. *Medical Economics*, pp. 172–174, 177–179, 183–184, 189–190.
21. Qui Tam FYI.
22. U.S. Department of Justice. (2009, October 30). *Texas hospital group pays U.S. $27.5 million to settle False Claims Act allegations.* Retrieved November 20, 2010, from http://www.justice.gov/opa/pr/2009/October/09-civ-1175.html. The relator (whistle-blower) in this *qui tam* lawsuit received $5.5 million from the proceeds of the settlement.
23. Tricia Bishop. (2010, November 10). Md. hospital to pay $22 million. *Washington Post*, p. B6.
24. Lawrence Blades. (1967, December). Employment at will vs. individual freedom: On limiting the abusive exercise of employer power. *Columbia Law Review 67*, p. 1407.
25. Westin, pp. 133–136.
26. Bowman et al., p. 4.
27. Westin, p. 144.
28. Stephen Barr. (1993, October 19). Whistleblowers sound alarm on their superiors' reprisals. *Washington Post*, p. A21.
29. U.S. Merit Systems Protection Board. (1998). *Adherence to the merit principles in the workplace: Federal employees' views* (p. 12). Washington, DC: Author.
30. John P. Keenan & C.A. Krueger. (1992, August). Whistleblowing and the professional. *Management Accounting 74*(2), pp. 21–24.
31. Laurie Larson. (1999, September). The right thing to do: An ethical framework helps trustees lead the way. *Trustee 59*(2), p. 10.
32. W. Edwards Deming. (1994). *The new economics for industry, government, education* (2nd ed.). Cambridge, MA: MIT-CAES, 1994.
33. Edward L. Hannan, Joseph E. O'Donnell, Harold Kilburn, Jr., Harvey R. Bernard, & Altan Yazici. (1989, July). Investigation of the relationship between volume and mortality for surgical procedures performed in New York State hospitals. *Journal of the American Medical Association 262*(4), pp. 503–510; Harold S. Luft, John P. Bunker, & Alain C. Enthoven. (1979, December). Should operations be regionalized? *New England Journal of Medicine 301*(25), pp. 1364–1369; Spencer Rich. (1984, April 26). Hospitals doing more operations lose fewer patients. *Washington Post*, p. A2.
34. Regionalizing cardiac surgery facilities contributes to improved outcomes and lower costs. (1996, January/February). *Research Activities 190*, pp. 1–2; Volume of procedures for physicians, hospitals, and geographic areas linked to

outcomes for angioplasty and bypass patients. (1995, July/August). *Research Activities 186*, pp. 1–3.

35. John D. Birkmeyer, Andrea E. Siewers, Emily V.A. Finlayson, Therese A. Stukel, F. Lee Lucas, Ida Batista, H. Gilbert Welch, & David E. Wennberg. (2002, April 11). Hospital volume and surgical mortality in the United States. *New England Journal of Medicine 346*(15), pp. 1128–1137; R. Adams Dudley, Kirsten L. Johanson, Richard Brand, Deborah J. Rennie, & Arnold Milstein. (2000, March 1). Selective referral to high-volume hospitals: Estimating potentially avoidable deaths. *Journal of the American Medical Association 283*(9), pp. 1159–1166; Philip P. Goodney, F.L. Lucas, & John D. Birkmeyer. (2003). Should volume standards for cardiovascular surgery focus only on high-risk patients? *Circulation 107*, pp. 384–387.

36. Recommendations for preventing transmission of human immunodeficiency virus and hepatitis B virus to patients during exposure-prone invasive procedures. (1991, July 12). *MMWR Recommendations and Reports.* Retrieved March 28, 2011, from http://www.cdc.gov/mmwr/preview/mmwrhtml/00014845. htm. An invasive procedure is defined as "surgical entry into tissues, cavities, or organs, or repair of traumatic injuries" associated with any of the following: 1) an operating or delivery room, emergency department, or outpatient setting, including both physicians' and dentists' offices; 2) cardiac catheterization and angiographic procedures; 3) vaginal or cesarean delivery or other invasive obstetric procedure during which bleeding may occur; or 4) the manipulation, cutting, or removal of any oral or perioral tissues, including tooth structure, during which bleeding occurs or the potential for bleeding exists.

37. *Ibid.*

38. American Medical Association. (2001, December). *Report 4 of the Council on Scientific Affairs (A-03): Consolidation of the AMA house policies on HIV/AIDS* (p. 8). Chicago: Author.

39. American Dental Association. (2003). *Resource manual for support of dentists with HBV, HIV, TB and other infectious disease.* Retrieved March 28, 2011, from http://www.ada.org/policiespositions.aspx.

40. How to balance interests of physician, patients, and your organization when physician is HIV-positive. (2003, August). *Credentialing & Peer Review Legal Insider,* p. 1.

41. Susan Okie. (1999, January 12). French surgeon gave a patient AIDS virus. *Washington Post*, p. 9.

42. Ronald Bayer. (1991, May). The HIV-infected clinician: To exclude or not exclude? *Trustee 44*(5), p. 17.

43. Rafael Harpaz, Lorenz von Seidlein, Francisco M. Averhoff, Michael P. Tormey, Saswati D. Sinha, Konstantina Kotsopoulou, Stephen B. Lambert, Betty H. Robertson, James D. Cherry, & Craig N. Shapiro. (1996, February 29). Transmission of hepatitis B virus to multiple patients from a surgeon without evidence of inadequate infection control. *New England Journal of Medicine 334*(9), pp. 549–554.

44. Juan I. Esteban, Jordi Gomez, Maria Martell, Beatriz Cabot, Josep Quer, Joan Camps, Antonio Gonzalez, Teresa Otero, Andres Moya, Rafael Esteban, & Jaime Guardia. (1996, February 29). Transmission of hepatitis C virus by a cardiac surgeon. *New England Journal of Medicine 334*(9), pp. 555–559.

Biomedical Ethical Issues

S ection IV analyzes consent and issues at the end of life, the biomedical ethical issues commonly confronted by health services managers and their organizations. Myriad other biomedical ethical issues affect some managers, including genetic engineering, screening, and counseling; reproductive technologies; psychosurgery and behavior control; the right to healthcare; personhood, fetal rights, and abortion; implants and transplants; and mental illness and involuntary commitment.

The thorny issue of consent is addressed in Chapter 9. Consent affects managers in all types of health services organizations. The law defines acceptable relationships between provider and patient; for managers this is but a starting point, one that builds on their moral agency and the organization's expected philosophy.

Chapter 10 addresses ethical issues arising at the end of life, often called the *ethics of dying and death*. Changes since the 1970s, many caused by technology, raise new questions. The chapter addresses the definition of death, application of life-sustaining treatment (using the example of infants with impairments), withholding or withdrawing treatment, futile care guidelines, and the ethics of terminal illness. Health services organizations are affected by some or all of the ethical issues that arise at the end of life. As with consent, these have major implications for managers.

Chapter 11 explores the relationships among physician-assisted suicide (PAS), autonomy, and the organization. PAS is an ethical issue with deep historical roots in medicine, even though it is prohibited by the Hippocratic tradition. European views and actions regarding PAS are explored and contrasted with developments in the United States.

CHAPTER 9

CONSENT

C onsent is an ethical imperative of great importance to managers and clinicians. It is clear that patients want to be more involved in medical decision making. The issues that consent raises suggest both a problem and a goal for health services providers.

The concept of consent in medical care evolved to protect patients from nonconsensual touching. Although the ethical and legal dimensions overlap, the legal requirements of consent are the minimum expected. The ethics of consent are grounded in the principle of respect for persons, specifically the element of autonomy, which reflects a view of the equality and dignity of human beings. In addition, the ethics of consent reflect the special relationship of trust and confidence between physician and patient and between organization and patient. This fiduciary relationship is supported by the principles of beneficence and nonmaleficence. The manager's virtues of trustworthiness, honesty, integrity, and candor also support the ethics of consent.

According to the law, failure to obtain consent can support a legal action for battery, an intentional tort. Beyond this, an action for negligence can be brought if the physician breaches the duty to communicate information necessary for the patient to give informed consent.

Paternalism stems from beneficence and is the ethical value that competes with patient autonomy in implementing consent. Paternalism arises naturally from the relationship between physician and patient because psychologically, technically, and emotionally, the physician is in a position of superior knowledge and is expected to help choose the best course of action for the patient. This reflects the ethics of care discussed in Chapter 1. The paternalism inherent in the physician–patient relationship was first described in the Hippocratic oath. Beneficence, nonmaleficence, and paternalism continue to be important and are implicit elements of the practice of medicine. The revisions of the Principles of Medical Ethics adopted by the American Medical Association (AMA) in 1980 moved organized medicine from paternalism toward autonomy and patient rights, themes that continued in the 2001 revision. The AMA's Council on Ethical and Judicial Affairs amplified these themes in its Fundamental Elements of the Patient–Physician Relationship statement. This document and the 2001 Principles of Medical Ethics are reproduced in Appendix B.

Specialized codes that guide biomedical research (e.g., the Declaration of Helsinki) also recognize the importance of consent. The emphasis on patients' rights or sovereignty in documents such as these are ideals toward which managers and organizations should strive.

LEGAL ASPECTS

Legally, consent must be voluntary, competent, and informed. The law presumes that persons unable to give consent in an emergency want to receive treatment. The presumption of wanting treatment can be rebutted if a competent patient declines it or if the person requiring treatment has an advance directive, such as a nonhospital do-not-resuscitate order. In addition, if that person's attorney-in-fact (e.g., someone who holds a durable power of attorney) is present, consent must be obtained. If minors or persons considered mentally incompetent are patients and those who speak for them refuse to give consent, and withholding treatment is not in the patient's best interests, the organization is usually successful in persuading a court to order treatment.

Even in nonemergencies, general consent for treatment is implied by the patient's presence in the outpatient department, for example, which shows the patient's apparent desire to be treated. Noninvasive elective treatment of a routine nature requires only general consent. Special consent is necessary, however, for invasive, surgical, or special procedures, or when the patient is part of an experiment. Consent for the invasive procedures common in intensive care units is problematic, for example, especially because they are often performed as emergencies and patients may not be able, or their surrogates may not be available, to give informed consent.[1] Oral consent is legally binding, but staff changes, faulty memories, and prudence dictate that consent is written. The George Washington University Medical Center's general and special consent forms are shown in Figures 7 and 8, respectively.

To be *voluntary*, consent must be given free of duress. Duress can be subtle and its presence depends on the facts. Threats or force are clearly duress. Persons with diminished autonomy cannot make voluntary choices; military personnel or prisoners are examples. Historically, the military and prisoners were important sources for research involving human subjects. Negative publicity and public indignation have virtually eliminated experimentation in such settings.

Competent consent means that the person has the capacity to understand the nature and consequences of the treatment or nontreatment. The law presumes minor children to be incompetent. In addition, persons whose mental illness or cognitive disability have resulted in a legal determination of incompetence may not decide about medical treatment or experimentation; others must make such decisions for them. Judging mental competence is complex when patients are terminally ill, depressed, or suicidal; expert opinion is required.

Consent must be *informed*. The law requires full disclosure of the nature of the patient's condition and treatment proposed, available alternatives, and consequences and difficulties that may likely result from treatment or nontreatment. The courts are about evenly split between those holding that patients should receive as much information as a reasonable physician would provide under the same or similar circumstances, and those using a standard based on what a reasonable patient would want to know. A legal criterion used by a few courts—and one oriented to patient sovereignty—is what that specific patient would want to know.

Historically, cases involving Jehovah's Witnesses, a religion that prohibits even homologous (self-donation) transfusions of whole blood or components, have been problematic for hospitals. Potential legal liability for transfusing or not transfusing the patient has resulted in numerous court cases. In early cases, courts often overrode the patient's wishes and ordered transfusion when patients, especially mothers, had significant family responsibilities. These cases showed that judges considered more than liberty rights (autonomy) when important societal interests such as caring for children were present. Developments in bloodless medicine and surgery in the 1960s and 1970s were spurred in the mid-1980s by problems with the blood supply, such as transmission of hepatitis and the human immunodeficiency virus. These developments have caused a rethinking of the use of blood and blood products; transfusion is avoided, if possible. New evidence suggests that transfusion requirements are often overestimated and that there are several modalities to treat Jehovah's Witnesses with acute blood loss, for example.[2]

The right of competent persons to refuse treatment is well established in the law:

GENERAL POLICY: All patients shall be treated, admitted and assigned accommodation without distinction to race, religion, color, national origin, sexual orientation, age or handicapping condition.

CONSENT TO TREATMENT: I have come to The George Washington University Hospital for medical treatment. I ask the health care professionals at the Hospital to provide care and treatment for me that they feel is necessary. The undersigned consents to the procedures, which may be performed during this hospitalization, or on an outpatient basis including emergency treatment or services. I consent to undergo routine tests and treatment as part of this care. These may include but are not limited to laboratory, radiology, medical or surgical tests, treatments, anesthesia or procedures as directed under the general and special instruction of the physician or surgeon. I understand that I am free to ask a member of my health care team questions about any care, treatment or medicine I am to receive. Because The George Washington University Hospital is a teaching hospital, I understand that my health care team will be made up of hospital personnel (to include nurses, technicians, and ancillary staff) under the direction of my attending physician and his/her assistants and designees (to include interns, residents, fellows and medical students). I am aware that the practice of medicine is not an exact science and admit that no one has given me any promises or guarantees about the result of any care or treatment I am to receive or examinations I am to undergo.

PHYSICIANS NOT AS EMPLOYEES: I understand that each physician is an independent contractor who is self employed and is not the agent, servant or employee of the hospital. I understand that I may receive separate billing from each of these providers for services rendered. _____Initials

RELEASE OF INFORMATION: The George Washington University Hospital is authorized to release any information necessary, including copies of my hospital and medical records, to process payment claims for health care services which have been provided, and to duly authorized local and federal regulatory agencies and accrediting bodies as required or permitted by law. George Washington University Hospital is further authorized to release demographic information to organizations performing patient satisfaction surveys. Such records may include information of a psychological or psychiatric nature, pertaining to my mental condition or treatment for conditions relating to the use of alcohol or drugs. In addition, I authorize my insurance carrier, employer or person otherwise responsible for payment to provide The George Washington University Hospital information necessary to determine benefits or process a claim. This release will be valid for the period of time to process the claim or until consent is revoked by myself. I release and forever discharge The George Washington University Hospital, its employees and agents, and my attending physician from any liability resulting from the release of my medical records or information from them for payment purposes. I understand that my name will be displayed in the signage system outside my hospital room.

PERSONAL VALUABLES: THE GEORGE WASHINGTON UNIVERSITY HOSPITAL WILL NOT BE RESPONSIBLE FOR LOSS OR DAMAGE TO CLOTHES, PERSONAL PROPERTY OR VALUABLES.

NON-SMOKING POLICY: In accordance with regulatory agency standards, the Hospital is a non-smoking facility.

FINANCIAL AGREEMENT/ASSIGNMENT OF BENEFITS: I assign any and all insurance benefits payable to me to The George Washington University Hospital. I understand that I am responsible for payment for services rendered at the Hospital including excluded services from my insurance either because the plan deems such services not medically necessary, or for any other reason including pre-certification requirements, second opinions or preexisting conditions. Should the account be referred to any attorney or collection agency for collection, I understand that I will be responsible for attorney or collection expenses. I give permission to my insurance provider(s), including Medicare and Medicaid, to directly pay The George Washington University Hospital for my care instead of paying me. I understand that I am responsible for any health insurance deductibles and co-insurance and non-covered services.

I certify that the information I have provided is true and accurate to the best of my knowledge. I understand that the information that I submit is subject to verification, including credit agency scoring, and subject to review by federal and/or state agencies and other as required, I authorize my employer to release to The George Washington University Hospital proof of my income. I understand that if any information I have given proves to be untrue, The George Washington University Hospital will re-evaluate my financial status and take whatever action becomes appropriate. I acknowledge by my signature that I have read and received a copy of this statement. I understand that by signing it, I am agreeing to it.

X_____

Signature of patient or responsible party

Unable to sign
( ) Serious Condition
( ) _____

_____   _____
Date   Witness

_____   _____
Hospital Representative   Date

Section 1:	By my signature below, I consent to laboratory studies (HIV, HBV, HCV) in the event a health care worker is exposed to my blood or body fluids. I consent to the appropriate disposal of any tissue or part removed from my body and to the taking of photographs during the procedure/operation/treatment for research, teaching, or scientific purposes as long as my identity is not disclosed.
Did you bring an Advance Directive (Living Will/Health Care Power of Attorney) **form with you?** ☐ Yes ☐ No	
(If YES, place a copy in the front of the patient's chart / If NO, go to Section 2)	
Section 2:	
1. I was given information on formulating an Advance Directive (including how to obtain assistance with completing the Advance Directive form). _____initials	
OR	
2. I do not have an Advance Directive and do not wish to formulate one. _____initials	Signature _____ Date _____

THE GEORGE WASHINGTON UNIVERSITY HOSPITAL

UHS
Universal Health

CO0010

PATIENT AUTHORIZATION FORM

80-010 (10/10)

Patient Label

WHITE - MEDICAL RECORD   YELLOW - BUSINESS OFFICE   PINK - PATIENT COPY

Figure 7. A general consent form. (From The George Washington University Medical Center. Copyright © 2011. Reprinted by permission.)

1. I, _____ (, or
   _____ as ☐ Parent   ☐ Representative
                                                       ☐ Guardian   (Check One)
   acting on his/her behalf,) request the procedure/operation/treatment set out below.

2. I have requested Dr(s). _____ perform
   and supervise my procedure/operation/treatment which has been explained to me to be:
   _____
   _____

   My doctor's explanation informed me about my medical condition as well as the common foreseeable benefits and risks of the
   procedure/operation/treatment as well as of its reasonable alternatives, if any.

3. I know, too, that during my procedure/operation/treatment it may become apparent to my doctor that in his/her professional judgement further
   procedures, operations, or treatments may be necessary. I therefore authorize modification or extension of this consent to include those
   additional procedures which in my doctor's professional judgement are medically necessary under these special circumstances and for my
   benefit with the exception of (check one): ☐ type of procedure _____ ☐ no exceptions

4. I understand that if a member of the Department of Anesthesiology is to participate in my care, for general, regional, or monitored anesthesia
   care, a separate consent will be obtained for these services.

5. If my doctor has indicated to me that I will require a local anesthetic as part of my procedure/operation/treatment, I authorize its administration. I
   acknowledge that my doctor has explained the benefits and risks of my receiving a local anesthetic as well as a reasonable alternative, if any.
   Potential risks may include but are not limited to pain at the injection site, or very rarely allergic reaction to the anesthetic. Further, I understand
   that during my procedure/operation/treatment, unforeseen circumstances may require alternative methods of anesthesia, such as general, and I
   therefore authorize modification of anesthesia administration which my doctor's professional judgement indicates to be necessary under the
   circumstances.

6. If it is anticipated that I may require transfusion of blood or blood products during my procedure, I will be required to sign a separate INFORMED
   CONSENT TO BLOOD TRANSFUSION AND/OR BLOOD COMPONENT ADMINISTRATION form. If in the event of an unanticipated emergency
   during my operative care and based on the medical judgement of my physician, I require the transfusion of blood or blood products, I
   understand they will be administered and agree to such action being taken.

7. Knowing that the George Washington University Hospital is a teaching institution, I understand that along with my doctor and his/her assistants
   and designees, other Hospital personnel such as residents, trainees, nurses, and technicians will be involved in my procedure/operation/
   treatment and care. I understand and agree to the presence of appropriate observers for the advancement of medical education and care.

8. I consent to appropriate routine tests and treatment as part of my medical care associated with this procedure/operation/treatment.

9. I agree to the appropriate disposal of any tissue or part removed from my body, to the taking of photographs during the procedure/operation/
   treatment for research, teaching, or scientific purposes as long as my identity is not disclosed, and to participate in the
   _____ research protocol/program.

| PATIENT AFFIRMATION | By signing this request form, I am indicating that I understand the contents of this document and agree to its provisions. I know that if I have concerns or would like more detailed information, I can ask more questions and get more information from my attending physician. I am also acknowledging that I know that the practice of anesthesiology, medicine and surgery is not an exact science and that no one has given me any promises or guarantees about the designated procedure/operation/treatment or its results. I fully understand what I am now signing of my own free will. |

WITNESS TO AFFIRMATION AND SIGNATURE | DATE | TIME | PATIENT SIGNATURE (or Parent, Guardian or Representative) | DATE/TIME

Signature of physician obtaining consent if other than physician performing procedure _____ Date _____ Time _____

| PHYSICIAN ATTESTATION | I attest that this patient or the representative named above has been informed about the common foreseeable risks and benefits of undergoing the procedure as well as its reasonable alternative(s), if any. Further questions with regard to this procedure have been answered to his/her apparent satisfaction. |

PHYSICIAN'S NAME - PRINTED | PHYSICIAN SIGNATURE | DATE/TIME

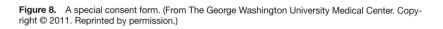

THE GEORGE WASHINGTON UNIVERSITY HOSPITAL

UHS
Universal Health

Patient Label

CO0024

**PATIENT'S REQUEST FOR
PROCEDURE, OPERATION
AND TREATMENT**
76-519 (07/06)

Figure 8. A special consent form. (From The George Washington University Medical Center. Copyright © 2011. Reprinted by permission.)

On the basis of either the common law liberty right to be free from unwanted treatment or by statute, competent adults, incompetent adults who have clearly expressed their wishes, and even older minors with adult-like decision-making capacity can legally refuse unwanted blood transfusions. As for minor children generally, although parents may not deprive their children of necessary care, if the parents have a choice between two or more effective treatment options, the state has no *parens patriae* interest in mandating treatment entailing the use of blood simply because it is the popular or standard approach. If the child's health problem can be effectively managed without the use of homologous blood, the parents should be free to choose that treatment option without governmental interference.[3]

An ethic that emphasizes autonomy and respect for persons can significantly affect the patient–caregiver relationship. Fully expressed, patients alone choose the level of involvement they want. In the early 1980s, the President's Commission stated that patient sovereignty with complete participation in the process is a desirable, if not a readily achievable, goal.[4] The principle of respect for persons cannot be realized, nor participation achieved, absent truthfulness and the organization's consistent efforts. Autonomy means patients may not agree with caregivers' recommendations and assessments. Sometimes, clinicians and organizations find this concept threatening.

Some patients choose not to participate in decision making. Explicitly or implicitly, they want to remain ignorant of their medical problems and exclude themselves from decision processes. They prefer paternalism and choose to delegate decision making to caregivers to do what they think is best. This relationship between patient and caregivers is neither the one envisioned as ideal by the President's Commission nor that demanded by contemporary patient rights advocates. Autonomy is also violated if the patient is forced to participate, however. Caregivers and managers should consider a decision not to participate to be acceptable and work to make it a reality. Delegating to others the authority to make decisions may be the ultimate expression of autonomy.

More Serious than She Knows[5]

Lilah is 6-months pregnant with her first child. Her husband, a member of the U.S. Army, is currently deployed to a combat zone. During his absence, Lilah has moved back to her hometown, where she has the emotional support of her tight-knit family and access to basic medical care at a small-town community hospital. Lilah's mother is excited at the prospect of being her daughter's birthing coach.

In anticipation of her due date, Lilah has signed releases authorizing the hospital and her obstetrician to share her medical information with her mother.

At her 6-month office visit, Lilah's blood pressure was slightly elevated. This prompted her obstetrician, Dr. Campos, to refer her to the hospital for outpatient testing to rule out preeclampsia, which is a potentially deadly complication of pregnancy. She was released after three hours with a clean bill of health and given instructions to avoid strenuous activity and to watch her diet. When Lilah and her mother returned to Dr. Campos's office three days later for a regularly scheduled ultrasound, the nurse noted that her blood pressure was even higher than before. Lilah told the nurse that she had followed the hospital's discharge instructions and suggested that the rise in blood pressure was caused by anxiety over her husband's safety, since his unit had suffered several casualties recently.

The ultrasound revealed that the baby's growth was unexpectedly retarded. Suspecting that Lilah and her child needed resources beyond the scope of the local hospital, Dr. Campos, immediately referred her to a perinatologist in a large city three hours away. "It's probably nothing serious, but it's better to err on the side of caution," he assured Lilah. "You and your mother can make a vacation of it. You could stay overnight and shop for the baby after the appointment."

As the nurse and Lilah completed paperwork in another room, Dr. Campos turned to Lilah's mother and said, "I don't want to cause Lilah additional stress, but this could be far more serious than she knows."

The law and medical ethics include the concept of therapeutic privilege, which permits physicians to withhold information from patients when the physician believes it serves the patient's best interests. States recognize therapeutic privilege in several ways; a general rule is difficult to formulate. Some reference the danger that full disclosure may cause to the patient's physical or mental health; others focus on patient best interests. Such paternalism is supported by the principles of beneficence and nonmaleficence and the virtue of caring. The therapeutic privilege exception is pragmatic and avails physicians of a range of actions. It is desirable that physicians possess the latitude to make such judgments, especially if the alternative is probable harm to the patient. If so, beneficence and nonmaleficence take precedence. Lilah's case is an expression of therapeutic privilege. Dr. Campos is concerned that apprizing Lilah as to the potential risks of her pregnancy may cause further stress and aggravate her condition. Telling Lilah's mother may assuage Dr. Campos's reluctance to communicate vital information to Lilah. Also, it makes her mother more alert to changes that may require emergency attention.

ETHICAL ASPECTS

The premise for a discussion of the ethics of consent is that the ethical standard is significantly higher than the legal standard. This expectation arises from exercising the principles of respect for persons (autonomy) and nonmaleficence—which are based on Kantian deontology (see Chapter 1), natural law, and rule utilitarianism—and is supported by virtue ethics as expressed by virtuous managers acting as moral agents.

The nuances inherent in duress and inducement are important in determining whether consent is *voluntary*. In these cases, ethical considerations and duties extend well beyond the standard in the law. Can patients suffering from a fatal disease make medical decisions voluntarily? Are patients' decisions free of duress if they fear losing their physicians' friendship and loyalty because they prefer an option the physician opposes? Clinical staff talk about "bad" patients, usually defined as uncooperative patients. Such patients are not intentionally harmed or mistreated, but they may not receive the same attention as "good" or pliable patients. Patients sense this attitude and it affects their volition. Patients are also heavily influenced by family and friends and may make decisions because of them. Similarly, family members may ask clinicians to act in ways that may be unwanted by a patient who is considered incompetent or that, under the principles of beneficence or nonmaleficence, do not serve the patient's interests.

Such considerations suggest that consent may never be entirely voluntary. Some have argued that patients' personal freedom to accept or reject medical treatment has been so reduced that it is only a right to veto unwanted procedures.[6] This argument is bolstered by the increasingly complex relationships in medical care and its delivery, all of which preclude simple answers and easy determinations as to the voluntariness of consent. Managerial and clinical staff must understand the difficulties of consent and make all efforts to further patient autonomy and control of medical decision making.

In determining the voluntariness of consent, some groups present special problems. As noted, in the past healthy persons with diminished autonomy, notably military service members and prisoners, participated in experimentation that was nontherapeutic—meaning that it had no direct benefit for them. The consent of persons in such groups is seen as nonvoluntary, and their use as healthy subjects is rare. Voluntariness may also be reduced because inducements are so significant that prudence is cast aside. Money or other incentives may be offered to those who participate in high-risk experimentation; for example, some persons may be persuaded by payments that, for them, are significant. Students who participate in experiments are unique in this regard and may fit into several categories. Often, they are economically disadvantaged. In addition, some faculty encourage students to participate in experiments by exempting them from other, seemingly more onerous requirements, such as research papers or examinations. Occasionally, there is implicit, or even explicit, coercion by faculty who control the students' academic (and sometimes economic) destiny, and who unethically use this position to "encourage" consent and participation in research.

Usually, the ethical aspects of whether one is *competent* to consent are easier than the ethics of whether consent was voluntary. Competence is assumed in adults. Typically, clinical staff can determine if a patient's mental status is questionable and then seek consultation. Absent evidence of questionable mental status, the organization's policies should include an explicit assumption that patients are autonomous for the purposes of decision making. It is incumbent on managers to assist in this process through staff education and the support provided by appropriate systems and procedures.

The third element of consent is that it must be *informed*. Some commentary suggests that being "informed" is the only criterion for consent. Because of the complexity of informed consent, whether the patient was *adequately informed* receives the most attention. Some states have statutes designed to ensure that patients obtain sufficient information to make informed medical decisions. A Virginia law regarding consent, for example, resulted from reports that physicians performed radical mastectomies (even though removal of the malignancy would have sufficed) and that women were not given enough information to make an informed decision.[7]

Wait a Little Longer, We'll Do It Then

The emergency department at County Hospital has a typical caseload: some true emergencies and urgent medical conditions, but many sniffles and other non-emergencies. The hospital contracts with an emergency medicine group, but administrative activities, including systems, procedures, and personnel, are the hospital's responsibility. The process for obtaining consent is typical: Unconscious patients are treated as their conditions necessitate. Competent patients who are able to communicate sign a consent form authorizing treatment. Parents and other family members are involved as needed and as available.

Early one afternoon, a conscious, middle-aged man who had been in a car accident was brought in. He was diagnosed with internal injuries that required immediate exploratory surgery. He was asked to sign the consent form but refused because, as a Christian Scientist, receiving medical treatment violated his religious beliefs. He asked for a Christian Science practitioner.

The physician-director of the emergency department was paged, and, after reviewing the chart, she felt certain she could obtain his consent for surgery. She discussed the situation with the patient, who clearly understood that without surgery he was likely to die. He continued to refuse and repeatedly asked for a Christian Science practitioner. The physician-director left the treatment area very agitated; her mouth and chin shook in anger. She said, "This man is throwing his life away, all in the name of some religion that denies scientific medicine to its followers. I can't believe he's doing it!" She turned to the nurse and whispered, "Let me know when he's unconscious and we'll save his life, despite his silly ideas."

Such deception rides roughshod over the patient's clearly expressed wishes. The patient is competent and informed; his refusal is voluntary. In addition to violating the principle of respect for persons (autonomy), the physician is ignoring the AMA's Principles of Medical Ethics and the AMA's Council on Ethical and Judicial Affairs's Fundamental Elements of the Patient–Physician Relationship. Such methods are unconscionable.

The organizational philosophy should prospectively consider the issues in this case. The discussion of Baby Boy Doe in Chapter 1 suggested that the organization might have intervened by petitioning a court to order life-saving surgery. Such intervention gives less weight to the principle of respect for persons (autonomy) and more to beneficence (and its corollary, utility) and paternalism. Increasing focus by courts on liberty rights such as autonomy make it unlikely that the Christian Scientist will be forced to undergo surgery, even if he has a family dependent on him. The principle of nonmaleficence supports action by the hospital. However, forcing treatment is paternalistic and greatly diminishes autonomy. The competing ethical principles in such cases pose true ethical dilemmas for organizations and managers.

ROLE OF THE ORGANIZATION

What is the organization's role in consent? Patients should give informed, voluntary, and competent consent before treatment—a simple ethical concept. As is often true, difficulties arise in operationalizing the concept; it is in instances such as these that the criteria for consent may be more often violated than met. Since the 1970s, organizations have focused greater attention on consent, an emphasis that likely reflects fear of legal problems more than a desire to do what is ethically right. Before the 1970s, organizations were less concerned about consent because they adopted and amplified the historic, paternalistic view of the patient, a view consistent with the Hippocratic concept of the physician–patient relationship.

At minimum, policies and procedures consistent with the organizational philosophy must be established for obtaining consent, and their application must be systematically monitored. If, as it should, the philosophy emphasizes patients' rights, actions and efforts to perfect those rights will be encouraged while actions and efforts that contravene them will be restricted. There are specific means that allow patients to assert their rights, but these means are costly and can result in adversarial relationships. One is to provide an advocate for each patient. Another establishes an ombudsman office to review problems and prevent them in the future.

Often, the circumstances of consent are complicated because many parties are involved.

When Is Consent Consent?

Henry Franklin was an emergency admission to University Hospital. He was diagnosed with mild cardiac failure by an attending physician. Because he was 78 years old and had complicating medical conditions, a dispute arose as to the proper course of treatment. The consulting cardiologist recommended that Franklin be treated medically and given the best quality of life possible. The cardiologist estimated that Franklin had 6 months to live.

The cardiac surgeons who also consulted on the case saw things differently. They recommended replacing the aortic and mitral valves and estimated that this procedure would provide at least 2 years of useful life. When the options were described to Franklin, he was told the probability of surviving the surgery was 50%. He decided he would work with the cardiologist.

After hearing his decision, the surgeons intervened directly with Franklin's family, with whom they had had previous conversations. The family agreed with the surgeons and pressured Franklin to consent, which he did. Franklin's body could not withstand the rigors of surgery; he died in the operating room.

Even if informed and competent, Franklin's final decision was made under duress. The coercive circumstances greatly reduced his autonomy. In such situations, family and physicians press for what they assert are the patient's best interests. However, sometimes both groups are driven by motives that conflict with the patient's self-expressed decision. Family may have various psychological and financial motives; physicians may act out of technological daring or hubris.

The challenge managers face is ensuring patient autonomy. Patients may choose a course of action that is not their first choice or even in their best interests (as the patient views them) because they defer to the wishes of others. They may fear abandonment or caregivers' anger if they choose a course of action other than what caregivers suggest or what they think caregivers want. An added complexity is that patients are often uncertain about what to do; they vacillate between wanting and not wanting aggressive treatment. Preserving patient autonomy in these circumstances is difficult, perhaps impossible, but must be attempted nonetheless.

The surgeons were important in the Franklin case. They may have allowed bravado to cloud their judgment, especially given the probability of success. Franklin's family was also important. Health services organizations interfere at their peril in situations that reflect family dynamics, even though their duty clearly lies with the patient. Involvement of the institutional ethics committee could provide an important buffer for the patient.

What is the role of the organization in determining that patients have consented in a way that meets ethical criteria? Obvious coercion will likely be noticed by staff. A patient advocate program may minimize duress. Complicating efforts to ensure consent is that the private attending physician has an independent ethical duty to inform patients about the procedure's nature, consequences, risks, and alternatives. The attending physician determines that the patient is competent to give consent and does so voluntarily. Some health services organizations see their ethical duty as independently determining or verifying that the criteria of consent have been met. Others ask only that patients sign an authorization verifying that their physician has informed them about the procedure and that the hospital may participate in rendering the care to which the patient has previously consented.

Unless it is certain that patients have been informed about the treatment in a way that meets organizational criteria, the ethically preferred course is that staff be involved, at least to the extent of verifying that the patient is informed and competent. The manager must fulfill the organization's positive ethical duty to monitor consent, which includes processes and procedures to assist and guide staff, as necessary. Physician and nonphysician staff will also benefit from education about the ethical (and legal) dimensions of consent.

The case of Henry Franklin is distinguishable from that of the Christian Scientist. Franklin had more time to consider his decision, which was likely influenced by his age. The other patient was middle-aged, with the potential for decades of life remaining. Beyond these apparent differences, both cases raise questions about patient autonomy and its relationship to the principles of beneficence and nonmaleficence. The weight given these principles in the organizational philosophy and the personal ethic of the actors determines the outcome.

Managers of nursing facilities face ethical issues regarding consent similar to those of their counterparts in acute care hospitals. Decision making in nursing facilities is more likely to be complicated by factors such as competence or abandonment of patients. Thus, the process requires special attention.

I Intend to Be Independent

Oliver Harris is 82 years old and has been a resident at Five Oaks Nursing Home for 7 years. When he first sought admission, Harris had been evaluated and found to be only marginally in need of the care provided at Five Oaks. Because he was a private-pay patient, management decided to admit him. For 5 years his health was such that he needed minimal nursing care. In the sixth year, he began to show evidence of dementia. Medical evaluation found that he had experienced several small strokes. Harris likes to visit with other residents as he walks around the facility. His declining physical condition has resulted in several falls, which caused cuts and bruises but no broken bones.

Harris's case was discussed at a staff conference. It was the consensus to physically restrain him so that he could not ambulate independently. Under federal guidelines, this was possible only with an order from Harris's physician. Staff doubted the physician would agree, but they believed that if Harris continued to walk unassisted, it was only a matter of time before he fell and sustained a fracture. Staff also believed that even if his physician ordered restraints, Harris would fight them. When the issue was discussed with Harris, he was adamant that he not be restrained. His daughter, however, agreed that physical restraint was wise.

Staff and management face a dilemma: How can they meet their duty of nonmaleficence to Harris while maximizing his autonomy under the principle of respect for persons? Harris is competent to decide about restraints. It is clear to staff (and to Harris) that his well-being is at risk. Major injury will likely cause deterioration of his general health. Staff does not seem very creative in finding a way to allow him to ambulate safely. Such options should be explored first. Alternatively, various possibilities should be tested for short periods. If Harris cannot be persuaded to accept restraints, he should be allowed to ambulate freely in the facility. But is Harris's choice to walk untethered different from a younger person who chooses to skydive, bungee jump, or extreme ski?

MEDICAL EDUCATION

The case of Richard Weidner in Chapter 7 involved problems of consent in the context of medical education. Weidner was admitted to the hospital for a cardiac catheterization following recurrent chest pain. His cardiologist allowed him to think that she would perform the procedure, but a cardiology resident actually did the catheterization. The misrepresentation violated Weidner's right to autonomy and informed decision making and angered him greatly. There is significant tension between medical education's legitimate needs and the rights of patients to be treated with dignity and respect. The two are not incompatible, however.

Medical education is a major source of problems in consent, especially as to patient knowledge about who will provide treatment. The conclusions of a New York State Assembly task force were based on interviews with chiefs of surgery, attending surgeons, residents, and anesthesiologists at 34 hospitals in the state. It reported:

- Private surgical patients in teaching hospitals are usually not operated on by the attending surgeon they retained, but rather by residents. Between 50% and 85% of the surgery in teaching hospitals is done by residents.
- Although most residents operated only under the close supervision of attending surgeons, some residents performed surgery without supervision, and some attending surgeons left the room while the operation was still in progress or before the incision was closed.
- Most patients are unaware of the degree to which residents participate in their surgery, and consent forms that name the attending surgeon and "such assistants as he shall select" do not give patients meaningful notice that a resident may do the actual cutting or suturing.[8]

The authors of the report stressed that there was no evidence that allowing residents to be active participants in surgery caused harm to patients. However, other researchers were less certain, suggesting that harm to patients from care rendered by physicians in training may be much more common than is generally known.[9] Whether harm occurs is a utilitarian measure. Kantians do not consider outcomes, but rather determine only whether actions meet the criterion of respect for persons. Misleading patients or lying to them violates this principle.

The report addressed the disclosure necessary for informed consent and sufficient supervision to ensure patient safety. It also recommended that physicians be required to obtain the patient's consent for each person who participates in the surgery and that vague phrases (e.g. "such assistants as the surgeon may select") be deleted from consent forms. The recommendations encouraged adequate supervision by limiting the number of patients a surgeon could treat and the number of operating rooms surgeons could reserve at one time.[10]

The AMA and the American College of Surgeons (ACS) have addressed the question of medical education and consent. They agree that if a resident—rather than the surgeon retained by the patient—actually performs the surgery, the patient must be made aware of that fact and consent to the substitution. The *Report of the Council on Ethical and Judicial Affairs of the AMA* states

> A surgeon who allows a substitute to operate on his or her patient without the patient's knowledge and consent is deceitful. The patient is entitled to choose his or her own physician and should be permitted to acquiesce in or refuse to accept the substitution.
>
> Under the normal and customary arrangement with patients, and with reference to the usual form of consent to operation, the operating surgeon is obligated to perform the operation but may be assisted by residents or other surgeons. With the consent of the patient, it is not unethical for the operating surgeon to delegate the performance of certain aspects of the operation to the assistant provided this is done under the surgeon's participatory supervision, i.e., the surgeon must scrub. If a resident or other physician is to perform the operation under nonparticipatory supervision, it is necessary to make a full disclosure of this fact to the patient, and this should be evidenced by an appropriate statement contained in the consent. Under these circumstances, the resident or other physician becomes the operating surgeon.[11]

The ACS devotes the second part of its Statements on Principles to "Relation of the Surgeon to the Patient"; in the section titled "The Operation—Responsibility of the Surgeon," it states

> The surgeon is personally responsible for the patient's welfare throughout the operation. . . . The surgeon may delegate part of the operation to associates or residents under his or her personal direction, because

modern surgery is often a team effort. If a resident is to perform the operation and is to provide the continuing care of the patient under the general supervision of the attending surgeon, the patient should have prior knowledge. However, the surgeon's personal responsibility must not be delegated or evaded. It is proper to delegate the performance of part of a given operation to assistants, provided the surgeon is an active participant throughout the key components of the operation. The overriding goal is the assurance of patient safety. . . .

It is unethical to mislead a patient as to the identity of the surgeon who performs the operation. This principle applies to the surgeon who performs the operation when the patient believes that another physician is operating ("ghost surgery") and to the surgeon who delegates a procedure to another surgeon without the knowledge or consent of the patient.[12]

These statements are unambiguous. The patient must be informed about a resident's participation in the operation. The evidence suggests, however, that these principles are often violated. Learning by doing is most apparent in surgical training. There is no ethical difference, however, between a surgical resident wielding a scalpel and a medical resident ordering a treatment or medication under the general supervision of an attending physician if patients have not given consent for them to participate in their care.

Patient consent in medical education settings generally receives inadequate attention. Examples range from conducting pelvic examinations on anesthetized women without their consent (37% of medical schools taught pelvic exams in this manner) to performing procedures (for educational purposes) on dead bodies without family members' consent. Almost half of accredited emergency medicine programs permitted physicians in training to perform procedures on dead bodies; three quarters admitted that they almost never obtained consent from family members.[13] Such breaches are all the more unacceptable because there is no therapeutic benefit derived by the "patient."

Similar ethical breaches occur in nonsurgical settings. Examinations and participation by physicians in training pose less risk to patients than those by surgeons in training. Nonetheless, the same ethical principles are violated if patients do not consent to participate in medical education.

Role and Status Uncertain

An internationally known medical center has a large number of physicians on staff. Consultants are ranked highest, are board-certified, and have achieved preeminence in the organization. Below them are fellows and residents, both of

whom see patients with general supervision from the consultant to
have been assigned. Fellows and residents hold state licenses and hav
uated through a credentialing process. Fellows work more independer
residents. Residents may be at various points in their post–medical sc   .ւ ain-
ing. Residents report to fellows or to the consultant, depending on the clinical
service and the wishes of the consultant.

The three categories of physicians wear the same type of name badges. The
badges do not identify their category or position in the organization's hierarchy.
Typically, a resident or fellow sees the patient first. Only rarely do they identify
themselves to patients other than to state something such as "Hello, I'm Dr. . . . "
Sophisticated patients and returning patients understand that a fellow or resident usually performs the preliminary examination or has the first interaction
with the patient. The consultant follows after, conferring with the fellow and/or
resident.

One patient was bold enough to ask the consultant, whom she had seen on
a previous visit, about the roles of the other two physicians who had already examined her. She wondered aloud why she had not been told that they were physicians in training and, as she stated, "were not fully qualified to be her doctors."

There is evidence that the problem described above is widespread. One
study[14] found that

> Residents introduced themselves as a doctor 82% of the time, but
> identified themselves as a resident only 7% of the time. While attend-
> ing physicians introduced themselves as a "doctor" 64% of the time,
> only 6% identified themselves as the supervising physician. Patients
> felt it was very important to know their physicians' level of training,
> but most did not.

In addition to the ethical and legal expectations incident to informed consent, the information about training status is important to patients. Patients in emergency departments prefer not to be seen by trainees; those
informed about physicians' credentials were less willing to be seen by more
junior trainees.[15]

Failure to obtain patient (or family) consent for purposes of medical
education occurs despite the work of accreditors such as the Joint Commission on Accreditation of Healthcare Organizations and the Liaison
Committee on Medical Education, both of whom emphasize proper consent. This issue raises questions about the adequacy of consent for treatment and emphasizes the need for increased attention by the organization
and its managers.

Medical education and patient consent are compatible, but medical
educators may fear that obtaining explicit consent will diminish educational

opportunities and therefore the quality of the educational program. Patients and families are likely to cooperate if asked to help with teaching needs.[16] In addition, patients will likely cooperate if they know that physicians in training will play a role in their care.[17] Patients who do not consent to residents' participation in their care should have their decision respected, or they should be encouraged to seek care elsewhere. Ignoring their autonomy shows that an ethical commitment to patient rights is lacking, that the organization and staff violate their moral obligations to patients, and that managers violate the virtues of honesty and trustworthiness.

CONCLUSION

This chapter addressed the ethical issues of consent. Health services organizations and their managers should consider legal requirements a minimum. Ethical principles should be the basis for a strong relationship with the patient. This independent relationship stems from autonomy and the respect owed the patient.

Operationalizing the desire of and need for patients to be fully involved in consent requires managerial attention to the consent process—itself not an easy task. More involvement means overcoming a history of medical paternalism and educating patients as well as encouraging and assisting them to become involved.

A significant ethical problem is that of providing information about treatment to patients in health services organizations in which clinical education occurs. Managers face many barriers in convincing attending staff and trainees that fully informing patients will not lead to less "clinical material" for teaching. Evidence suggests that few patients will refuse to participate after they have been informed; there is reason to believe that patients will overwhelmingly agree to having medical and surgical residents participate in their treatment. Regardless, the needs of medical education must be secondary to the right of patients to consent.

NOTES

1. Nicole Davis, Anne Pohlman, Brian Gehlbach, John P. Kress, Jane McAtee, Jean Herlitz, & Jesse Hall. (2003, April 16). Improving the process of informed consent in the critically ill. *Journal of the American Medical Association 289*(15), pp. 1963–1968.
2. Duncan B. Hughes, Brant W. Ullery, & Philip S. Barie. (2008). The contemporary approach to the care of Jehovah's Witnesses. *Journal of Trauma, Injury, Infection, and Critical Care 65*(1), pp. 237–247.

3. Donald T. Ridley. (1995, February). Working with Jehovah's Witnesses on treatment issues. *Hospital Law Newsletter 12*(4), p. 6.

4. President's Commission for the Study of Ethical Problems in Medicine and Biomedical and Behavioral Research. (1982). *Making health care decisions: A report on the ethical and legal implications of informed consent in the patient–practitioner relationship. Volume 1: Report.* Washington, DC: U.S. Government Printing Office.

5. Case authored by Carey Lafferty, MHSA, Washington, D.C. Used by permission. (2011).

6. Jay Katz. (1977, Winter). Informed consent—A fairy tale. *University of Pittsburgh Law Review 39*, pp. 137–174.

7. Breast cancer law opposed in Richmond. (1983, August 12). *Washington Post,* p. A4.

8. Margaret Keller Holmes. (1980, May). Ghost surgery. *Bulletin of the New York Academy of Medicine 56*(4), p. 414.

9. Toby Cohen. (1983, September 20). The high cost of bad medicine. *Washington Post,* p. A15.

10. Holmes, p. 415.

11. American Medical Association Council on Ethical and Judicial Affairs. (1994, June). *Code of medical ethics: Opinion 8.16—Substitution of surgeon without patient's knowledge or consent.* Retrieved December 26, 2010, from http://www.ama-assn.org/ama/pub/physician-resources/medical-ethics/code-medical-ethics/opinion816.shtml.

12. American College of Surgeons Board of Regents. (2004, March). *Statements on principles.* Retrieved December 19, 2010, from http://www.facs.org/fellows_info/statements/stonprin.html. Emphasis added.

13. Robin Fretwell Wilson. (2008). "Unauthorized practice": Regulating the use of anesthetized, recently deceased, and conscious patients in medical teaching. *Idaho Law Review 44*(432).

14. Sally A. Santen, Tricia S. Rotter, & Robin R. Hemphill. (2007, December 21). Patients do not know the level of training of their doctors because doctors do not tell them. *Journal of General Internal Medicine 23*(5), pp. 607–610.

15. Daniel J. Pallin, Rachel Harris, Camille I. Johnson, & Ediza Giraldez. (2008, December). Is consent "informed" when patients receive care from medical trainees? *Academic Emergency Medicine 15*(12), pp. 1304–1308.

16. Wilson.

17. Martin L. Kempner. (1979). Some moral issues concerning current ways of dealing with surgical patients. *Bulletin of the New York Academy of Medicine 55*(1), pp. 62–68.

CHAPTER 10

DYING
AND DEATH

Dying and death are intrinsic to human existence. As with abortion, the ethical questions involved often prompt emotional responses from the public and many health professionals. Ethical issues in dying and death arise in ways such as treating neonates with severe disabilities who are unlikely to survive, and caring for children or adults who are terminally ill and unable to be autonomous.

Technology is at the heart of the matter. Since the 1970s, renal dialysis, mechanical ventilation, cardiac medications, and intensive care units (ICUs) have made it possible to postpone the end of life. Similar developments allow neonates who would have died in the 1980s to survive. A great deal has been written about the questions such technology raises, but there are few widely accepted courses of action. Sometimes an ethical dilemma occurs when a person asks the health services organization to assist in achieving pain-free death.

Adding complexity to these ethical issues is that many are poorly developed in the law. Deliberately shortening a patient's life raises important ethical and legal questions. Juries are reluctant to convict perpetrators, even when violent means have been used to end the painful life of someone terminally ill.

Chapter 9 noted that in the early 1980s, the President's Commission for the study of Ethical Problems in Medicine and Biomedical and Behavioral Research recommended a physician–patient relationship that maximizes patient sovereignty, with the patient fully participating in the decision process. Often, by the time crucial medical decisions must be made, the patient can no longer participate effectively, however, and may not be competent. If available, advance medical directives are helpful, but families and caregivers may disregard them. A medical ethic dedicated to preserving life and staving off death controls, and it is typical that the technological imperative results in expending all efforts, many times with marginal results. The economic, emotional, and psychological costs are obvious.

Managers may feel uneasy discussing dying and death. They may think that decision making at the end of life is clinical, a situation in which they play no role. Certainly, physicians are the lead actors in these dramas, but the effect of such issues on the organization requires that managers are knowledgeable about them and participate in developing and implementing policies and procedures. Managers must also be involved in the work of relevant committees.

In the mid-1980s, a distinction was drawn between treatments that were life prolonging and those that were life sustaining. Since then, however, the two concepts have merged and are simply called *life-sustaining treatments*. Life-sustaining treatment is "any treatment that serves to prolong life without reversing the underlying medical condition. Life-sustaining treatment may include, but is not limited to, mechanical ventilation, renal dialysis, chemotherapy, antibiotics, and artificial nutrition and hydration."[1]

DEATH DEFINED

Historically, death was defined as the stoppage of blood circulation and the cessation of circulation-dependent animal and vital functions, such as respiration and pulsation. New technology proved this definition inadequate. Table 3 summarizes definitions of death. Definitions based in law and theology provide limited guidance for contemporary clinicians.

In 1968, a Harvard Medical School committee defined *irreversible coma*, which solved some problems but created others. The Harvard criteria were accompanied by a report stating that only a physician can determine the patient's condition, and that when the condition is found to be hopeless certain steps are recommended:

> Death is declared and *then* the respirator is turned off. The decision to do this and the responsibility for it are to be taken by the physician-in-charge, in consultation with one or more physicians who have been directly involved in the case. It is unsound and undesirable to force the family to make the decision.[2]

This quote is noteworthy because of changes in society's attitudes and perceptions that have occurred since 1968, including emphasis on patient autonomy and natural death statutes, family involvement in decision making,

Table 3. Definitions of death

Concept of death (Philosophical or theological judgment of the essentially significant change at death)	Locus of death (Place to look to determine whether a person has died)	Criteria of death (Measurements physicians or other officials use to determine whether a person is dead—to be determined by scientific empirical study)
1. Irreversible loss of flow of vital fluids (i.e., the blood and breath)	Heart and lungs	Visual observation of respiration, perhaps with the use of a mirror Feeling of the pulse, possibly supported by electrocardiogram
2. Irreversible loss of the soul from the body	Pineal body (?) (according to Descartes) Respiratory tract (?)	Observation of breath (?)
3. Irreversible loss of the capacity for bodily integration	Brain	Unreceptivity and unresponsivity No movements or breathing No reflexes (except spinal reflexes) Flat electroencephalogram (to be used as confirmatory evidence) All tests to be repeated 24 hours later (excluded conditions: hypothermia and central nervous system depression by drug)
4. Irreversible loss of consciousness or the capacity for social interaction	Probably the neocortex	Electroencephalogram

Adapted from Veatch, R.M.S. (1976). *Death, dying, and the biological revolution: Our lost quest for responsibility* (p. 53). New Haven: Yale University Press. Used with permission. Copyright © Yale University Press. Used with permission. This table has been modified using material from the 1989 second edition.

Note: Death is defined as a complete change in the status of a living entity characterized by the irreversible loss of those characteristics that are essentially significant to it. The possible concepts, loci, and criteria of death are much more complex than the ones provided here. These concepts are simplified models used to define death. It is obvious that those who believe that death means the irreversible loss of the capacity for bodily integration (3), or the irreversible loss of consciousness (4), have no reservations about pronouncing death when the heart and lungs have ceased to function. This is because they are willing to use loss of heart and lung activity as shortcut criteria for death, believing that once the heart and lungs have stopped, the brain or neocortex will necessarily stop, as well.

Note: In the table, (?) signifies uncertainty.

and establishment of institutional ethics committees (IECs). These changes have reduced the physician's primacy in decision making.

Near the time that the Harvard criteria were developed, a Virginia court issued one of the first rulings accepting brain death.[3] The case raised issues of consent, appropriate criteria and process for determining death, conflicts of interest, beneficence, nonmaleficence, and organizational philosophy and managerial ethics. The physicians involved tried to use a brain death standard but failed to meet the Harvard criteria because there was no electroencephalogram to verify brain activity and the respirator was turned off *before* the patient was pronounced dead. Despite the lapses, the court made legal history by accepting a determination that the patient was dead using a brain death criterion.

The National Conference on Uniform State Laws developed the Uniform Determination of Death Act (UDDA) in 1980 in cooperation with the American Medical Association (AMA) and American Bar Association (ABA). The AMA and ABA officially approved the UDDA in 1980 and 1981, respectively.[4] It provides alternative definitions of death. One uses the traditional definition—that is, irreversible cessation of pulsation (circulatory and respiratory functions); the other uses whole brain death. By 2008, a version of the UDDA had been enacted in 50 states and the District of Columbia.[5] The uniform act states:

> An individual who has sustained either (1) irreversible cessation of circulatory and respiratory functions, or (2) irreversible cessation of all functions of the entire brain, including the brain stem, is dead. A determination of death must be made in accordance with accepted medical standards.[6]

The UDDA has been endorsed by the National Kidney Foundation, the North American Transplant Coordinators Association, and the American Nephrology Nurses' Association.[7]

Brain death, as shown in the preceding UDDA definition, or some variation, as stated below, is now a commonly used alternative criterion for death:

> The three cardinal findings in brain death are coma or unresponsiveness, absence of brainstem reflexes, and apnea. The clinical examination of the brainstem includes testing of brainstem reflexes, determination of the patient's ability to breathe spontaneously, and evaluation of motor responses to pain.[8]

Definitions vary slightly, but the concept of whole brain death—defined as irreversible cessation of all functions of the brain, including the cortex and the brainstem—has been endorsed by the AMA, the ABA, and the

American Academy of Neurology. Efforts continue to make the clinical determination of brain death more precise and standardized.[9] Use of the whole brain death concept is law in 46 states.[10, 11]

As scientific developments permit increasingly sophisticated assessments of a patient's condition, especially prognosis, brain death criteria may be superseded by those that incorporate psychosocial factors. Prominent among the criteria proposed is the capacity or potential capacity for social interaction. This definition raises ethical issues and jeopardizes persons with no capacity for typical social interaction (e.g., persons with significant cognitive disabilities). A definition that includes a lack of the potential for typical social interaction was applied when infants with mental retardation, such as Baby Boy Doe, were allowed to die. Federal regulations since the 1980s specifically prohibit applying quality of life criteria to infants with disabilities who have life-threatening medical conditions, but there is evidence that quality of life criteria are commonly, if implicitly, used in decision making for other types of patients.

ADVANCE MEDICAL DIRECTIVES

When the federal Patient Self-Determination Act (PSDA) of 1989 took effect December 1, 1991, efforts to achieve patient participation in and control of their healthcare decisions gained a significant impetus. PSDA requires that hospitals, nursing facilities, hospice, home health agencies, and managed care organizations that participate in Medicare and Medicaid give all patients written information about their rights under state law to accept or refuse medical or surgical treatment and to formulate advance medical directives (AMDs). Adult patients must also be given the provider's written policies about implementing these rights. Medical records must document whether a patient has executed an AMD. Providers must also educate their staffs and communities about AMDs. Despite PSDA and the fact that all 50 states have laws authorizing some type of AMD (e.g., living wills, healthcare agents, medical powers of attorney),[12] problems continue in operationalizing patient involvement in decision making about AMDs; relatively few patients execute them. It is estimated that only 20% of Americans have AMDs.[13] As few as 5% of individuals older than age 65 may have AMDs.[14] A Maryland study found that about one-third of respondents had AMDs; those over 65 were more likely than younger adults to have an advance directive.[15]

The Joint Commission on Accreditation of Healthcare Organizations requires accredited hospitals to address the wishes of patients relating to end-of-life decisions. Adults must be given written information about their right to accept or refuse medical or surgical treatment, including forgoing or withdrawing life-sustaining treatment or withholding resuscitative services.[16] The decisions that patients should consider in their AMDs include specific types of life-sustaining treatment that they want used, withheld, or withdrawn. Examples include cardiopulmonary resuscitation (CPR), elective intubation, mechanical ventilation, surgery, dialysis, blood transfusions, artificial hydration and nutrition (AHN), diagnostic tests, antibiotics, and other medications and treatments, as well as future admission to the ICU. Patients tend to choose more restrictions on treatment as diseases progress.[17]

Living Wills

The living will was developed long before passage of the PSDA so that persons unable to participate in decision making could guide caregivers. The words *living* and *will* seem contradictory. Wills are the legal mechanism by which a deceased person's wishes as to disposition of real and personal property are known. Living wills allow persons unable to communicate with caregivers to express their wishes about the extent of treatment they want. Living wills allow persons to specify what is done for and to them and to control the technological imperative, regardless of its potential benefit. Absent state legislation or case law, living wills have no legal status; patients must rely on the willingness of caregivers to follow the directives in them. Generic living wills are useful in states without specific legal requirements.

State Statutes

Interest in living wills and public reaction to cases in which seemingly excessive treatment was provided led to rapid enactment of state laws recognizing the patient's right to control treatment processes. These laws are variously known as living wills laws, advance medical directives, natural death acts, or death with dignity laws. In early 1983, 14 states had such laws; by 1985, there were 35 states and the District of Columbia.[18] In 2009, all states and the District of Columbia had a medical directive law.[19] The Virginia Advance Medical Directive form is shown in Figure 9.

Generally, these statutes recognize a patient's right to direct physicians to withhold or withdraw life-sustaining treatment. When statutory requirements are met, the directives are legally binding on caregivers. The laws tend to be drafted narrowly and apply when a physician has determined that the patient who signed the declaration is terminally ill and has no prospect of recovery. Some statutes require that the directives must be reaffirmed when patients know they are terminally ill. Some include

VIRGINIA ADVANCE MEDICAL DIRECTIVE

I, _____, intentionally and voluntarily make known my wishes in the event that I am incapable of making an informed decision, as follows:

I understand that my advance directive may include the selection of an agent in addition to setting forth my choices regarding health care. The term *"health care"* means: the furnishing of services to any individual for the purpose of preventing, alleviating, curing or healing human illness, injury or physical disability, including but not limited to medications; surgery; blood transfusions; chemotherapy; radiation therapy; admission to a hospital, nursing home, assisted living facility or other health care facility; psychiatric or other mental health treatment; and life-prolonging procedures and palliative care.

The phrase *"incapable of making an informed decision"* means: unable to understand the nature, extent and probable consequences of a proposed health care decision; unable to make a rational evaluation of the risks and benefits of a proposed health care decision as compared with the risks and benefits of alternatives to that decision; or unable to communicate such understanding in any way.

This advance directive shall not terminate in the event of my disability.

(YOU MAY INCLUDE IN THIS ADVANCE DIRECTIVE ANY OR ALL OF SECTIONS I THROUGH V BELOW.)

SECTION I: APPOINTMENT OF AGENT
(CROSS THROUGH SECTION I AND SECTION II BELOW IF YOU DO NOT WANT TO APPOINT AN AGENT TO MAKE HEALTH CARE DECISIONS FOR YOU.)

I hereby appoint the following as my primary agent to make health care decisions on my behalf as authorized in this document:

Name of Primary Agent   Telephone   Fax if any

Address   E-mail if any

If the above-named primary agent is not reasonably available or is unable or unwilling to act as my agent, then I appoint the following as successor agent:

Name of Successor Agent   Telephone   Fax if any

Address   E-mail if any

I hereby grant to my agent named above full power and authority to make health care decisions on my behalf as described below whenever I have been determined to be incapable of making an informed decision. My agent's authority is effective as long as I am incapable of making an informed decision.

In exercising the power to make health care decisions on my behalf, my agent shall follow my desires and preferences as stated in this document or as otherwise known to my agent. My agent shall be guided by my medical diagnosis and prognosis and any information provided by my physicians as to the intrusiveness, pain, risks and side effects associated with treatment or nontreatment. My agent shall not make any decision regarding my health care which he or she knows, or upon reasonable inquiry ought to know, is contrary to my religious beliefs or my basic values, whether expressed orally or in writing. If my agent cannot determine what health care choice I would have made on my own behalf, then my agent shall make a choice for me based upon what he or she believes to be in my best interests.

My agent shall not be liable for the costs of health care that he or she authorizes, based solely on that authorization.

—page 1 of 4—

Figure 9. An example of an advance medical directive. (Retrieved April 4, 2011, from www.vsb.org//sections/hl/VA-2010-Basic.pdf)

penalties against caregivers and the organization if directives are ignored. In addition to statutes, state court decisions affect how the laws are interpreted and their effect on use of life-sustaining treatment.

These laws solve some of the issues of control (autonomy), patient role, and, to an extent, organizational and provider efforts to comply with the patient's wishes. Even when there is an AMD, caregivers may not

Figure 9.   continued

SECTION II: POWERS OF MY AGENT

(CROSS THROUGH ANY POWERS IN THIS SECTION II THAT YOU DO NOT WANT TO GIVE YOUR AGENT AND ADD ANY POWERS OR INSTRUCTIONS THAT YOU DO WANT TO GIVE YOUR AGENT.)

The powers of my agent shall include the following:

A. To consent to or refuse or withdraw consent to any type of health care, treatment, surgical procedure, diagnostic procedure, medication and the use of mechanical or other procedures that affect any bodily function, including, but not limited to, artificial respiration, artificially administered nutrition and hydration, and cardiopulmonary resuscitation. This authorization specifically includes the power to consent to the administration of dosages of pain-relieving medication in excess of recommended dosages in an amount sufficient to relieve pain, even if such medication carries the risk of addiction or of inadvertently hastening my death.

   My agent's authority under this Subsection A shall be limited by any specific instructions I give in Section IV below regarding my health care if I have a terminal condition.

B. To request, receive and review any oral or written information regarding my physical or mental health, including but not limited to medical and hospital records, and to consent to the disclosure of this information.

C. To employ and discharge my health care providers.

D. To authorize my admission to or discharge (including transfer to another facility) from any hospital, hospice, nursing home, assisted living facility or other medical care facility. If I have authorized admission to a health care facility for treatment of mental illness, that authority is stated in Subsections E and/or F below.

E. To authorize my admission to a health care facility for the treatment of mental illness for no more than 10 calendar days provided that I do not protest the admission and provided that a physician on the staff of or designated by the proposed admitting facility examines me and states in writing that I have a mental illness, that I am incapable of making an informed decision about my admission, and that I need treatment in the facility; and to authorize my discharge (including transfer to another facility) from the facility.

F. To authorize my admission to a health care facility for the treatment of mental illness for no more than 10 calendar days, **even if I protest**, if a physician on the staff of or designated by the proposed admitting facility examines me and states in writing that I have a mental illness, that I am incapable of making an informed decision about my admission, and that I need treatment in the facility; and to authorize my discharge (including transfer to another facility) from the facility.

   (If you give your agent the powers described in this Subsection F, your physician must complete the following attestation.)

Physician attestation: I am the physician or licensed clinical psychologist of the declarant of this advance directive. I hereby attest that I believe the declarant to be presently capable of making an informed decision and that the declarant understands the consequences of this provision of this advance directive.
Physician Signature   Date
Physician Name Printed

G. To authorize the following specific types of health care identified in this advance directive **even if I protest**.
   (Specifically cross-reference any applicable sections of this advance directive.)

   (If you give your agent the powers described in this Subsection G, your physician must complete the following attestation.)

Physician attestation: I am the physician or licensed clinical psychologist of the declarant of this advance directive. I hereby attest that I believe the declarant to be presently capable of making an informed decision and that the declarant understands the consequences of this provision of this advance directive.
Physician Signature   Date
Physician Name Printed

H. To continue to serve as my agent even if I protest the agent's authority after I have been determined to be incapable of making an informed decision.

I. To authorize my participation in any health care study approved by an institutional review board or research review committee according to applicable federal or state law if the study offers the prospect of direct therapeutic benefit to me.

—page 2 of 4—

comply. Fragmentation of care among several providers and organizations further complicates patients' use of AMDs and poses a special challenge to managers in the organization to which the patient has been transferred. For example, an AMD in a nursing facility medical record may not accompany the patient to the hospital, especially in an emergency. A study of

Figure 9.   continued

J.   To authorize my participation in any health care study approved by an institutional review board or research review committee pursuant to applicable federal or state law that aims to increase scientific understanding of any condition that I may have or otherwise to promote human well-being, even though the study offers no prospect of direct benefit to me.

K.   To make decisions regarding visitation during any time that I am admitted to any health care facility, consistent with the following directions:

_____

_____

_____

L.   To take any lawful actions that may be necessary to carry out these decisions, including the granting of releases of liability to medical providers.

(Add below any additional powers you give your agent, limits you impose on your agent or other information to guide your agent.)

I further instruct my agent as follows:

_____

_____

_____

SECTION III: HEALTH CARE INSTRUCTIONS

(CROSS THROUGH SUBSECTIONS A AND/OR B BELOW IF YOU DO NOT WANT TO GIVE ADDITIONAL SPECIFIC INSTRUCTIONS ABOUT YOUR HEALTH CARE.)

A.   I specifically direct that I receive the following health care if it is medically appropriate under the circumstances as determined by my attending physician:

_____

_____

B.   I specifically direct that the following health care not be provided to me under the following circumstances:
    (You also may specify that certain health care not be provided under any circumstances.)

_____

_____

SECTION IV: INSTRUCTIONS ABOUT END-OF-LIFE CARE ("LIVING WILL")

(CROSS THROUGH THIS SECTION IV IF YOU DO NOT WANT TO GIVE SPECIFIC INSTRUCTIONS ABOUT YOUR HEALTH CARE IF YOU HAVE A TERMINAL CONDITION.)

If at any time my attending physician should determine that I have a terminal condition where the application of **life-prolonging procedures** – including artificial respiration, cardiopulmonary resuscitation, artificially administered nutrition and artificially administered hydration – would serve only to artificially prolong the dying process, I direct that such procedures be withheld or withdrawn and that I be permitted to die naturally with only the administration of medication or the performance of any medical procedure deemed necessary to provide me with comfort care or to alleviate pain.

In the absence of my ability to give directions regarding the use of such life-prolonging procedures, it is my intention that this advance directive shall be honored by my family and physician as the final expression of my legal right to refuse health care and my acceptance of the consequences of such refusal.

(Cross through Subsections A and/or B below if you do not want to give additional instructions about care at the end of your life.)

A. OTHER DIRECTIONS ABOUT LIFE-PROLONGING PROCEDURES

(If you wish to provide your own directions about life-prolonging procedures, or if you wish to add to the directions you have given above, you may do so in this Subsection A. If you wish to give specific instructions regarding certain life-prolonging procedures, such as artificial respiration, cardiopulmonary resuscitation, artificially administered nutrition and artificially administered hydration, this is where

older patients hospitalized for acute illnesses found that in 75% of cases the medical record did not indicate that physicians had consulted the patient's living will or designated proxy before making treatment decisions, including whether to resuscitate. The problem was attributed to several factors: nursing facilities failed to transfer the information, patients were not asked

Figure 9.   continued

you should write them. If you give specific instructions in this Subsection A, cross through any of the language above in this SECTION IV if your specific instructions that follow are different.)

I direct that:

_____

_____

_____

B. DIRECTIONS ABOUT CARE OTHER THAN LIFE-PROLONGING PROCEDURES

(You may give here any other instructions about your health care if you have a terminal condition aside from your instructions about life-prolonging procedures, which are addressed in Subsection A above.)

I direct that:

_____

_____

_____

SECTION V: APPOINTMENT OF AN AGENT TO MAKE AN ANATOMICAL GIFT OR ORGAN, TISSUE OR EYE DONATION

(CROSS THROUGH THIS SECTION V IF YOU DO NOT WANT TO APPOINT AN AGENT TO MAKE AN ANATOMICAL GIFT OR ANY ORGAN, TISSUE OR EYE DONATION FOR YOU.)

Upon my death, I direct that an anatomical gift of all of my body or certain organ, tissue or eye donations may be made pursuant to Article 2 (§ 32.1-291.1 et seq.) of Chapter 8 of Title 32.1 of the Code of Virginia and in accordance with my directions below, if any. I hereby appoint as my agent to make any such anatomical gift or organ, tissue or eye donation following my death *(choose one)*:

○   the same agent (and alternate) named in SECTION I above; **OR**

○   _____

Name of Agent   Telephone   Fax if any

_____

Address   E-mail if any

I further direct that:

_____

_____

(Declarant's directions, if any, concerning anatomical gift or organ, tissue or eye donation.)

(You must sign below in the presence of two witnesses.)

AFFIRMATION AND RIGHT TO REVOKE: By signing below, I state that I am emotionally and mentally capable of making this advance directive and that I understand the purpose and effect of this document. I understand that I may revoke all or any part of this document at any time (i) with a signed, dated writing; (ii) by physical cancellation or destruction of this advance directive by myself or by directing someone else to destroy it in my presence; or (iii) by my oral expression of intent to revoke.

_____   _____

Signature of Declarant   Date

The declarant signed the foregoing advance directive in my presence.

_____   _____

(Witness)   (Witness)

or did not volunteer the information, and the hospital staff failed to ask or to ensure that such documents were part of the record. Once documented in the hospital medical record, AMDs influenced treatment decisions in 86% of cases involving patients who were judged incompetent.[20]

There are other problems with AMDs, including determining mental status and whether the patient comprehends the effect of what is being done and establishing the presence of a terminal illness. Of course, ethical issues arise for organizations when the patient has not met statutory requirements or there is no statute or AMD.

The challenge for the organization is to provide processes that promote the completion of AMDs. Completion rates for AMDs can be markedly improved by altering the time when information is distributed to patients entering hospitals for planned admissions. Patients were far more likely to complete an AMD at a hospital that distributed information several days before admission rather than only on the day of admission. The most common reason given for not completing an AMD was that it was not seen or was not read, a problem more common in hospitals that did not provide information in advance.[21] Other data suggested that providing reminders, education, and feedback to attending physicians and a new documentation form used by physicians for AMDs can greatly increase the percentage of patients with AMDs. The study also found that 87% of physician-attested directives agreed with the treatment preferences of patients interviewed. Other results showed that physicians' attitudes and interest in AMDs improved.[22] Research suggested, too, that changes in the care of dying patients may not have kept pace with national recommendations, in part because many physicians and nurses disagreed with and may have been unaware of some key guidelines, such as the permissibility of withdrawing treatment.[23]

Surrogate Decision Making

Surrogate decision making occurs when someone other than the patient makes decisions about healthcare. A form of surrogate decision making called *substituted judgment* occurs when someone makes decisions for a patient who is unable to do so, and the surrogate's decisions are based on what the surrogate believes the patient would want were the patient able to make a decision. Surrogates are needed to make decisions when patients are too young or otherwise legally incompetent or have a physical or mental infirmity and no AMD. Historically, surrogates have been appointed by courts upon a petition that a person was incompetent to make healthcare decisions. To avoid the cost and delay of court proceedings, some states enacted laws that established a priority list of relatives who could make decisions for someone with no AMD. In 2009, 43 states and the District of Columbia had statutes specifically authorizing surrogate decision making.[24]

Powers of attorney are another type of surrogate decision making. Powers of attorney are prepared before the fact and are a delegation of decision-making authority by a competent person, who is called the *principal*.

Powers of attorney may be *general* (broad powers to act for the principal) or *limited* (authority to act for the principal for a specific purpose). Powers of attorney are *durable* when the grant of authority extends beyond the principal's incapacitation. Capacity (competence) is an important issue in healthcare decision making. Healthcare agents are persons who have been granted durable powers of attorney to make healthcare decisions for the principal. States may use different names for these limited, durable powers of attorney. By the end of 2001, all 50 states had statutes recognizing appointment of healthcare agents.[25] Figure 9, the Virginia Advance Medical Directive form, includes appointment of a healthcare agent. State advance directive laws vary.

Do-Not-Resuscitate Orders

The do-not-resuscitate (DNR) order is a type of AMD that is used at the point of service delivery. As noted, many patients have neither living wills nor AMDs complying with state requirements. This emphasizes the organization's need to have policies and processes about resuscitating patients who are terminally ill and patients for whom life continuation decisions must be made (e.g., a patient in persistent vegetative state [PVS]*). Health services organizations usually have DNR policies affirming the legal right of a patient (or surrogate, as appropriate) to direct caregivers. The DNR policy should identify the chemical and mechanical technologies included and the specific instances in which they will be applied. Patients who are DNR may require surgery and anesthesia management for palliative care, for relief of pain or distress, or to improve the patient's quality of life. DNR orders present unique ethical problems that should be addressed prospectively by the organization.[26]

In the 1990s, state laws began to recognize nonhospital DNR orders that allow persons to refuse resuscitation when medical emergencies occur. By 2003, more than half the states had such laws;[27] in 2011, the number was 47.[28] These are known as emergency medical services do-not-resuscitate (EMS DNR) orders. EMS DNR orders make the patient's wishes legally binding in the home or a similar setting and supersede state laws that require EMS technicians to undertake CPR.

A study of three Houston teaching hospitals without DNR policies reported inconsistent application of DNR orders.[29] The study found that some patients with DNR orders underwent chemotherapy and surgery

---

Permanent is used instead of *persistent* after a vegetative state has continued longer than one year.

and were admitted to the ICU unit while others received inadequate hydration and nutrition. Staff are often confused about what types of care DNR patients should receive, perhaps because they disagree with such decisions. The study found that in 10% of cases, no decision had been reached about keeping the patient alive. This finding indicates that efforts to decide about resuscitation before a crisis commonly fail. In most no-decision cases, the subject of DNR had not been broached with the patient or family. Other studies of DNR orders report similar findings.[30] A key aspect of DNR is whether patient wishes about CPR are clear to physicians. One study found that in nearly one of three cases, the patient's preference not to be given CPR was at odds with the doctor's perception of what the patient wanted.[31]

Summary

It has been suggested that the widespread use of AMDs, such as natural death act declarations, may encourage systematic rationing of healthcare to older adults. If a right to die becomes a duty to die, the living will and its progeny, the natural death act declaration, will become a Frankenstein monster. Indeed, the suggestion by former Governor Richard Lamm of Colorado, as well as by officials at the U.S. Department of Health, Education, and Welfare (now called the Department of Health and Human Services [DHHS]), that older people should be required to have living wills raised a storm of protest. Regardless of true motives, such suggestions are often seen as motivated by economics.

It has been suggested that treatment may end because physicians assume it is not in a patient's interest or because physicians believe the patient would not want it.[32] Others, however, assert that physicians are caught up in the same ethos of "death as failure" as patients and family; these commentators are focusing on what has been called the riddle—physicians' determination to diagnose and cure the disease. When there is no longer a riddle —when death is inevitable—physicians' interest may decline or be lost entirely, and having lost the major battle, they may try to maintain some authority by controlling the dying process of their patients.[33] If correct, these views neither consider patients as independent decision makers nor as involved participants, and thus physicians may be acting other than in the patients' best interests, as determined by the patient. Both suggest significant ethical problems in meeting the wishes of terminally ill patients.

It would seem that surrogate decision makers will accurately reflect patient's wishes about life-sustaining treatments. That appears not to be true, however. Even those who know patients well are not highly accurate in predicting their life-sustaining treatment preferences. Chronically ill patients are more satisfied with their primary care physicians and the care they deliver when AMDs are discussed.[34] Neither AMDs nor discussion of directives significantly improved the accuracy of substituted judgment, however.[35] Family members were more accurate in making substituted judgments than were physicians, but even they still fell short of complying with patients' wishes. The presence of AMDs assisted hospital-based physicians but not primary care physicians in their actions as surrogate decision makers.[36] Significant work remains if health services organizations are to provide health services consistent with AMDs and patients' wishes regarding end-of-life care. Furthermore, end-of-life care needs improvement both in meeting patients' wishes to die at home (rather than in an institution) and in the quality of palliative care.[37] The role of palliative care is discussed in Chapter 13.

The organization must be alert to the ethical issues of AMDs, which are present regardless of a natural death act statute or a living will. Health services organizations and their managers must consider these issues prospectively and develop policies that respect patients' wishes, consistent with the organizational philosophy.

Improving care of the dying in health services organizations should include the following: reaffirming patients' rights to palliative care, providing adequate pain and symptom management, improving policies and procedures to ensure that AMDs are available as needed, ensuring a well-functioning IEC, improving access by all concerned to the IEC, enhancing community outreach education, ensuring timely referrals to hospice and family support services, and encouraging medical education in dying and ethics.[38]

EUTHANASIA

Euthanasia comes from the Greek *eu* (good) and *thanatos* (death). In the context of the Hippocratic tradition, which prohibits physicians from administering a deadly drug, euthanasia describes care that makes an inevitable death pain-free.

In contemporary parlance, however, euthanasia describes situations in which active steps cause death. Such word use blurs important distinctions. Providing comfort care and pain control without purposefully hastening death allows persons to die with dignity and free of pain. This discussion uses the contemporary definition of euthanasia as active steps to cause death—that is, mercy killing. Actively ending life is illegal in all states.[39]

Morphia Somnolence

Henrietta Morrow was diagnosed with inoperable cancer 18 months ago. Chemotherapy was ineffective. The lymph system had spread the disease throughout her body, and Morrow was in severe pain. Initially, she received care through a home hospice program. As the disease worsened, she became an inpatient at the hospice. She was expected to live less than 3 months.

Morrow received nutrition, hydration, and comfort care. The morphine used for pain control was increased as the disease progressed and her pain worsened. A staff member asked the medical director about the depressant effect that morphine would have on Morrow's respiration. She worried about depressing respiration so much that death would result. Her concern was expressed in both legal and ethical contexts. The medical director assured her that there were no legal problems and described the ethical considerations, including ordinary versus extraordinary care, active and passive euthanasia, voluntary versus involuntary euthanasia, and the rule of double effect.

Ordinary versus Extraordinary Care

Hastening or bringing about death by increasing the morphine beyond that needed to control pain would be euthanasia, an unethical and illegal act. For Morrow, comfort care and pain relief will have the benefit of providing a comfortable and pain-free dying process—defined as ordinary care. Because the hope of benefit for recovery from the cancer is virtually nil, further chemotherapy is defined as extraordinary care. Natural hydration and nutrition are always ordinary care. Artificial hydration and nutrition (AHN) is ordinary care, too, if there is hope of benefit from administering it. AHN becomes extraordinary when a patient's condition is such that there is no hope of benefit. Some assert that AHN is never extraordinary, however. The principle of nonmaleficence provides a distinction:

> Ordinary means are all medicines, treatments, and operations which offer reasonable hope of benefit and which can be obtained and used without excessive expense, pain, or other inconvenience. Extraordinary means are all medicines, treatments, and operations which cannot be obtained or used without excessive expense, pain, or inconvenience, or which, if used, would not offer a reasonable hope of benefit.[40]

Simply put, continuing a course of treatment (including AHN) that offers no hope of benefit only prolongs the dying process and inflicts unnecessary suffering and discomfort on the patient.

Ordinary and *extraordinary* are not defined as usual and unusual, respectively. This definition could be confusing because there is variation even among similar hospitals as to which treatments are usual or unusual. The usual emergency treatment in a shock trauma unit is different from that provided in a community hospital emergency room. Instead, the criterion is hope of benefit as compared with excessiveness of expense, pain, or other inconvenience. Absent hope of benefit, any medicine, treatment, or operation is extraordinary. If there is hope of benefit, use of the same medicines, treatments, and operations is ordinary care if they can be obtained and used without excessive expense, pain, or inconvenience.

Some ethics literature uses benefits to, and burdens on, the patient— the proportionality of treatment. It is suggested that proportionate and disproportionate are more clear and descriptive than ordinary and extraordinary. The criteria used to measure proportionate and disproportionate care are like those used for ordinary and extraordinary but are stated somewhat differently. The type of treatment and its complexity or risk, cost, and appropriateness are studied and compared with results to be expected, taking into account the state of sick persons and their physical and moral resources.[41] Using this calculus, it is ethical to provide the treatment if the potential benefit justifies the burden. Like ordinary and extraordinary, proportionate and disproportionate are primarily qualitative measures of the ethical appropriateness of treatment. Crudely summarized, ordinary/ extraordinary and proportionate/disproportionate mean "Does the benefit justify the burden?"

Types of Euthanasia

Euthanasia has four permutations: voluntary active, voluntary passive, involuntary active, and involuntary passive. *Voluntary* means that the person has freely consented. *Involuntary* means that the person either has not freely consented, or cannot freely consent, but is presumed to want to die. *Active* means that positive steps are taken to bring about death, an action that should be called killing. *Passive* means that nothing is done to hasten death; it is only the natural course of the disease that causes death. All types of euthanasia include providing comfort care and pain control.

Active or Passive Euthanasia   The case of Henrietta Morrow raises questions about the concept of euthanasia: Does increased morphine for pain control constitute euthanasia that is active or passive or voluntary or involuntary? Active euthanasia occurs when someone's death is purposely hastened. Intentionally giving Morrow more morphine than needed to control pain is active euthanasia, an act that is both unethical and illegal. Passive euthanasia occurs when the patient is allowed to die and no extraordinary means are used to sustain life, or when extraordinary means

for sustaining life are withdrawn and the patient dies as the result of the natural course of the disease. Withholding or withdrawing life-sustaining treatment does not preclude providing comfort care and pain control. AHN are extraordinary (disproportionate) care, however, if they offer no reasonable hope of benefit.

Voluntary or Involuntary Euthanasia   Voluntary and involuntary euthanasia refer to patient decisions about treatment. It is unknown whether Morrow is aware that increasing the amount of morphine may shorten her life, and if she agrees to hazard a shortened life. It is reasonable to assume that she prefers to live pain-free despite morphine's side effects. Organizations emphasizing patient autonomy will involve competent patients in decisions regarding all treatment, including pain control, to the fullest extent possible.

Rule of Double Effect   Morrow's situation suggests application of the moral rule of double effect (RDE). Like ordinary and extraordinary care, double effect is a subset of nonmaleficence.

> Classic formulations of the RDE identify four conditions or elements that must be satisfied for an act with double effect to be justified. Each is a necessary condition, and together they form sufficient conditions of morally permissible action.
> 1. *The nature of the act*—The act must be good, or at least morally neutral (independent of its consequences).
> 2. *The agent's intention*—The agent intends only the good effect. The bad effect can be foreseen, tolerated, and permitted, but it must not be intended.
> 3. *The distinction between means and effects*—The bad effect must not be a means to the good effect. If the good effect were the direct causal result of the bad effect, the agent would intend the bad effect in pursuit of the good effect.
> 4. *Proportionality between the good effect and the bad effect*—The good effect must outweigh the bad effect. That is, the bad effect is permissible only if a proportionate reason is present that compensates for permitting the foreseen bad effect.[42]

The rule of double effect allows ethical use of morphine, even in increasing quantities, to ease Morrow's pain.

PATIENT DECISION-MAKING PROCESS

Competent Persons

Persons who are competent have an ethical and a legal right to decide what treatments they will accept. This precept applies equally to withholding and withdrawing treatment. Consent is discussed in Chapter 9. Anecdotal evidence suggests that staff find it easier to withhold than withdraw treatment. Reluctance to discontinue treatment may be driven by fear of legal liability as well as by uncertainty as to the ethically correct choice.

The Henninger Case   The case of 85-year-old G. Ross Henninger was decided by the New York State Supreme Court. Henninger was confused, depressed, and irritable when he was hospitalized for treatment of fever and infection. His medical problems were compounded by a stroke, arthritis, heart disease, and hardening of the arteries. The court stated it would not "go against [Henninger's] wishes and order this 85-year-old person to be operated on, or be force fed, or to be restrained for the rest of his natural life."[43] The decision followed a hearing in which attorneys for Henninger and the nursing facility where he lived petitioned the court to determine the legality of the facility allowing him to starve to death, which was his wish. Henninger died the day following the decision.

The case of Henrietta Morrow suggests the similarity of decisions about dying and death in various types of health services organizations. Nursing facilities, hospice, and home health agencies must prospectively address the ethical issues that end-of-life decisions raise. This focus entails a review from organizational philosophy down to operational policies. The philosophy and policies regarding matters such as life-continuation decisions and AHN must be communicated to patients and potential patients and their families.

Somebody Changed the Rules!

In 1996, Ruth Mittlemann was admitted to the Hebrew Home, a nursing facility. Mittlemann suffered from amyotrophic lateral sclerosis, or Lou Gehrig's disease. Her condition deteriorated gradually. By late 1999, it was clear that she would soon be unable to swallow and thus could not take food and water by mouth. Before entering the facility, Mittlemann had executed a living will expressly stating that she did not want to receive artificial hydration or nutrition; she wished to be kept comfortable and treated for pain when she could no longer swallow. At the time Mittlemann entered the Hebrew Home, her living will posed no problem because the facility had no organizational policy on this issue.

In early 1998, the Hebrew Home's board of trustees began work on a policy regarding artificial nutrition and hydration. It was the most rancorous issue the board ever considered. Several members resigned because of the intense debate, which sometimes degenerated into personal attacks. The result was a policy adopted in late 1998 stating that the sanctity of life had to be respected and that only if death were imminent could patients or their surrogates direct that such basic human care as food and water be stopped.

Mittlemann learned of this new policy only when she was informed that it would be necessary to place a nasogastric tube so that she could be hydrated and fed. She protested vehemently and reaffirmed her living will. She did not want to move to another nursing facility in the area; she liked where she was. She only objected to being forced to receive treatment that she did not want.

On its face, this change is fundamentally unfair to Mittlemann. She is caught in a situation not of her making and beyond her control. The organization also faces a dilemma: acceding to Mittlemann's wishes causes the organization to violate its new values statement about the sanctity of life.

The principle of respect for persons—specifically, fidelity (promise keeping)—governs the Mittlemann case. The organization is obliged to apprize patients of policies that affect them. Because the Hebrew Home had no written policy on AHN when Mittlemann was admitted, the trust she placed in the organization when she chose it is being violated. Moving her elsewhere does not eliminate the home's duty. As distasteful as it may be to the organization and its board, Mittlemann's wishes must be an exception to the policy.

Formerly Competent Patients

In theory, patients retain the right to determine what care they receive and when it will be discontinued. However, treatment decisions, even for competent inpatients, often become psychologically and physically overwhelming. The processes and the persons who apply them dominate; the patient loses control. Patients (or their advocates) may be forced to bring legal action to reassert their autonomy.

Instructions from a Formerly Competent Patient

Constance Emerson had lived a full life. She had been active in the community. She worked as a volunteer at Homer House, a noted settlement house, where she developed educational programs for children of working mothers. Emerson is 92 and lives in a nursing facility. In 1995, she fell and sustained a cerebral hemorrhage. Her mental faculties remain impaired even after extensive therapy.

After her injury, Emerson's husband cared for her until his own health deteriorated and it became impossible for him to continue. Emerson has long had diabetes. She requires a special diet and insulin. She eats only soft foods or liquids and is bedridden, blind, and deaf. Emerson experiences occasional respiratory infections that respond well to treatment. Her heart is strong. Except for mild arthritis, she has no pain. She sometimes recognizes her husband when he visits, but her speech is often unintelligible.

Three years before her injury, Emerson gave a talk on the miseries of prolonging life for older adults who are dying. Having experienced the agony of deterioration in her relatives, she made an eloquent plea for a "dignified and simple way to choose death." She showed the manuscript to her husband and mentioned publishing it, but since then she had not done so. Her husband now fears speaking to her about what she had written or how she feels about her life because she might infer that he wants her to die. The Emersons' son visits her weekly and feels they should not disturb the care she is receiving.[44]

This case illustrates the ethical problems of caring for older people who are infirm and no longer mentally competent. The care provided to Emerson maintains her life; her brain injury is irreversible. The evidence as to Emerson's views about people in a situation like hers is several years old. Her mental state precludes knowing her current wishes. Even if Emerson could direct her care or had an AMD, she could not force the organization to help her end her life.

Applying the criteria of ordinary and extraordinary care to Constance Emerson, who needs a special diet, insulin, and occasional antibiotics, leads to the conclusion that nothing being done is extraordinary. All care offers reasonable hope of benefit without excessive expense, pain, or inconvenience. Reasonable hope of benefit is not based on an expectation that she will regain her former cognitive and physical condition, but that she will have the life of a 92-year-old woman who has sustained a brain injury. She is not terminally ill; discontinuing treatment is unethical.

It is instructive to apply the last definition of death in Table 3 (see above) to Emerson. Is she "alive" if a social interaction criterion is applied? The case notes that she sometimes recognizes her husband when he visits. Whether she has the capacity for social interaction could be determined. If she is not capable of social interaction, this definition of death would allow the organization to withhold antibiotics or insulin, thus rapidly hastening her death. Given the facts in this case, however, the only ethical action is to continue hydration, nutrition, and medication.

Noncompetent Adult Patients

The Quinlan Case   Karen Ann Quinlan was 21 years old in mid-1975 when she became comatose after overdosing on alcohol and tranquilizers. On appeal, the New Jersey Supreme Court permitted Karen's father to be appointed her guardian.[45] The court authorized Quinlan to discontinue all extraordinary measures to sustain life if the family and physicians agreed that there was no reasonable possibility that Karen would emerge from her vegetative state and if there was consultation with the hospital ethics committee. This ruling was among the earliest recognitions of an ethics committee and stimulated New Jersey hospitals to establish more of them. It is clear from the opinion that the court intended to reference a prognosis committee, whose role is very different from that of contemporary ethics committees.

After her father ordered the respirator disconnected, Karen was successfully weaned and able to breathe unaided. She was discharged to a nursing facility, where she remained until her death in mid-1985. When she died, she weighed 66 pounds and her body was locked in a fetal position.

In addition to New Jersey, courts in Massachusetts and New York have been especially active in cases like Quinlan. The cases have been brought by families seeking to regain control from the organization or by managers wanting protection from legal claims. Not all like cases follow Quinlan, however. Some patients continue to receive treatment absent hope of benefit. In others, painful treatment of little benefit was withheld. With court guidance, health services organizations are attempting to solve the problem of when to withdraw life-sustaining treatment. The courts are a necessary final arbiter in settling legal questions that arise, especially when there is dissonance in the ethics of those involved (including the organization). Court decisions aid persons and organizations in developing and refining their ethic. They should be a last resort, however.

The Cruzan Case   A landmark legal case on withdrawing life-sustaining treatment was handed down by the U.S. Supreme Court in 1990. Nancy Cruzan was a young adult who sustained severe injuries in a 1983 automobile accident. She was subsequently diagnosed as being in PVS. A permanent gastrostomy tube provided hydration and nutrition. When it became apparent that Cruzan had virtually no chance of regaining her cognitive faculties, her parents asked the Missouri state hospital caring for her to end AHN. The staff refused to do so without court approval. A state trial court found that someone in Cruzan's condition had a fundamental right under state and federal constitutions to refuse treatment or direct the withdrawal of "death-prolonging procedures."

The Missouri Supreme Court reversed the trial court's decision and ruled that the state constitution included no right to privacy that would support an unrestricted right to refuse treatment. The court found that

Missouri's living will statute embodied a policy strongly favoring preservation of life, and that Cruzan's statements to her housemate that she would not want to continue her life unless she could live "halfway normally" were unreliable in determining her intent.[46] The court concluded that her parents could not withdraw medical treatment because no one can make that choice on behalf of an incompetent person absent the formalities required by the state's living will statute or clear and convincing evidence of the patient's wishes.

In mid-1990, the U.S. Supreme Court affirmed the Missouri decision.[47] It held that the U.S. Constitution does not forbid Missouri to require that an incompetent person's wishes about withdrawing life-sustaining treatment be proved by clear and convincing evidence. The Court distinguished the rights of competent persons, who it assumed have a constitutionally protected right to refuse life-sustaining hydration and nutrition, from those of incompetent persons. It noted that the state had established procedural safeguards to ensure that a surrogate's action conforms as closely as possible to wishes expressed while the person was competent. The Court granted broad latitude to the states to protect and preserve human life, and recognized their right to require a standard of clear and convincing evidence as to a person's intentions regarding life-continuation decisions. It noted that the state is entitled to guard against potential abuses by surrogates who may not act to protect the patient's interests. In addition, states may decline to judge the quality of a person's life and simply assert an unqualified interest in preserving human life, to be weighed against the constitutionally protected interests of the individual. The Cruzan case makes it clear that the U.S. Supreme Court is unwilling to extend to incompetent persons (through surrogates) the same constitutional right of self-determination available to competent persons.

In November 1990, Cruzan's parents were granted a second hearing in state court, which Missouri did not oppose. New evidence convinced the judge that Nancy Cruzan would not have wanted to live in PVS. In late 1990, he ordered the feeding tube removed. Anti-euthanasia groups unsuccessfully sought to intervene, but the state did not appeal the decision. Cruzan died of dehydration 2 weeks later, 8 years after her accident.[48]

The Cruzan decision granted the states broad latitude to legislate in such situations. State law guides health services organizations. In addition, they shoulder a special burden: advising patients about their legal rights regarding AMDs, as directed by federal law. The organization must go beyond informing and assisting patients to actually ensuring that the guidance is part of the medical record and is applied in the process of care.

Health services organizations meet that challenge as part of their commitment to the principles of beneficence, nonmaleficence, and respect for persons.

Cases such as Henninger and Cruzan have not settled the issue of withdrawing life-sustaining treatment for those in PVS. The case of Terri Schiavo in Florida[49] and similar situations are fueling a debate about whether health services organizations and their clinical staff are ethically and legally obliged to provide AHN to patients in PVS. When patients must be sedated or restrained to endure tube feedings or intravenous lines, the burdens are significant and it must be asked whether care in this context is required.[50] Another way to state the issue is whether life-sustaining hydration and nutrition for this type of patient is extraordinary (disproportionate) care, although under usual circumstances nutrition and hydration are ordinary (proportionate) care.

Some may question whether feeding and hydrating patients who are terminally ill or in PVS should ever be considered extraordinary (disproportionate) care. The AMA addressed this issue in the mid-1980s when it stated that it was not unethical for physicians to discontinue "life-prolonging" medical treatment for patients with terminal illness or irreversible coma when the physician determined that the burdens of treatment outweighed its benefits. Treatment was defined to include medication and artificially or technologically supplied respiration, nutrition, or hydration.[51] There were protests from those who feared that the new policy might cause physicians to discontinue nutrition and hydration when they considered it in the patient's best interests, even though patients believed their interests were furthered by continuing these treatments but could not communicate this decision. The AMA maintains this position but with greater emphasis on patient autonomy and surrogate decision making, where necessary, rather than on a physician determination of benefits and burdens.[52]

The goals of AHN are often unclear. When initiated, the hope is that AHN will sustain the patient until improvement or recovery occurs. Subsequently, however, the situation is often allowed to drift so that AHN continues without an identified end point. Here, the greater reluctance of clinicians (and family) to withdraw treatment than withhold it has been identified. Furthermore, AHN for dying patients may prolong life but simultaneously worsen suffering. Of the many potential complications of AHN, the largest risk is fluid overload. It is recommended that a defined therapeutic goal for AHN is firmly stated and agreed on before intervention; family members should be part of the decision process and the evaluation of the results of AHN.[53]

A common question regarding patients denied hydration and nutrition has been whether it is inhumane because of the pain they are believed to experience. The issue may not be entirely settled, but the weight of evidence is that prolonged dehydration and starvation produce no pain and that ice chips or swabs will relieve the limited discomfort from a dry mouth. Problems with excessive secretions, edema, or incontinence can be alleviated.[54] As Sullivan[55] stated,

> In the setting of dehydration and starvation, death can occur from a multitude of causes. Arrhythmia, infection, and circulatory system collapse due to volume depletion are common terminal events. The clinical course of each should be rapid and, ideally, not associated with perceived discomfort by the patient.

Sullivan's conclusion is supported by nurses' assessments that patients who refused food and water had "good deaths," generally within 2 weeks, with little pain or suffering, thus refuting the popular assumption that such a death is painful and gruesome.[56] Some organizations insist on continuing hydration even though nutrition is stopped, an action that seems pointless and only prolongs the dying process.

Objections to this ethic are heard less often now than in the mid-1990s. Most people are likely to find themselves greatly discomforted if food and water are not provided. Regardless of debate at the theoretical level, an ethic must be applied at the bedside. What is the ethically correct action for a particular patient? This may begin the debate anew.

Infants

The Baby Doe cases added an important dimension to what began with the Quinlan case in the mid-1970s. The name Baby Doe derives from court proceedings in several states in the early 1980s. All cases involved parents who decided to forgo life-sustaining treatment of their newborn infants with treatable genetic anomalies. Publicity surrounding the subsequent deaths of two such infants prompted the DHHS to issue regulations in April 1982 prohibiting hospitals that receive federal funds from withholding life-sustaining treatment from infants with disabilities. Authority for this action was claimed under Section 504 of the Rehabilitation Act of 1973 (PL 93-112), which prohibits discrimination on the basis of disability. The regulations were challenged by health services organizations on procedural grounds, and a court injunction suspending implementation was issued. Another attempt to promulgate a modified version of the regulations followed in 1983. Like the first regulations, they mandated telephone hotlines to report alleged cases of withholding life-sustaining treatment from newborns with serious illnesses. Signs with information about the need to treat such newborns had to be posted. For providers, the hotlines were the most hated and controversial requirement. Opponents claimed the regulations turned providers into spies. An important modification in the 1983 revision was that impossible or futile acts or therapies that merely prolong the dying of an infant born terminally ill are not required. Opponents of the regulations successfully obtained judicial relief preventing implementation.

In June 1985, the U.S. Supreme Court agreed to hear a U.S. Justice Department appeal of a lower court decision that invalidated the Baby Doe regulations. This was surprising because the actions of Congress and the DHHS had eliminated the need for the first regulations. In June 1986, the high court agreed with the lower court in an opinion that struck down the Baby Doe rules. It agreed that Section 504 of the Rehabilitation Act of 1973 did not empower the DHHS to force hospitals to treat infants with severe disabilities over parental objections. The Court's decision displeased some disability advocacy groups, who claimed that there are major enforcement problems with the Child Abuse Prevention and Treatment Act Amendments of 1984 (PL 98-457), both procedurally and because of a basic antidisability bias held by some physicians and child protective services agencies. They contended that these biases will result in do-not-treat decisions in large numbers of cases.

Child Abuse Amendments

The original controversy surrounding the Baby Doe cases prompted Congress to address the question of newborns with serious disabilities in the Child Abuse Amendments of 1984. Subsequent regulations established treatment and reporting guidelines for care of newborns with significant disabilities. Withholding medically indicated treatment from infants with disabilities is illegal except when

> In the treating physician's (or physicians') reasonable medical judgment any of the following circumstances apply:
> (i) the infant is chronically and irreversibly comatose; or
> (ii) the provision of such treatment would merely prolong dying, not be effective in ameliorating or correcting all of the infant's life-threatening conditions, or otherwise be futile in terms of the survival of the infant; or
> (iii) the provision of such treatment would be virtually futile in terms of the survival of the infant and the treatment itself under such circumstances would be inhumane.[57]

The definition of *medically indicated treatment* includes appropriate care, such as nutrition, hydration, and medication.[58] The regulations do not allow decisions based on subjective opinions about the future quality of life of a person with mental retardation or another disability.[59]

Under the law, affected health services organizations must designate persons who will report suspected problems to state child protective services agencies. The agencies coordinate and consult with those persons and, after notification of suspected medical neglect, may initiate legal action.

CONCLUSION

Ethical issues arising from end-of-life decisions are among the most common that health services organizations and their clinical and managerial staffs encounter. Technology is central to the ethical and legal problems surrounding dying. New technology may solve some problems, but if history is prologue, technology will likely create as many ethical dilemmas as it solves. For treatments such as tube feedings, which extend life using low technology, the issue is more basic. Food and water are fundamental to human existence. It is likely, however, that both will be seen as extraordinary treatment when their continued provision offers no reasonable hope of benefit.

NOTES

1. American Medical Association. (1994, June). *E-2.20: Withholding or withdrawing life-sustaining medical treatment.* Retrieved March 15, 2004, from http://www.ama-assn.org/ama/pub/category/8457.html.
2. A definition of irreversible coma: Report of the Harvard Medical School Ad Hoc Committee to Examine the Definition of Brain Death. (1968, August). *Journal of the American Medical Association 205*(6), pp. 337–338.
3. Robert M. Veatch. (1972, November). Brain death: Welcome definition or dangerous judgment? *Hastings Center Report 2*(6), p. 10.
4. National Conference of Commissioners on Uniform State Laws. (1980). *Uniform Determination of Death Act.* Retrieved December 2, 2003, from http://www.law.upenn.edu/bll/ulc/fnact99/1980s/udda80.htm.
5. Eun-Kyoung Choi, Valita Fredland, Carla Zachodni, J. Eugene Lammers, Patricia Bledsoe, & Paul R. Helft. (2008, Winter). Brain death revisited: The case for a national standard. *Journal of Law, Medicine, and Ethics 36*(4), p. 825.
6. National Conference of Commissioners on Uniform State Laws.
7. *Ibid.*
8. Eelco F.M. Wijdicks. (1995, May). Determining brain death in adults. *Neurology 45*, p. 1005.
9. Eelco F.M. Wijdicks, Panayiotis N. Varelas, Gary S. Gronseth, & David M. Greer. (2010, June 8). Evidence-based guideline update: Determining brain death in adults. Report of the Quality Standards Subcommittee of the American Academy of Neurology. *Neurology 74*, pp. 1911–1917.

10. Ascension Health. (2003, October 17). *Brain death*. Retrieved March 2, 2011, from http://www.ascensionhealth.org/index.php?option=com_content&view =article&id=117&Itemid=172.

11. The American Academy of Neurology (AAN) adopted the Uniform Law Commissioners' definition of whole brain death in 1978. "For legal and medical purposes an individual with irreversible cessation of all function of the brain, including the brain stem, is dead. Determination of death under this act shall be made in accordance with reasonable medical standards." American Academy of Neurology, personal communication, May 17, 1996.

12. Partnership for Caring. (2001, February). *Facts about surrogate decision making law*. Retrieved October 28, 2003, from http://www.partnershipforcaring.org/ Resources/pdf/surrogate.pdf.

13. *Ibid.*

14. Center for Bioethics at the University of Minnesota–Twin Cities. (2003, October 21). *Advance directives*. Retrieved March 15, 2004, from http://www.bioeth ics.umn.edu/resources/topics/advance_directives.shtml.

15. Keshia M. Pollack, Dan Morhaim, & Michael A. Williams. (2010, June). The public's perspectives on advance directives: Implications for state legislative and regulatory policy. *Health Policy 96*(1), pp. 57–63.

16. Joint Commission on Accreditation of Healthcare Organizations. (2004). Ethics, rights, and responsibilities. In *Hospital accreditation standards* (p. 109). Oakbrook Terrace, IL: Author.

17. Richard J. Ackermann. (2000, October 1). Withholding and withdrawing life-sustaining treatment. *American Family Physician 62*, p. 1556.

18. Choice in Dying. (1996, March). *State statutes governing living wills and appointment of health care agents*. New York: Author; Partnership for Caring. (2001, December 31). *Summary of state statutes: State statutes governing living wills and appointment of health care agents*. Retrieved March 15, 2004, from http://www .partnershipforcaring.org/Resources/developments_set.html.

19. Dahm, Lisa. (2008, August). Medical futility and the Texas medical futility statute: A model to follow or one to avoid? *Health Lawyer 20*(6). Retrieved March 1, 2011, from http://www.americanbar.org/groups/health_law/resources/re sources_for_law_students/V20_6_Marc_Meyer.html.

20. R. Sean Morrison, Ellen Olson, Kristan R. Mertz, & Diane E. Meier. (1995, August 9). The inaccessibility of advance directives on transfer from ambulatory to acute care settings. *Journal of the American Medical Association 274*(6), pp. 478–482.

21. Anna Maria Cugliari, Tracy Miller, & Jeffery Sobal. (1995, September 25). Factors promoting completion of advance directives in the hospital. *Archives of Internal Medicine 155*, pp. 1893–1898.

22. Brendan M. Reilly, Michael Wagner, C. Richard Magnussen, James Ross, Louis Papa, & Jeffrey Ash. (1995, November 27). Promoting inpatient directives about life-sustaining treatments in a community hospital. *Archives of Internal Medicine 155*, pp. 2317–2323.

23. Mildred Z. Solomon, Lydia O'Donnell, Bruce Jennings, Vivian Guilfoy, Susan M. Wolf, Kathleen Nolan, Rebecca Jackson, Dieter Koch-Weser, & Strachan Donnelley. (1993, January). Decisions near the end of life: Professional views on life-sustaining treatments. *American Journal of Public Health 83*(1), pp. 14–21.

24. American Bar Association Commission on Aging. (2009, November). *Default surrogate consent statutes*. Retrieved November 28, 2010, from http://new.aba net.org/aging/PublicDocuments/famcon_2009.pdf.
25. Partnership for Caring, 2001 (December).
26. Bonnie S. Jacobson. (1994, September). Ethical dilemmas of do-not-resuscitate orders in surgery. *AORN Journal 60*(3), pp. 449–452; Proposed AORN position statement on perioperative care of patients with do-not-resuscitate (DNR) orders. (1994, October). *AORN Journal 60*(4), pp. 648, 650; Statement of the American College of Surgeons on advance directives by patients: "Do not resuscitate" in the operating room. (1994, September). *ACS Bulletin*, p. 29; Judith O. Margolis, Brian J. McGrath, Peter S. Kussin, & Debra A. Schwinn. (1995). Do not resuscitate (DNR) orders during surgery: Ethical foundations for institutional policies in the United States. *Anesthesia and Analgesia 80*, pp. 806–809.
27. Partnership for Caring. (2003, November 25). *States are creating a new form called a "nonhospital DNR order": Here's why*. Washington, DC: Author.
28. Charles P. Sabatino. (2011). *Deciding for others: A shifting legal landscape*. Retrieved January 5, 2011, from http://www.abanet.org/aging/cle/docs/Boston _Unbefriended-CS.pdf.
29. Andrew L. Evans & Baruch A. Brody. (1985, April). The do-not-resuscitate order in teaching hospitals. *Journal of the American Medical Association 253*(15), pp. 2236–2239.
30. Susanna E. Bedell & Thomas L. Delbanco. (1984, April). Choices about cardiopulmonary resuscitation in the hospital: When do physicians talk with patients? *New England Journal of Medicine 320*(17), pp. 1089–1093.
31. Joan M. Teno, Rosemarie B. Hakim, William A. Knaus, Neil S. Wenger, Russell S. Phillips, Albert W. Wu, Peter Layde, Alfred E. Connors, Neal V. Dawson, & Joanne Lynn, for the SUPPORT Investigators. (1995, April). Preferences for cardiopulmonary resuscitation: Physician–patient agreement and hospital resource use. *Journal of General Internal Medicine 10*, pp. 179–186.
32. Susan Morse. (1985, July 15). Final requests: Preparing for death. (Quoting ethicist Robert Veatch.) *Washington Post*, p. B5.
33. Sherwin B. Nuland. (1995). *How we die: Reflections on life's final chapter* (pp. 248, 258–259). New York: Vintage Books.
34. William M. Tierney, Paul R. Dexter, Gregory P. Gramelspacher, Anthony J. Perkins, Xiao-Hua Zhou, & Frederic D. Wolinsky. (2001, January). The effect of discussions about advance directives on patients' satisfaction with primary care. *Journal of General Internal Medicine 16*(1), pp. 32–40.
35. Peter H. Ditto, Joseph H. Danks, William D. Smucker, Jamila Bookwala, Kristen M. Coppola, Rebecca Dresser, Angela Fagerlin, R. Mitchell Gready, Renate M. Houts, Lisa K. Lockhart, & Stephen Zyzanski. (2001, February 12). Advance directives as acts of communication: A randomized controlled trial. *Archives of Internal Medicine 161*(3), pp. 421–430.
36. Kristin M. Coppola, Peter H. Ditto, Joseph H. Danks, & William D. Smucker. (2001, February 12). Accuracy of primary care and hospital-based physicians' predictions of elderly outpatients' treatment preferences with and without advance directives. *Archives of Internal Medicine 161*, pp. 431–440.

37. Andis Robeznieks. (2002, December 9). End-of-life care receives failing grades. *American Medical News.* Retrieved November 14, 2003, from http://www.ama-assn.org/amednews/2002/12/09/prsd1209.htm.

38. Lois LaCivita Nixon & Lori Roscoe. (1999, June). How can you improve end-of-life decision making? *Trustee 52*(6), p. 12.

39. Carrie Gordon Earll. (2001, February 27). Status of physician-assisted suicide law. *CitizenLink: Focus on Social Issues.* Retrieved November 4, 2003, from http://www.family.org/cforum/fosi/bioethics/euthanasia/a0028006.cfm.

40. Gerald Kelly. (1951, December). The duty to preserve life. *Theological Studies 12*, p. 550.

41. Vatican Congregation for the Doctrine of the Faith. (1980, June 26). *Declaration on euthanasia.* Vatican City: Author.

42. Tom L. Beauchamp & James F. Childress. (2001). *Principles of biomedical ethics* (5th ed., p. 129). New York: Oxford University Press.

43. Patient's right to starve upheld. (1984, February 3). *Washington Post,* p. A20.

44. Robert M. Veatch. (1977). *Case studies in medical ethics* (pp. 340–341). Cambridge, MA: Harvard University Press.

45. In re Quinlan, 70 NJ. 10, 355 A.2d 647 (1976).

46. Susan M. Wolf. (1990, January/February). Nancy Beth Cruzan: In no voice at all. *Hastings Center Report 20*(1), p. 39.

47. Cruzan v. Director, Missouri Department of Health et al. 110 S. Ct. 2841 (1990).

48. Malcolm Gladwell. (1990, December 27). Woman in right to die case succumbs. *Washington Post,* p. A3.

49. Terri Schiavo's case was more complex, emotional, and public than Nancy Cruzan's. Schiavo's diagnosis as being in PVS was disputed. Her husband, Michael, and her parents, Robert and Mary Schindler, were locked in a legal dispute regarding control of decision making for Schiavo. Michael sought to withdraw life-sustaining AHN; the Schindlers opposed him. Numerous advocacy groups supported each side in their efforts. Dozens of hearings, trials, and appeals were held in state and federal courts over a 10-year period. The case became politicized, eventually involving the Florida legislature and governor and the U.S. Congress and president. Michael prevailed in the contest for control of Terri's future; she died approximately 2 weeks after life-sustaining AHN was withdrawn. The autopsy found that the direct cause of Schiavo's death was dehydration; other autopsy findings were consistent with persistent vegetative state (PVS). A thorough review and chronology of the Schiavo case can be found in Chad D. Kollas & Beth Boyer-Kollas. (2006). Closing the Schiavo case: An analysis of legal reasoning. *Journal of Palliative Medicine 9*(5), pp. 1145–1163.

50. Joanne Lynn & James E. Childress. (1983, October). Must patients always be given food and water? *Hastings Center Report 13*(5), pp. 17–21; John J. Paris & Anne B. Fletcher. (1983, October). Infant Doe regulations and the absolute requirements to use nourishment and fluids for the dying infant. *Law, Medicine & Health Care 11*, pp. 210–213.

51. American Hospital Association. (1986, March 15). *Withholding and withdrawing life-prolonging medical treatment.* Chicago: Author.

52. American Medical Association, Council on Ethical and Judicial Affairs. (1994). *Code of medical ethics: Current opinions with annotation* (pp. 36–38). Chicago: Author.
53. Michael E. Frederich. (2002, Fall). Artificial hydration and nutrition in the terminally ill. *AAHPM Bulletin 4*(1), pp. 8–9, 13.
54. Robert J. Sullivan, Jr. (1993, April). Accepting death without artificial nutrition or hydration. *Journal of General Internal Medicine 8*, p. 222.
55. *Ibid.*
56. Donald G. McNeil, Jr. (2003, July 1). First study on patients who fast to end lives: Survey says starving isn't painful or grisly. *New York Times*, p. A19.
57. Child Abuse and Neglect Prevention and Treatment, 45 C.F.R. §1340.15(b)(2). (1999).
58. *Ibid.*
59. Child Abuse and Neglect Prevention and Treatment, 45 C.F.R. §1340.20 (Appendix to Part 1340—Interpretation of Guidelines Regarding 45 C.F.R. 1340.15.) (1999).

CHAPTER 11

PATIENT AUTONOMY AND THE PARADIGM OF PHYSICIAN-ASSISTED SUICIDE

Physician-assisted suicide (PAS) became a prominent ethical and legal issue in the United States in 1990, thrust into the public's consciousness by the machinations of Jack Kevorkian, MD, a Michigan pathologist. Though seldom discussed, it is widely understood that the preeminent role of the physician is to "comfort always," a role especially important when hope of benefit from further treatment has faded. This ethic has never included assisting in suicide. Sometimes, eliminating pain necessitated large amounts of morphine, but an unintended death in pursuit of comfort care raised few ethical (or legal) concerns. Doubtless, physicians and other caregivers (e.g., nurses) have sometimes heeded the pleas of pain-wracked patients to help them die, or solely from humanitarian instincts they have occasionally performed involuntary active euthanasia on a medically hopeless patient who could no longer communicate. The Hippocratic tradition prohibits physicians from giving a deadly drug and considers it unethical for physicians to deliberately cause death, whether requested by the patient or for the noble purpose of pain relief. Patient wishes are given no weight. The Hippocratic ethic is reflected in the illegality of homicide and the laws in almost all states that prohibit assisting in suicide.

PAS is one of three types of aid in dying or physician-assisted death. The three are sometimes incorrectly treated as synonymous. Strictly defined, PAS fits none of the types of euthanasia described in Chapter 10. It has characteristics of voluntary (patient desired), active (specific steps) euthanasia, but it differs in a critical aspect. PAS occurs when a physician provides the means and medical advice that enable someone to commit suicide. In some manifestations, the physician's assistance is such as to provide assurance that the suicide will be successful. In all manifestations of PAS, however, patients perform the act that directly causes their deaths.

Broadly defined, it is a good death because it is intended to be pain-free. It is not, however, euthanasia, as defined previously. Physical disability prevents some from engaging in an act that would cause death. They are candidates for voluntary active euthanasia should it become legal. The mental competence of those wishing to be assisted in suicide or to be euthanized is always an issue.

LEGAL ASPECTS OF PAS IN THE UNITED STATES

Legalizing PAS was considered in ballot initiatives in Washington State (1991) and California (1992). Both initiatives were rejected. In 1994, Oregon voters narrowly (52% to 48%) approved an initiative to enact the Death with Dignity Act, which legalized PAS. Court challenges delayed implementation. The legislature asked voters to repeal the law, but this request was soundly defeated (60% to 40%). PAS became available for terminally ill Oregonians in late 1997.

In 2011, PAS was legal in Oregon, Washington State, and Montana. In 2009, the Montana Supreme Court held that PAS did not violate state law or contravene supreme court precedent, and therefore was not unlawful.[1] PAS legislation has been considered in more than a dozen other states.[2] PAS is illegal by specific statute or common law precedent in almost all states. In 2011, statutes in 36 states prohibited assisted suicide; in 7 states, the common law achieved the same purpose. Four states and the District of Columbia had neither statutory nor common law prohibitions against assisted suicide.[3] This legal context is resoundingly inconsistent with the polls that show that a large majority of Americans favor physician help in ending lives of the terminally ill (see the section below titled "Issues for Health Services Managers").

In March 1996, the California-based federal 9th Circuit Court of Appeals ruled in *Washington v. Glucksberg* that the Washington State law making physician-assisted suicide a felony was a denial of due process of law under the 14th Amendment to the U.S. Constitution. Its reasoning relied heavily on the Supreme Court's abortion cases, which the circuit court found to have compelling similarities.[4] A month later, the New York–based federal 2nd Circuit Court of Appeals ruled in *Vacco v. Quill* that terminally ill people have the same right to hasten death by taking drugs as they do by refusing artificial life support, thus striking down a New York law. Its ruling was based on the equal protection clause of the 14th Amendment.[5]

In 1997, the U.S. Supreme Court agreed to hear appeals of these two cases. A unanimous U.S. Supreme Court ruled in *Washington v. Glucksberg*[6] and *Vacco v. Quill*[7] that states may ban assisted suicide without violating either the due process or equal protection clauses of the 14th Amendment to the U.S. Constitution, respectively. The Court did not decide whether states could pass laws permitting assisted suicide. In a companion case, the Court declined to review a lower court ruling in *Lee v. Harcleroad*,[8] holding that a group of terminally ill persons and their physicians had no standing to challenge the constitutionality of Oregon's PAS law because it posed no personal danger to them.[9] Thus, the issue of physician assistance in suicide remains firmly within the purview of the states.

The Case of "Dr. Death"

In 1990, 54-year-old Janet Adkins, who suffered from early-stage Alzheimer's disease, feared losing her memory and the ability to engage in normal activities. She sought the help of Dr. Jack Kevorkian, a retired pathologist, to assist her in committing suicide before her mental abilities became so impaired that she could no longer make a rational decision.[10] Kevorkian had gained national prominence earlier that year at a press conference in which he showed a device he had designed that enabled persons who wanted to die to self-administer toxic chemicals, after initial assistance from a physician. Kevorkian's help to Adkins was criticized as procedurally flawed, and Adkins's competence was questioned because of her diagnosis.[11] The case starkly focused the public's attention on the issue of active, voluntary euthanasia and the right to assisted suicide.

In early assisted suicides, Kevorkian played an active role by starting a saline IV. The patient then initiated the flow of potassium chloride and barbiturates that caused death. Kevorkian's role changed as he continued to assist in suicides. After his medical license was revoked, Kevorkian, or "Dr. Death" as his critics called him, could no longer legally obtain the chemicals used previously. He began using carbon monoxide, which was breathed through a mask placed on the face of the patient, who then initiated the flow of gas. Kevorkian began videotaping conversations with "patients" held before assisting their suicide, in which they answered questions that documented their state of mind as well as their desire to die. By the end of 1996, Kevorkian had assisted in more than 40 suicides. All of his assisted suicides occurred in Michigan, which initially had no law banning it. Hastily passed legislation outlawing assisted suicide did not stop him and he continued the practice.

The numerous criminal proceedings against Kevorkian for assisting in suicide were unsuccessful for various reasons: the Michigan Court of Appeals ruled that the ban on assisted suicides was passed illegally; judges dismissed charges against Kevorkian, ruling that assisted suicide is a constitutional right; and juries acquitted him.[12] Kevorkian was finally convicted of second-degree murder in 1998, a conviction substantially based on a videotape that he made. It showed him administering a lethal injection to a person with amyotrophic lateral sclerosis (ALS, or Lou Gehrig's disease). Kevorkian called it a mercy killing (euthanasia); prosecutors and a jury disagreed. He was sentenced to a term of 10–25 years in prison. Kevorkian was paroled in 2007, after serving 8 years. He promised to continue working to legalize assisted suicide.[13] By his own count, Kevorkian assisted in at least 130 suicides.[14] Of 69 persons known to have died with Kevorkian's assistance or intervention, only 25% had been diagnosed as terminally ill.[15] The majority were suffering from early stages of degenerative disease, a fact that raises significant ethical issues.

Kevorkian has been criticized on professional and ethical grounds, including assertions that he did not know his "patients," was unqualified to diagnose or understand illnesses because he is a pathologist, had a conflict of interest because of his desire to publicize himself and his suicide machine, assisted persons who did not have terminal illness, and was not qualified to judge the mental competence of the persons he assisted. Kevorkian had hoped to establish an obitorium, a clinic where terminally ill persons wanting to commit suicide could be assisted to do so.

One of Kevorkian's stated goals was to test the limits of patient autonomy. His primary defense was that the law criminalizing assisted suicide is an unconstitutional interference in the right to privacy. This defense used reasoning like that in *Roe v. Wade*, the U.S. Supreme Court decision that found a constitutional right to privacy protected a woman's decision to abort her pregnancy in the first trimester, free from state interference. Assisted suicide presents an even stronger case for individual autonomy as expressed in the right to privacy because no other life (i.e., a fetus) is involved. Experts disagree on the constitutionality of assisted suicide, however.[16,17] In mid-1995, the U.S. Supreme Court declined to review Kevorkian's appeals from his criminal conviction.[18]

The Oregon Experience

Several states have introduced bills to legalize PAS. At this writing, however, only Oregon and Washington have enacted PAS. Their statutes have many similarities. The Oregon statute has a longer history and is the focus of this discussion.

Oregon law permits physicians to prescribe but not administer medications to end life. To request a prescription for lethal medications, a person must be 18 years of age or older, a resident of Oregon, capable (able to make and communicate healthcare decisions), and diagnosed with a terminal disease that will lead to death within 6 months. Having met that threshold, a series of steps must be followed to receive the prescription:

- Patients must make two oral requests to their physician, separated by at least 15 days.
- Patients must provide a written request to their physician, signed in the presence of two witnesses.
- A prescribing physician and a consulting physician must confirm the diagnosis and prognosis.
- If either physician believes the person's judgment is impaired by a psychiatric or psychological disorder, the patient must be referred for a psychological examination.
- The prescribing physician must inform the patient of feasible alternatives to assisted suicide, including comfort care, hospice care, and pain control.
- The prescribing physician must request, but may not require, the patient to notify their next of kin of the prescription request.[19]

The law was amended in 1999 to require that pharmacists must be informed of the ultimate use of a prescription involved in PAS.[20] The physician may attend the patient when medication is taken, but is not required to do so.[21] Physicians must report their participation to the state health division; those who act in good faith within the law are protected from both professional discipline and legal liability.[22]

Results   The first suicide under the Oregon law was reported in March 1998.[23] The Blue Cross and Blue Shield plans of Oregon began covering PAS in early 1998.[24] In late 1998, the Oregon Health Plan (which covers Medicaid patients) added PAS to end-of-life comfort care services, alongside such measures as pain medication and hospice care.[25] By the end of 2010, a total of 525 Oregonians had been assisted in suicide since the law passed.[26]

Patient Characteristics   Oregonians who choose PAS continue to be concerned about loss of autonomy, loss of dignity, and a decreasing ability to engage in activities that make life enjoyable. In 2010, most participants were over 65 years of age (70.8%), white (100%), well educated (42.2% had at least a baccalaureate degree), and had cancer (78.5%). Overwhelmingly, they had some form of insurance (96.7%); 92.6% were enrolled in hospice. Approximately one-third (36.7%) had no insurance other than Medicare or Medicaid.[27] These data should allay fears that the law will be used primarily by Oregonians who are poor, uneducated, mentally ill, or socially isolated. As in the Netherlands, however, older adults may begin to believe that they are at special risk because of an express or implied utilitarian calculus that they have less social and economic value than younger persons do. Chapter 14 addresses this aspect of PAS in the context of equity and allocation decisions.

Physician Characteristics   In 2010, 55 physicians wrote 96 prescriptions for lethal doses of medication; the number of prescriptions written by individual providers ranged from 1 to 11. One physician was referred to the Oregon Medical Board for failing to wait the required 48 hours between the time of the patient's written request and provision of the prescription.[28]

Summary   In previous annual reports, Oregon's Department of Human Services noted that availability of PAS may have led to improved end-of-life care using other modalities. For example, most major hospitals have established effective pain management programs to give patients an alternative to assisted suicide.[29] Also, a request for PAS offers an opportunity for physicians to explore patients' fears and wishes about end-of-life care and the options available. Reportedly, physicians have sought to learn more about pain medications for the terminally ill, improve their recognition of psychiatric disorders, and refer patients more frequently to hospice care.[30] Few complications of the suicide process are being reported in Oregon—a result inconsistent with data from the Netherlands discussed below. No complications were reported in 2009. The time from ingestion to death ranged from 2 minutes to 4 1/2 days.[31] One wonders if lingering for days after ingesting a "fatal" dose of medication can be anything other than a complication.

One possible conclusion of the Oregon data is that physicians are using the law prudently and cautiously. Another explanation is that there are too few data for a true picture to emerge. The findings may also suggest a high level of tentativeness on the parts of both physicians and those who might seek assistance in suicide—tentativeness likely to diminish over time and as PAS becomes more common and socially acceptable. Given the evolution of PAS in the Netherlands, this latter explanation warrants attention.

PHYSICIAN-ASSISTED SUICIDE AND
EUTHANASIA IN THE NETHERLANDS

International comparisons are instructive. Assisted suicide has been available in parts of Switzerland since 1942; increasingly, that country is a destination for "suicide tourists."[32] In 2002, Belgium legalized voluntary euthanasia and assisted suicide with a law similar to that of the Netherlands (the Dutch law is discussed below).[33] In mid-2003, a year after passage of the original law, Belgian lawmakers proposed expanding euthanasia to children younger than 18 years of age.[34] PAS and euthanasia are being debated elsewhere in Europe, notably in Spain and France. A 2002 survey in France showed that 88% favor or would tolerate euthanasia.[35] Assisted suicide is illegal in Britain; however, prosecutors there have indicated that they will be less likely to charge someone who was wholly motivated by compassion and reported a suicide to the police than someone who was paid to assist in a suicide or was acting as a medical or healthcare professional. The distinction is stated as "compassionate support versus malicious encouragement."[36] Such prosecutorial discretion adds ambiguity and may cause inconsistent applications of the law. Regardless, it signals a move toward greater tolerance of assisting in suicide.

The vanguard of assisted dying, however, is the Netherlands, where euthanasia and PAS have been practiced since the 1980s—despite their illegality at the time—and where 92% of the population supports the practice.[37] Before they were made legal in 1993, a 1990 government study found that 2% of deaths were the result of euthanasia and PAS.[38] It was found that in 1,000 other cases, a patient's life was ended without an explicit recent request to die.[39] The data also showed that in 1990, death was hastened for 16,850 patients, of whom 8,750 died by withholding or withdrawing treatment and 8,100 died by administering pain-killing drugs. Consent was obtained from only 3,100 of the 8,100 patients in the second group. Thus, the majority of patients from whom treatment had been withdrawn or withheld or who had died from administration of painkilling drugs (5,000) had not consented.[40] Data from a 1995 Dutch government study showed 3,600 deaths from assisted suicide and euthanasia, of which 900–1,000 were officially acknowledged to have been involuntary. Another 2,000 patients were given large doses of painkilling drugs with the primary aim of ending their lives, but these cases were not classified as euthanasia.[41] These data show that even after voluntary euthanasia and PAS became legal, involuntary euthanasia continued—a practice that may have stimulated passage of another revision of the law in 2001.

The revision of the 1993 law that first legalized voluntary active euthanasia and PAS went into effect in 2002.[42] It expanded the categories of persons who may use euthanasia and PAS. Physicians who provide these "services" are required to use due care in terminating a life (euthanasia) or assisting in suicide. By performing the procedure in a medically appropriate manner, the crimes of euthanasia and assisted suicide are legally defined as medical treatments.

The statute specifically allows euthanasia for incompetent patients. Persons 16 years and older can make an advance written statement containing a request to terminate their lives, which a physician may carry out. The written statement need not be made in conjunction with a specific medical condition and it could have been written years before, based on views that may have changed. The physician can administer euthanasia based on the prior written statement.[43]

In addition, the law allows other categories of persons to request and receive euthanasia or assisted suicide: teenagers (with varying degrees of parents' or guardians' approval, depending on age), and persons for whom the doctor "holds the conviction that the patient's suffering is lasting and unbearable."[44]

The 2002 Dutch law requires physicians to meet specific criteria to be immune from criminal prosecution. The following must be considered:

- *Voluntary*—The physician must be convinced that the patient has made a voluntary, persistent, and carefully considered request to die.
- *Suffering*—The physician must be convinced that the patient's suffering is unbearable and that there is no prospect of improvement of the patient's situation. (There is no requirement that the suffering must be physical or that the patient must be terminally ill.)[45]
- *Informed*—The physician has informed the patient about his or her medical situation and medical prospects.
- *Alternatives*—The physician, together with the patient, must be convinced that there is no reasonable alternative.
- *Consultation*—The physician has consulted at least one other physician with an independent viewpoint who has seen the patient and given a written opinion on the due-care criteria [*sic*].
- *Due care and attention*—The physician must have assisted the patient to die with due medical care and attention.[46]

These criteria are similar to the 1993 law. The review of assisted deaths in the 2002 law, however, is very different.

All oversight of euthanasia and assisted suicide is done by a regional review committee for termination of life on request and for assisted suicide. The committees comprise a legal specialist, a physician, and an expert in philosophical issues, specifically with expertise as to the requisites for meaningful life. Significantly, the 2002 law shifts the burden of proof. No longer must the physician justify the need to terminate life. It is the prosecutor who must show that terminating a life failed to meet the requirement of due care. Prosecutors will only learn about termination of a life if the regional committee sends information to them. The law does not prohibit physicians from administering euthanasia to a nonresident.[47] It is hoped that the law will bring into the open euthanasia that historically has been hidden. New concerns about "hidden euthanasia" surfaced only a year after the 2002 law went into effect. Terminal sedation, for example, occurs when physicians give to patients in severe pain quantities of morphine large enough to also hasten death. Because euthanasia is defined as the active termination of life on request, such overdoses are not reportable—it is not clear that the death was intended. The death is considered a natural death.[48]

Some argue that, in effect, the Netherlands will "be issuing retrospective licenses for consensual killing."[49] Legally sanctioning active euthanasia for various groups of "patients" (with varying degrees of consent from parents or guardians for certain of them) is a significant change and moves euthanasia from the exceptional to an accepted way of dealing with medical conditions beyond serious or terminal illness. Palliative care is one casualty of the Netherlands's history of PAS, and hospice care use there lags behind other countries.[50]

The technical aspects of PAS appear to be simple. Data from the Netherlands suggest, however, that problems occur even when a physician is present. Problems include medications not working as expected, technical difficulties, or unexpected side effects. In 16% of cases in which patients tried to kill themselves using doctor-prescribed drugs, the medication did not work as expected. Furthermore, 7% of the time technical problems or unexpected side effects occurred. Physicians witnessing the attempted suicide felt compelled to intervene and ensure death in 18% of cases. Even when a doctor directly performed euthanasia, the researchers found that there were complications 3% of the time. In another 6% of attempts, patients took longer to die than expected or went into a drug-induced coma that was supposed to be fatal but from which they later awoke.[51] Thus, it appears that assisted suicide and euthanasia do not necessarily result in the easy and peaceful death that they promise, and that they can in fact add to the patient's misery and suffering. Rather than showing that they are absent, the lack of reported complications in Oregon data suggests inadequate reporting and follow-up.

The 1993 law may have only recognized existing practice—de facto became de jure. That a western European democracy was willing to acknowledge this development, however, raises important ethical questions. Seemingly begun as a way to enhance individual self-determination, the Dutch experience shows that active euthanasia is not limited to persons who request it. The continuing and troubling scenario of large numbers of persons being involuntarily, actively euthanized highlights the slippery slope, defined as one exception leading to other, more easily accepted exceptions.

That there is no requirement for suffering to be physical or that the patient must be terminally ill suggests a significant new dimension for active euthanasia and assisted suicide—persons tired of living and choosing to end their lives. Persons who are in various states of aging, have a disability, or have health problems now face the prospect that they will have to justify their continued existence. Given that Dutch physicians historically have been willing to actively euthanize persons without their consent, the persons at risk fear that their lives will be ended against their will.[52] This fear has caused many of those most vulnerable—individuals with disabilities and older adults—to carry cards specifying their desire to continue to stay alive.[53]

Dutch health services organizations participate in euthanasia-assisted suicide (EAS) and physician-assisted suicide. The 2002 euthanasia act and national guidelines are the most commonly cited sources of institutional policy statements and practice guidelines. About one-quarter of Dutch healthcare institutions do not have policy statements on EAS. Physicians reported that written guidelines for EAS supported them in their decision making after a patient's request for EAS.[54] Only a minority of patients in a cross section of healthcare settings requested EAS at the end of life; of these requests, more than half were not granted.[55]

SUICIDE AND THE ORGANIZATION: THE CASE OF ELIZABETH BOUVIA

In late 1983, a dramatic case began in California that highlights several of the concepts described in this chapter. Elizabeth Bouvia, a 26-year old with cerebral palsy, entered the county-owned Riverside General Hospital and asked that the staff aid her in fasting until she died. Unable to move, she required assistance in all physical activities. She wanted the hospital to provide hygienic care and the drugs necessary to give her a painless death by starvation. A court injunction prevented the hospital from discharging her. To ensure adequate nutrition, hospital staff inserted a nasogastric tube, allegedly against her wishes. She asserted that she had reached a competent and rational decision, one her lawyer argued was protected by the constitutional right to privacy and self-determination. Her mental competence was confirmed by several psychiatrists.

California has criminal penalties against aiding and abetting a suicide. After a hearing on whether the hospital could be forced to assist Bouvia in her suicide, the court ruled that "despite her right to commit suicide, which is not illegal in California, she could not ask society in the person of the hospital staff to help her because she was not a terminal patient."[56] The court distinguished Bouvia from individuals with terminal illnesses. In January 1984, the California Supreme Court refused to hear her appeal.[57]

The decision permitted the hospital to force-feed Bouvia. She was discharged from Riverside General on April 7, 1984, and was hospitalized in Tijuana, Mexico.[58] It was reported that she had reconsidered her demand to die and would return to the United States for medical treatment. Her lawyer maintained that she still wished to die, despite the fact that she had been accepted for care somewhere in California on the condition that she not stop eating.[59]

After a year in the new institution and a subsequent stay of several months at an acute care hospital, where a morphine pump was installed for pain control, Bouvia was admitted to Los Angeles County–High Desert Hospital in late 1985. As at Riverside General Hospital, and against her wishes, the staff inserted a permanent feeding tube. Court action by Bouvia initially resulted in the court's refusal to order discontinuation of the forced feeding. On appeal, however, the case was remanded, with instructions to consider her request further. As a result, tube feeding was discontinued and Bouvia was discharged. Her attorney stated, "She's promised to continue to eat her liquid diet. I know she would welcome death . . . but she has renounced [suicide]."[60] In May 1986, Bouvia was hospitalized at Los Angeles County University of Southern California Medical Center, where she was treated for chronic pain.[61] In June 1986, the California Supreme Court affirmed a lower court decision allowing her to die by refusing force-feeding (at the time she was accepting a liquid diet). The hospital had argued that removing the tube would officially endorse suicide.[62] Elizabeth Bouvia was reported alive in 2005.[63] Since then, she has shunned publicity.

Ethical Issues and Legal Considerations

In addition to highlighting the problems of situations that do not involve terminal illness, the Bouvia case delineates the clash between organizational philosophy (here with both ethical and legal justification) and
patient autonomy. Bouvia's problem was not that the health services organization where she was treated refused to discharge her; instead, it was
difficult to find a facility that would admit her. Those that agreed to admit
her insisted on doing everything they could to maintain or improve her
physical condition—thus the force-feeding. Several state courts have specifically addressed this issue. A number of states have statutes that permit
withholding or withdrawing tube feeding, but several prohibit such actions
under certain circumstances.[64]

The Bouvia case suggests the limit of what patients can legally (and
ethically) ask of health services organizations. As shown by Bouvia, the law
determines what the organization and its managers can do, and the obligation to obey the law is a minimum performance. The ethics reflected in the
organization's philosophy determine the extent to which it uses a higher
standard. The law is different in other states (e.g., New York, New Jersey),
and this difference reinforces the organization's need to be aware of state
law and, more important, to address such issues prospectively.

If assistance in suicide gains wider social acceptability and becomes
legal in more states, health services organizations will have to address the
ethical issues it raises. Nursing facilities, hospice, and acute care hospitals
have patients with degenerative neurological diseases and those who are
terminally ill or in a persistent vegetative state (PVS). Traditional conscience clause protections will likely be available to providers who find
assistance in suicide morally repugnant. Further, various federal laws protect those who refuse to provide medical services that they find morally
unacceptable.[65] This reinforces the need for health services organizations
to address issues such as end-of-life care in their values statements. A long-
term, clearly enunciated position lends credence to the organization's position. The values statements of most organizations will likely take patients'
rights and reasonable expectations into account.

Perhaps the most important reason for traditional health services organizations to decline to provide assistance in suicide is that the members of the public may find it inconsistent that providers they trust to help
them regain and maintain their health also assist in suicide. The public
may distrust providers because their role at any one time may be unclear.
This suggests that establishing specialized facilities—such as the obitoria

suggested by Kevorkian—and even commercialization of assistance in suicide, are possible.

ISSUES FOR HEALTH SERVICES MANAGERS

Public opinion polls in the United States consistently show a high and increasing level of support for legalizing and regulating PAS. Polls taken before and after the conviction of Jack Kevorkian showed an increase in public support of PAS from 70% to 75%.[66] In 2007, 53% of Americans surveyed thought Kevorkian should not have been jailed; more than two-thirds believed that there are circumstances when a patient should be allowed to die.[67]

As noted, there are ethical distinctions between providing comfort care and pain control to allow a pain-free, dignified death and hastening death through active intervention. Kevorkian's uses of PAS did not occur in health services organizations, nor could an organization have legally assisted him. Even under Oregon law, the assistance provided is only that of a physician who writes a prescription. Kevorkian's "patients" were ambulatory. They were not in skilled nursing facilities or hospitals, for example, when questions of assistance in dying arose. He assisted them to die by various means and in settings that included a motel room and a minivan.

Nonetheless, the opinion poll cited above should strongly encourage health services organizations to prospectively address assisted suicide. In this effort, managers are a vital resource. As moral agents and the organization's conscience, health services managers play a crucial role in identifying, reinforcing, modifying, and monitoring the organization's values. To be effective in these activities, the manager must have a well-defined personal ethic that is consistent with the organization's values, and a clear understanding of its application in strategic and tactical management decision making. The importance of the manager's role in setting the ethical tone for the organization and leading by example cannot be overstated.

Economics of Physician-Assisted Suicide

Developments in Oregon suggest that third-party payers and managed care organizations will offer assistance in suicide as a covered benefit soon after it becomes legal. They may even urge enactment of such laws. Covering PAS, however, raises significant issues of duality of interests. The savings of early death may produce economic benefits for insurers, regardless of any reduction in discomfort and lessened suffering for the insured.

Traditionally, physicians who advocated for their patients and were not pressured to control costs or prioritize services tended to counterbalance system efforts to limit services. Traditional relationships in the private sector are changing, however. This change will make more prominent the questions of aid in dying as arrangements that economically bind physicians and organizations, especially hospitals, become increasingly common. Physician networks and alliances are the logical extension, and the private sector is establishing them.

Psychological or economic oneness between physician and organization raise significant ethical issues, including the risk that a focus on the interests of patients will diminish. Economic incentives in traditional private, fee-for-service medicine reward too much care, and the physician's and organization's interests in voluntary or involuntary passive euthanasia are limited to questions of the futility, or hope of benefit, from continued treatment. Newer forms of payment and organizational arrangements will change the incentives for health services organizations, even as they become less able to meet the costs of services. Since the early 1980s, hospitals have had a form of capitation. The incentive of diagnosis-related groups (DRGs)—the payment scheme for Medicare and Medicaid—is to limit services. Cost shifting is increasingly difficult for health services organizations. Thus, they must either reduce costs through greater productivity (achieving the same results with fewer resources) or change the content of care.

Fixed-sum payment schemes such as capitation or DRGs have the incentive to minimize the number and range of services, especially those that are more costly. Such incentives cause an inherent conflict of interest between providing services that might be in the patient's best interests and holding to a fixed monetary limit. The implications are the same for private insurers and government. Although government is likely to use euphemisms such as "quality of life" and insurers are likely to focus more overtly on costs, the issue is the same for both: How can costs be controlled? Certain services (especially costly ones) are likely to be withheld, and services will be withdrawn from persons who are deemed to have a poor quality of life or prognosis (e.g., cases of futile care). Here, the fact that earlier death is the ultimate cost reduction may provide an attractive economic alternative. Awareness that this duality of interests is present enables the manager to monitor utilization data to minimize potential harm to patients. Systems in the United States in which capitation or global budgets are used may not take positive steps to end life, but rather may simply deny certain types of care because they are uneconomic or have little effect on improving the quality of life. In such cases, Oregon's priority list of services for Medicaid beneficiaries, discussed in Chapter 13, is instructive.

Summary

Often, hospitals and nursing facilities have patients who are in PVS, bed-ridden with a terminal illness, or too ill to transfer. What are their rights compared with those of the organization? The importance of an organizational philosophy with specific attention to aid in dying is clear; legally and ethically, the organization cannot be forced to compromise its values.

International comparisons may help predict evolution of the issues of assisted suicide and euthanasia in the United States. The Dutch experience clearly shows that 30 years of debate led to a slippery slope. The rules governing assistance in suicide and euthanasia became less demanding and ever broader in their application. PAS—illegally performed in Michigan, and legally performed in Oregon—did not involve health services organizations. It seems a small step to involve them, however. As noted, health services organizations in the Netherlands are involved in euthanasia and PAS. This concern was raised in Belgium as its euthanasia law was debated.[68] Given the seemingly inevitable erosion of safeguards protecting those whom caregivers may consider to have an inadequate quality of life, health services organizations will be pressured to participate.

ISSUES FOR PHYSICIANS

A primary issue for many physicians is that their profession is being turned on its head. Traditionally, physicians have been guardians of life. Now they may be asked to assist in causing death. If physicians may legally euthanize their patients, the trust so important to the patient–physician relationship will end. Older adults, individuals with disabilities, and others with lives of perceived "diminished quality" will correctly fear that instead of helping them live, their doctors may hasten their deaths. To prove the assertion that physicians and nurses, like anyone, can become inured to what is essentially murder, one only need read media reports describing killing patients as common practice.[69] The extraordinary the case of Dr. Harold Shipman is chilling. Shipman was a general practice physician in Manchester who became England's most prolific serial killer. Early in his career, Shipman received psychiatric and drug treatment after the death of his first victim. Subsequently, he killed at least 215 of his patients during a 24-year medical career. Possible reasons for his actions include easing the burden on the National Health Service (England's government-run health system) and wanting to play God. Of great concern is that Shipman could elude detection for so long by issuing death certificates attributing his patients' deaths to natural causes.[70]

Proposals in the United States that physicians provide aid in dying have been roundly condemned by organized medicine. This condemnation, however, may overstate physicians' opposition; they may be more willing to provide aid in dying than the Hippocratic tradition allows. A national survey taken in the late 1990s, when physician assistance in suicide was illegal everywhere in the United States, found that 6% of physicians responding who regularly cared for the dying had either given at least one lethal injection or written a prescription so patients could kill themselves. The survey also found that a third of doctors would write prescriptions for deadly doses and a quarter would give lethal injections if these activities were legal.[71] Similarly, in 1995, 12% of responding physicians in Washington State reported receiving one or more explicit requests from patients for PAS; 4% had received one or more requests for euthanasia.[72] State surveys from the mid-1990s found that a majority of physicians in Michigan (Dr. Jack Kevorkian's home state) and in Oregon favored legalization of assisted suicide, although a sizable minority (31%) in Oregon objected to legalization and participation on moral grounds.[73] A 2007 survey of physicians in Washington State found that 50% supported PAS legislation similar to that in Oregon, while 42% opposed it.[74] Physicians in Vermont who cared for terminally ill patients were far less likely to support legislation for PAS, perhaps because they are more experienced with palliative care.[75]

Data from a survey of Oregon physicians not opposed to PAS help explain their concerns about assisting in suicide. Half feared that the attempt would fail and cause harm, half were not confident that their prognosis of 6 months to live was accurate, half were unsure which drug to prescribe, one-third feared someone other than the patient would take the drug, one-third were not confident they could recognize depression, and some did not want to become known as "suicide doctors."[76]

The willingness of physicians to perform euthanasia and PAS is reinforced by findings from the early 1990s that only 11% of Dutch physicians said they would not participate in euthanasia or assisted suicide.[77] Given legal developments in the Netherlands and apparent widespread public support, however, medical practice and public opinion will become inured to PAS and euthanasia and fewer and fewer physicians will be unwilling to provide aid in dying.

The question of aid in dying raises significant moral questions and necessitates a thorough reexamination of the physician–patient relationship.

To this point, physicians cannot be required to perform a procedure that they morally oppose. Our society's tradition of the overriding importance of personal conscience in such matters must govern. Perhaps thanatology, the study of death and dying, will be recognized as a new medical specialty.

CONCLUSION

As framed, the debate on decisions at the end of life focuses on negative rights. Freedom from unwanted health services is a negative ethical and legal right grounded in the right to freedom from unwanted interference. Simply stated, this is autonomy. Continued attention to the implications of technology for patient autonomy and the principle of nonmaleficence are necessary if the organization is to fulfill its mission in the context of its philosophy.

It is noteworthy that none of the legislation that allows physician assistance in suicide establishes a patient's positive right to assistance in dying. A physician willing to assist the patient must be found; as yet, physicians cannot be compelled to provide assistance in suicide. It is almost certain that if assistance in suicide and active euthanasia become more accepted, the number of physicians willing to perform such acts will increase. The dehumanization of provider and patient will become ever more common, and the hardening of the human beings involved will make such actions commonplace, even lauded.

Demedicalizing assistance in suicide reduces ethical problems for physicians, but it raises ethical issues for society in general. German law, for example, effectively makes it illegal for physicians to assist in suicides. Neither suicide nor assisting in the suicide of persons who are capable of exercising control over their actions and have freely made a responsible choice to commit suicide are illegal, however, so unique views about suicide and assistance in suicide have developed in Germany. One expression of these views is the development of societies organized to assist members to commit suicide.[78]

The incentives resulting from cost constraints and the increasingly interlocking economic and psychological interests of physicians and organizations, whether or not under healthcare reform, ensures a reassessment of aid in dying. Numerous questions must be answered. Must physicians meet the demands of their patients for aid in dying through active means? Is it reasonable (or wise) to ask those committed to preserving and extending life to become thanatologists? Do patients who cannot physically participate in assisted suicide have a legal (or moral) right to voluntary active euthanasia? For health services managers, does the organization have a role to aid in dying, regardless of how the current controversy is resolved? It is possible that like abortion, suicide will be defined by courts or legislatures as a privacy issue. If so, health services organizations and their managers will be forced to address assisted suicide solely from the perspective of its ethical implications. At minimum, health services managers are ethically obliged to ensure that in their organization, a right to die does not become a duty.

NOTES

1. Baxter v. Montana, 224 P.3d 1211 (Mont. 2009).
2. Death with Dignity National Center. (2010). *Death with dignity around the U.S.* Retrieved March 23, 2010, from http://www.deathwithdignity.org/2009/06/16/death-dignity-around-us/.
3. ProCon.org. (2010, January 1). *Assisted suicide laws by state.* Retrieved December 13, 2010, from http://euthanasia.procon.org/view.resource.php?resource ID=000132.
4. Henry Weinstein. (1996, March 7). Appeals court in West strikes down prohibition against doctor-aided suicides. *Washington Post*, p. A5.
5. Joan Biskupic. (1996, April 3). U.S. appeals court overturns New York assisted-suicide ban. *Washington Post*, p. A1.
6. 521 U.S. 702 (1997).
7. 521 U.S. 793 (1997).
8. 522 U.S. 927, certiorari denied (1997).
9. Joan Biskupic. (1997, October 15). Oregon's assisted-suicide law lives on. *Washington Post*, p. A3
10. Victor Cohn. (1990, June 12). An assisted suicide: Is it the first step toward euthanasia? *Washington Post.*
11. Nancy Gibbs. (1990, June 18). Dr. Death's suicide machine. *Time*, pp. 69–70.
12. Public Broadcasting Service. (1996, May). *Chronology of Dr. Jack Kevorkian's life and assisted suicide campaign.* Retrieved November 4, 2003, from http://www.pbs.org/wgbh/pages/frontline/kevorkian/chronology.html.
13. Monica Davey. (2007, June 4). Kevorkian speaks after his release from prison. *New York Times.* Retrieved March 28, 2011, from http://www.nytimes.com/2007/06/04/us/04kevorkian.html.
14. *Ibid.*
15. Howard Brody. (2001, January/February). Assisted suicide for those not terminally ill. *Hastings Center Report 31*(1), p. 7.
16. Yale Kamisar argued that assisted suicide is unconstitutional. See Yale Kamisar. (1993, May/June). Are laws against assisted suicide unconstitutional? *Hastings Center Report 23*(3), pp. 32–41.
17. Robert A. Sedler argued that assisted suicide is constitutional. See Robert A. Sedler. (1993, September/October). The Constitution and hastening inevitable death. *Hastings Center Report 23*(5), pp. 20–25.

18. Frank J. Murray. (1995, April 25). High court won't touch Michigan suicide aid ban. *Washington Times*, p. Al.

19. Oregon Department of Human Services. (n.d.) *The Oregon Death with Dignity Act: Oregon revised statutes.* Retrieved March 26, 2011, from http://public.health .oregon.gov/ProviderPartnerResources/EvaluationResearch/DeathwithDig nityAct/Documents/statute.pdf.

20. *Ibid.*

21. Charles H. Baron. (1999, July). Assisted dying. *Trial 35*(7), pp. 44, 46, 48–49.

22. Melinda A. Lee & Susan W. Tolle. (1996, January 15). Oregon's assisted suicide vote: The silver lining. *Annals of Internal Medicine 124*(2), pp. 267–269.

23. William Booth. (1998, March 26). Woman commits doctor-assisted suicide. *Washington Post*, p. A7.

24. Oregon health plans proceed with caution on suicide coverage. (1998, March 16). *AHA News 34*(10), p. 5.

25. Assisted-suicide coverage could be expanded. (1998, November 2). *AHA News 34*(43), p. 6.

26. Oregon Public Health Division. (n.d.) *Oregon's Death with Dignity Act—2010.* Retrieved March 27, 2011, from http://public.health.oregon.gov/Provider-PartnerResources/EvaluationResearch/DeathwithDignityAct/Documents/year13.pdf.

27. *Ibid.* Even health services organizations treating the terminally ill are reluctant to participate in PAS. Oregon data show that "no hospice is willing to assist in all phases of the physician-assisted death process." Courtney S. Campbell & Jessica C. Cox. (2010, September/October). Hospice and physician-assisted death: Collaboration, compliance, and complicity. *Hastings Center Report 40*(5), pp. 26–35.

28. Oregon Public Health Division.

29. Baron.

30. Oregon Department of Human Services, 2003; Linda Ganzini, Heidi Nelson, Melinda Lee, Dale F. Kraemer, Terri A. Schmidt, & Molly A. Delorit. (2001, May 9). Oregon physicians' attitudes about and experiences with end-of-life care since passage of the Oregon Death with Dignity Act. *Journal of the American Medical Association 285*(18), pp. 2363–2369.

31. Oregon Department of Human Services, 2009.

32. Alison Langley. (2003, February 4). "Suicide tourists" go to the Swiss for help in dying. *New York Times*, p. A3.

33. Derek Humphry. (2003, March 9). A twentieth century chronology of voluntary euthanasia and physician-assisted suicide. *Euthanasia Research & Guidance Organization.* Retrieved January 1, 2004, from http://www.finalexit.org/chron frame.html.

34. WorldNetDaily. (2003, June 21). *Belgian lawmakers propose euthanasia for children.* Retrieved November 17, 2003, from http://worldnetdaily.com/news/article.asp?ARTICLE_ID=33199.

35. Delphine Soulas. (2003, October 27). Euthanasia debate renewed: Mercy killing of Frenchman forces society to re-examine right to die. *Washington Times*, p. A14.

36. Karla Adam. (2010, February 26). Britain clarifies assisted-suicide law. *Washington Post*, p. A14.

37. Charles Truehart. (1999, August 15). Holland prepares bill legalizing euthanasia. *Washington Post*, p. A19.
38. Marlise Simons. (1993, February 10). Dutch parliament approves law permitting euthanasia. *New York Times*, p. A10.
39. *Ibid.*
40. John Keown. (1991, November 5). Dutch slide down euthanasia's slippery slope. *Wall Street Journal*, p. A18.
41. Herbert Hendin. (2003, July/August). The practice of euthanasia. *Hastings Center Report 33*(4), pp. 44–45.
42. International Task Force on Euthanasia and Assisted Suicide. (2003, November 4). *Holland's euthanasia law*. Retrieved December 5, 2003, from http://www.internationaltaskforce.org/hollaw.htm.
43. *Ibid.*
44. *Ibid.* Children as young as 16 may request termination of life in writing, which the physician can legally administer without parental or guardian approval (although they must be involved in the decision process); children as young as 12 may request and receive euthanasia or assisted suicide (with agreement of parents or guardians).
45. *Ibid.*
46. Joris Vos, Ambassador, Embassy of the Netherlands. (2001, May 3). The Netherlands' euthanasia law explained [Letter to the editor]. *Washington Times*, p. A18.
47. *Ibid.*
48. Keith B. Richburg. (2004, January 4). Death with dignity, or door to abuse? *Washington Post*, p. A1.
49. James Meek. (1999, November 21). Dutch wrestle with morality of mercy killings: Parliament is expected to legalize euthanasia, doctor-assisted suicide. *Washington Times*, p. C12.
50. Herbert Hendin, Chris Rutenfrans, & Zbigniew Zylicz. (1997, June 4). Physician-assisted suicide and euthanasia in the Netherlands. *Journal of the American Medical Association 227*, pp. 1720–1722.
51. Assisted suicide takes a hit. (2000, February 24). *Washington Times*, p. A7.
52. Jenny Nolan. (2001). *Dutch legalize euthanasia and assisted suicide*. Retrieved November 14, 2003, from http://www.nrlc.org/news/2001/NRL05/dutch.html.
53. Anne Allen. (2001, April 15). Euthanasia is threat to our freedom. *Express on Sunday*, p. 1.
54. Berniek A.M. Hesselink, H. Roeline W. Pasman, Gerrit van der Wal, Paul J. van der Maas, Agnes van der Heide, & Bregje D. Onwuteaka-Philipsen. (2010, March). Development and dissemination of institutional practice guidelines on medical end-of-life decisions in Dutch health care institutions. *Health Policy 94*(3), pp. 230–238.
55. Bregje D. Onwuteaka-Philipsen, Mette L. Rurup, H. Roeline W. Pasman, & Agnes van der Heide. (2010, July). The last phase of life: Who requests and who receives euthanasia or physician-assisted suicide? *Medical Care 48*(7), pp. 596–603.
56. Jay Matthews. (1983, December 17). Judge rejects palsy victim's bid to starve. *Washington Post*, p. A3.
57. California Supreme Court rejects appeal by Bouvia to starve. (1984, January 20). *Washington Post*, p. A15.

58. Patient repeatedly calls off her effort to starve to death. (1985, April 24). *New York Times*, p. B15.
59. The latest word. (1985, August). *Hastings Center Report 15*(4), p. 36.
60. Doctors stop force-feeding of quadriplegic who sued. (1986, April 18). *Washington Post*, p. A12.
61. Bouvia moves to another CA hospital. (1986, May 30). *Hospital Week*, pp. 21–23.
62. Right to refuse forced feeding upheld in court. (1986, June 6). *Washington Post*, p. A8.
63. Matt Schudel. (2005, April 23). GWU prodigy, doctor Habeeb Bacchus dies. *Washington Post*. Retrieved December 30, 2010, from http://www.washington post.com/wp-dyn/content/article/2005/04/22/AR2005042201478.html.
64. Tinker Ready. (1989, December 18). Medical groups back plaintiffs in right-to-die case. *Healthweek*, 6–8.
65. Ishmeal Bradley. (2009, May 28). Conscientious objection to medicine: A moral dilemma. *Clinical Correlations*. Retrieved December 16, 2010, from http://www.clinicalcorrelations.org/?p=1454.
66. Baron.
67. Americans still split on doctor-assisted suicide: Most believe in patient's right to die, but not doctor's role, AP poll shows. (2007, May 29). Associated Press. Retrieved March 3, 2011, from http://www.msnbc.msn.com/id/18923323/ns/health-health_care/#.
68. Elizabeth Bryant. (2001, August 13). Belgian left pushes vote on euthanasia law. *Washington Times*, A12.
69. Maggie Gallagher. (2001, April 14). Dutch death. *Washington Times*, A10.
70. Batty, David. (2003, July 15). Q&A: Harold Shipman. *Guardian*. Retrieved December 5, 2003, from http://www.guardian.co.uk/society/2005/aug/25/health.shipman.
71. Daniel Q. Haney. (1998, April 23). 6 percent of physicians in survey say they have assisted in patient suicides. *Washington Post*, p. A9.
72. Anthony L. Back, Jeffrey I. Wallace, Helene E. Starks, & Robert A. Pearlman. (1996, March 27). Physician-assisted suicide and euthanasia in Washington State: Patient requests and physician responses. *Journal of the American Medical Association 275*(12), pp. 919–925.
73. Jerald G. Bachman, Kirsten H. Alcser, David J. Doukas, Richard L. Lichtenstein, Amy D. Coming, & Howard Brody. (1996, February 1). Attitudes of Michigan physicians and the public toward legalizing physician-assisted suicide and voluntary euthanasia. *New England Journal of Medicine 334*(5), pp. 303–309; Melinda A. Lee, Heidi D. Nelson, Virginia P. Tilden, Linda Ganzini, Terri A. Schmidt, & Susan W. Tolle. (1996, February 1). Legalizing assisted suicide: Views of physicians in Oregon. *New England Journal of Medicine 334*(5), pp. 310–315.
74. Kevin B. O'Reilly. (2008, October 27). Polls show Washington voters favor physician-assisted suicide. *American Medical News*. Retrieved December 12, 2010, from http://www.ama-assn.org/amednews/2008/10/27/prsb1027.htm.
75. Alexa Craig, Beth Cronin, William Eward, James Metz, Logan Murray, Gail Rose, Eric Suess, & Maria E. Vergara. (2007). Attitudes towards physician-assisted suicide among physicians in Vermont. *Journal of Medical Ethics 33*, pp. 400–403.

76. Hilary Evans. (1997, September). Pitfalls of physician-assisted suicide. *Physician's News Digest*. Retrieved November 4, 2003, from http://www.physi ciansnews.com/commentary/997wp.html.

77. *Ibid.*

78. Margaret P. Battin. (1992, March/April). Assisted suicide: Can we learn from Germany? *Hastings Center Report 22*(2), pp. 44–51.

Ethical Issues on the Horizon

There have been numerous changes in the management of health services organizations since the early 1970s. Change is the future and seems to be occurring at an accelerating pace. New managerial challenges mean greater demands on organizational philosophies and cultures and on the manager's personal ethic. Managers with an ill-defined personal ethic will feel adrift in a world that seems to have few solid foundations.

Chapter 12 examines marketing and managed care in competitive environments, Chapter 13 addresses resource allocation, and Chapter 14 considers the social responsibility of health services organizations. These areas have become much more important, and their ethical implications require special attention.

The competitive environment has convinced health services mangers that marketing their organizations and programs is essential to their survival. Marketing is not new to these institutions; however, applying it in ways that are more commercial and entrepreneurial is. Many managers question the ethical implications, especially those who manage not-for-profit organizations.

Managed care has emerged as a primary means of organizing and financing health services delivery. Like marketing, managed care is not new to health services, but its prevalence, coupled with quality and cost pressures, raise complex ethical issues that will challenge management.

Health services managers are acutely aware of the struggle for resources that is occurring everywhere in society. The health services organization is a microcosm of this struggle. Given its importance in providing critical services to society, the health services organization and its managers play a central role as arbiters of resource allocation. The ethical implications to both managers and society are great.

CHAPTER **12**

ETHICS IN MARKETING AND MANAGED CARE

n the 1920s, President Calvin Coolidge stated that the business of America is business. This statement remains true and the United States is the bastion of free-market, democratic capitalism. Unique among its enterprises are health services organizations. These enterprises differ in purpose, type of service provided, orientation, and motives. Health services providers are often faith-based and have not-for-profit tax status. Health services organizations are unique because they are intimately involved with several professions and provide services that have significant emotional and psychological dimensions. Health services organizations are social enterprises with an economic dimension, rather than economic enterprises with a social dimension.

The elements of marketing—product, place, promotion, and pricing—have been applied to health services. Here, again, health services differ significantly. Unlike marketing in traditional business enterprises, which seeks to create demand, health services marketing seeks to meet a demand, perhaps unrealized, for its services. The distinction between business enterprise and health services has become less clear since the 1980s. Health services organizations have engaged in marketing for many years. Any type of community outreach is an implicit form of marketing. Historically, marketing occurs in several ways, including community health days, disease screening, well-baby clinics, and press releases from the provider. The milieu of the competitive marketplace, however, began to require that marketing become systematic, focused, and much more aggressive.

NEED VERSUS DEMAND

Opinions vary when the role of marketing in health services is assessed: Is demand being created or is it being met? Important to answering this question is disagreement about the types of health services demand that are meritorious (in itself a value-laden concept). Few would disagree that it is important to create consumer demand for hypertension or colorectal cancer screening. The desirability of such efforts is tempered by calculating costs and benefits. Depending on the population and the disease, screening may be unacceptably expensive when measured by the number of true positives found and the morbidity and mortality prevented. Screening may be done even when it is not cost-effective, for reasons of political correctness or to further a feeling of well-being in a population.

Both price and nonprice competition may increase demand. Competition in the business sector is generally deemed to be desirable, but its desirability is less clear in health services. This is true because services are duplicated and because competing for physicians, staff, and patients is costly. Despite acceptance of competition, disagreement continues as to whether the demand created is appropriate.

In addition, conditions requiring medical intervention may be treated with different therapies. Coronary artery bypass surgery or angioplasty for individuals who have had mild heart attacks is an example of an expensive therapy that patients may be able to avoid. One study found that patients given the most elaborate tests and treatments were two or three times more likely to suffer a second heart attack or die within 30 days than were those diagnosed and treated with noninvasive therapies, such as exercise stress tests and drugs that dissolved blood clots. It has been estimated that 400,000–600,000 Americans could avoid angioplasty each year at a cost of $20,000–$25,000 per procedure.[1] The benefits are obvious.

Similar treatment controversies are found in diagnoses such as prostate cancer. Following early detection using the prostate-specific antigen test, the standard therapy has been to treat all malignant prostate tumors aggressively with surgery or with radiation therapy. As a result, men who would neither die from nor likely even notice small prostate tumors endure treatment that often causes complications such as incontinence, impotence, injury, and sometimes death. Watchful waiting with active surveillance (WWAS) is a more desirable alternative. WWAS entails closely monitoring the progression of small, slow-growing tumors and initiating treatment only as necessary.[2] Added to quality of life benefits is that of a marked decrease in costs compared with active treatment. WWAS is especially desirable for men who may not live another 10 years, such as those older than age 75, or those with severe heart disease or diabetes.

More subjective situations contrast with the objective need to intervene when coronary artery disease is present. Cosmetic surgery is often cited as an example of an "unnecessary" medical service. It is claimed that face lifts, tummy tucks, silicone implants, and Botox waste medical resources—regardless of payment source—and that these "resources" should be used for other health problems. This is a subjective definition of need. Reasonable persons could differ as to what patients need and how or whether the demand that arises from that need should be met by the healthcare system. Perhaps interventions such as cosmetic surgery should not be defined as health services, but rather as consumer services similar to hair styling, exercise and yoga classes, laser vision correction, and bodybuilding.

Epidemiologic studies should be used to develop data about populations. These data reveal the incidence and prevalence of diseases as well as psychological and physical concerns of the population that may fall outside traditional definitions of disease. The real problem in terms of assessing need and demand arises when those judging such data apply their personal value systems to determine how important the "problem" is. These judgments cause the process to be less than objective, whether it affects decisions in determining what to study or what is to be done with the results. In turn, these decisions affect the choice of regimens and decisions about whether to provide treatment. More important, however, they diminish or thwart the autonomy and decision making of individuals.

The debate about need is most heated when the ethics of marketing is included. This is especially true when marketing is to be used to affect demand or to encourage persons to seek elective procedures. Physical or psychological conditions about which an individual is either unaware or unwilling to seek treatment represent potential demand. Conditions for which no help is sought because of financial barriers also represent potential demand; examples are dental care, hammertoes, hemorrhoids, and mental health services.

Troubling in this debate is the suggestion that meeting potential, consumer-driven demand is unethical. The constitution of the World Health Organization defines health as "a state of complete physical, mental, and social well-being and not merely the absence of disease or infirmity."[3] This broad definition includes as beneficial all efforts to improve physical, mental, and social well-being. It is instructive to consider wellness (prevention) activities. The possibilities for organizational involvement are almost limitless because every facet of life could be affected to improve general health and prevent medical problems. Beyond wellness activities are questions of how to treat demand for services that may seem foolish to some. Should persons be denied cosmetic surgery because others judge such procedures to be trivial or because what they seek to correct is not life threatening? Currently, such infringements on individual autonomy are greater than the public will accept.

It is not clear how and by whom need and demand are to be judged. Despite the presence of the occasional hypochondriac or patient with Munchausen's syndrome, demand for medical services should be accepted as rational. When typical patients hear about new medical problems or treatment and diagnostic possibilities, they respond rationally. The "worried well" are not clinically ill but are concerned about their health and quality of life. Their decisions about elective procedures are personal cost–benefit analyses. It is when publicly funded programs use cost–benefit analyses to make macroallocation decisions that services may become unavailable. Oregon's example of prioritizing health services in its Medicaid program is instructive and rational when political decisions determine the services available.

Responsible Marketing

How does the health services organization market to patients and potential patients in ways that are consistent with its ethical obligation to avoid creating unnecessary demand, but which simultaneously find and serve those who might need services? In its Principles and Practices for Marketing Communications in Hospitals and Health Systems, the Society for Healthcare Strategy & Market Development (SHSMD) of the American Hospital Association (AHA) includes a marketing communications checklist.[4] The checklist has 12 areas for organizations to consider in marketing communications. Examples include "Does the product or service being promoted add genuine value for the patient?," "Does the communication set realistic expectations?," "If quality measures are highlighted, are words such as *safe*, *high(est)*, *effective*, *painless*, *best*, and *top quality* used with caution and only when they can be verified and objectively substantiated?," and "Is the language in the communication readily understandable by the audience for which it is intended?" Separate sections provide guidance on price information, endorsements and testimonials, use of physicians in marketing, social media, and blogger advertising, among others. In sum, the SHSMD advisory encourages marketing communications that are truthful, fair, accurate, complete, and sensitive to the healthcare needs of the public.

The emergence and widespread use of social media has added a dramatically new and potentially problematic dimension to health services marketing. At this writing, it is estimated that 250 hospitals are using YouTube, Facebook, Twitter, or blogs in outreach to their service areas.

Some hospitals are using Twitter to show live surgical procedures. In one instance, the Twitter broadcast is enhanced by tweets from a physician observing the procedure and providing live commentary. Should a complication arise, the hospital will cut away from the live broadcast and substitute a video from a similar procedure. This raises ethical issues because it will mislead the public about the procedure's risks. In addition, concerns have been raised about patient privacy.[5] Social media offer great potential for service recovery, responding to and sharing positive feedback, and learning how other health services organizations use those same tools. An argument against using social media is that the organization cannot control what is being said about it on these various sites. But the comments are being made regardless and the organization will benefit from becoming part of the conversation. By knowing what is being said, the organization can improve its services and respond to concerns and complaints from users. Nonetheless, ethical issues abound in the interactions that can come from social media. The organization is obliged to ensure that responses to social media interactions meet basic requirements established by the AHA and are consistent with its own values.[6]

If profit and return on investment are their primary reasons for being, organizations will have a very different view of responsible marketing and appropriate competition. This is the difference between giving the public whatever it wants and tempering desires and potential demand with judgments about value and usefulness. This view of the patient includes elements of paternalism, but it should be consistent with the organization's mission statement.

Demarketing to Avoid Bankruptcy

Chief executive officer (CEO) Chris Hines had finally gotten down far enough in the stack of papers on her desk to get to last month's emergency department (ED) activity report. She had already digested the grim news about the continued financial hemorrhage affecting Community Hospital. The current deficit was $500,000—and it was only the fourth month of the fiscal year. Because Community Hospital served largely inner city patients, many of whom were uninsured or whose care was paid by a chronically underfunded Medicaid program, there seemed to be little hope that the financial situation would improve.

Hines knew that more than 40% of Community Hospital's admissions come through the ED and that about half of those admissions arrived by taxi, private automobile, or on foot. The other half arrived via the city-owned ambulance service. Hines had tried to implement a plan to increase elective admissions, and thus improve the payer mix, by encouraging her attending physicians to admit their private patients to Community. Her effort failed. Next, Hines tried to work with city officials to implement a new ambulance routing system that would give Community a chance to improve its financial condition. Unsympathetic city officials refused to help.

Hines knew that Community Hospital's endowment would carry the hospital for approximately 3 more years, but that the institution would have to close if it were not breaking even by then. Because the city was uncooperative, Hines concluded that the key to survival lay with reducing the number of uninsured and Medicaid patients admitted through the ED.

Hines spoke with several marketing consultants, one of whom offered to do pro bono work for Community Hospital. He seized on the idea of "demarketing" the ED. He reasoned that it was the fine reputation enjoyed by Community Hospital's ED that was largely responsible for the 50% of ED patients who arrived by means other than city ambulance. He listed the following ways the ED could be made less attractive to potential patients: reducing ED staffing to a minimum; closing the parking lot near the ED; reducing housekeeping services so that the physical plant would be dirty and unkempt; deferring nonsafety-related maintenance; changing triage policies, procedures, and staffing to increase waiting time for nonemergency patients; using staff who were most likely to be rude and inconsiderate; and encouraging rumors that closure of the ED was imminent.

The consultant knew that there might be repercussions beyond the ED, but Community was desperate, and he believed extreme action was necessary.

A first question is whether Hines and her managers ignored other steps to improve the financial condition of Community. Examples include closing the ED rather than demarketing it (a more honest solution); undertaking other, more remunerative medical care activities to offset ED losses; or opening less costly primary care clinics to care for the worried well and other nonemergent medical problems.

Even if such options were available, however, a demarketing strategy raises two ethical issues. First, the steps contemplated are likely to negatively affect the quality of care in the ED. Beyond staffing and the physical aspects directly affected, the psychological impact on ED staff, with its ripple effect on inpatient care, will reduce employee morale and ultimately the quality of care. Such actions violate the principles of beneficence and nonmaleficence and the virtues of caring and honesty.

A second ethical principle to be considered is justice. People in the community are caught between the city bureaucracy and the efforts of Community Hospital to remain financially viable. They may have little choice but to endure the indignities and reduction in quality of service resulting from the demarketing strategy. Deliberately adding insult to injury should give all concerned great discomfort. A dimension of justice and the virtue of fidelity deplore the unfairness associated with forcing ED staff to work under such conditions. They will bear the brunt of angry patients and the dilapidated, depressing environment of the ED.

That the declining financial condition of Community Hospital might eventually result in the same changes in the ED does not justify taking them as recommended by the consultant. Desperate managers may consider desperate acts, but the actions being recommended are not morally justifiable.

FUTURE OF COMPETITION

A theory in political science suggests that, over time, enemies begin to take on one another's attributes. This concern is troubling to the not-for-profit sector of the health services system, which views itself as holding and furthering values different from and superior to those in the for-profit sector. These individuals fear that competition for market share and the focus on financial considerations and economic survival will cause them to lose sight of their humanitarian and charitable motives.

In this regard, payment systems are especially significant. The advent of reimbursement using diagnosis-related groups for hospitalized Medicare beneficiaries was the opening round of what is proving to be a continuing reassessment of payment schemes. Competition and cost-cutting are furthering the shift from fee-for-service to various forms of fixed payment. Physician and organizational providers are becoming aligned in relationships that add a significant amount of complexity to traditional ethical problems and raise new ones as well. Physicians are beginning to push back against the various pressures on them, however. Many are limiting the number of Medicare and Medicaid patients in their practices, refusing to accept assignment from managed care and managed care organization (MCO) fee schedules, and establishing boutique practices to serve fee-for-service patients exclusively. Hospitals have less flexibility, but market conditions may allow them to negotiate better reimbursement schedules with MCOs.[7]

Some writers suggest that the pressures of fixed-fee reimbursement will lead to an adversarial relationship between patients and health services organizations (and, perhaps, physicians) and that the interests of patients will be subordinated to the demands of efficiency and economic survival. Such results are possible under any payment system or ownership, and they will occur whenever caregivers and managers lose sight of their reason for being. Doing more with less is not at variance with efforts to operational-ize the principles of respect for persons, beneficence, nonmaleficence, and justice, as well as several of the virtues. It remains for all who organize, plan, and deliver health services to keep these values in mind.

COMPETITION AND HUMAN RESOURCES POLICY

Highly competitive suburban and metropolitan markets bring with them a unique set of ethical issues, especially those that arise in hiring.

Hiring the Competition

The two nursing facilities in town are highly competitive. This competition has caused each to oppose the other's certificates of need applications to the point of suing each other. The chief operating officers (COOs) of the nursing facilities were friends long before they were first employed by their respective nursing facilities. They play golf monthly. When the COO of one nursing facility is fired because of political intrigue on the board of directors, the other COO offers to hire him as a consultant.

Professional codes of ethics do not cover such circumstances. The fired COO is privy to proprietary information that would likely give the other nursing facility an unfair competitive advantage. In theory, the fired COO could consult only on matters that do not require him to reveal or use proprietary information. Given the organizations' history, however, this is unlikely. The ethically superior answer is to not hire the former compet-ing manager. Short of that, it may be possible to avoid using the competi-tor's proprietary information, something that could be determined only by knowing what work the newly hired consultant will perform.

Does a fired manager have any duty to a former employer? Manag-ers have an ethical duty to keep proprietary information confidential after they sever relations with an employer. This duty of confidentiality contin-ues until events have overtaken the confidential information. Were there no duty of confidentiality, former employees could hold organizations hostage. Managers would be among the first to agree that this is an unde-sirable situation from both managerial and professional perspectives.

MANAGED CARE

Simply put, managed care is an organized effort to control the costs of health services through various means. The primary ethical issue that arises in managed care is the duality of interests that leads to conflicts of interest. Conflicts of interest are inherent in managed care because the goals, purposes, and objectives of management and personnel may be at variance with the interests of enrollees. The tension between the MCO and its enrollees and potential enrollees occurs as early as initial marketing when benefits packages and market segments are identified. The duality of interests that may become conflicts of interest are unavoidable, but their presence and consequent negative effects can be minimized if they are recognized by clinicians and managers. Enrollees are increasingly aware of this duality of interests.

The possibility that conflicts of interest will arise is exacerbated because many not-for-profit MCOs seek to establish and maintain a perception that they are more public service–oriented and on a higher moral plane than their for-profit competitors. Historically, not-for-profit health plans and health maintenance organizations (HMOs) have encouraged a perception that they are a "purer" delivery system, one untainted by profit motive and one through which members could gain access to high-quality medical services at reasonable cost. That perception is changing because of financial scandals in charitable organizations, disclosures of very generous compensation paid to their executives, and highly publicized denials of services to enrollees. Nonetheless, the historical perception generally remains. To the extent that marketing ignores or purposely excludes high-risk groups ("cream skimming"), there may be variance between historic and current missions. The duality of interests present when no relationship exists between providers and those toward whom marketing is directed can lead to conflicts of interest.

Adverse Selection and Marketing Managed Care

The marketing strategy must consider whether to minimize significant clinical strengths that provider components may have. If the MCO is or is perceived to be a leader in treating complex or high-cost medical conditions, adverse selection is likely and the MCO will be inundated with persons requiring that treatment. If higher quality results in higher costs, the MCO falls into a vicious cycle. An MCO's reputation for high-quality results encourages more high-risk persons who need that expensive care to join. Straining against this adverse selection may cause quality to decline for other enrollees, or the MCO may be forced to restrict benefits or increase premiums. Thus, to survive (and thrive), MCO marketers may have to minimize references to superb care of specific types and focus instead on developing a reputation that the MCO delivers general medical services of high quality but without centers of excellence.

I Want to See Dr. Nightengale

Dr. Nightengale is a pediatrician with HMO, Inc., located in a medium-size city. She has had no specialty training beyond her residency, but she has developed into an adept diagnostician, often diagnosing cases that baffle her colleagues.

At the last open enrollment, management noted that an unexpectedly large number of families with young children enrolled. As is typical, HMO, Inc., limits in-area, out-of-plan services and restricts referrals to subspecialists. Dr. Nightengale uses subspecialists more often than her colleagues do, but she achieves excellent results. The new member survey showed that for many families, the presence of excellent pediatric care was an important factor in making their decision to join HMO, Inc. A few named Dr. Nightengale specifically.

Management expressed fears that such perceptions might cause significant adverse selection. Management even suggested that to protect the organization's financial position, a special review of Dr. Nightengale's use of subspecialists should be undertaken. Some thought this was an overreaction. They agreed on a wait-and-see approach. If there were problems, they would talk to her.

Another example of adverse selection occurred in treating individuals who were HIV positive. An HMO in metro Washington, D.C., had achieved a well-deserved reputation for providing high-quality care to this group. Disseminated throughout the community, this knowledge caused high-risk individuals to enroll in larger-than-expected numbers. The HMO has not compiled data showing higher costs for enrollees with HIV. However, it is generally agreed that hospitalization and high-cost drug therapies as HIV progresses to frank AIDS will make care expensive, even though less expensive sources of care are increasingly available. Sicker enrollees require more care, which places an MCO with disproportionate numbers of high-cost patients at financial risk and, in terms of economic survival, at a competitive disadvantage.

Service Utilization in MCOs

Managers, staff, and clinicians in the MCO seek to maximize position, power, income, and rewards with the least disruption of the organization's homeostasis. Achieving these goals, especially maximizing income, may minimize service, whether or not that is consistent with the contract between MCO and payer. The bureaucratic response may even be at variance with the MCO's long-term survival needs. To regain or retain their health, enrollees want to pay as little as necessary but obtain all needed services—at the least, they want value for their premium. When enrollees use services efficiently and stay well at minimum cost, MCO and enrollee goals are congruent. The situation is rarely that simple, however.

A primary source of differing interests is in the utilization of services. Enrollees may be divided into two groups: light and moderate users of services and heavy users. The MCO's interests and the interests of light and moderate users are generally congruent; to be competitive, the MCO must control heavy users. Even moderate users are potential financial threats to MCOs in a competitive environment, and to cut costs, the MCO may seek to transform them into light users. The likelihood that conflicts of interest will arise is clear.

How do the differing interests, as shown by incongruent goals of MCO and enrollee, become conflicts of interest? The MCO's marketing will stress access to primary and specialty services and minimize limits on services. Enrollees may be constrained by limited hours, services, and having too few clinical staff to meet demand, thus purposely creating queues. Waits for appointments will reduce operating costs, especially for the 85% of medical complaints that are self-limiting. Enrollees are unlikely to endorse a deliberate strategy of deferring treatment, regardless of its clinical and economic soundness. MCOs have an escape valve for these pressures by providing advice nurse consultation and treating walk-ins during office hours. The furor that resulted when the CEO of a large East Coast HMO stated publicly that his HMO used a deliberate policy of allowing queues, noting their value in reducing demand for certain services (especially self-limiting conditions), was a lesson to all MCO managers. Such policies may cause disenrollment in the long term but are effective in the short term.

Physician Incentives and Disincentives

For the enrollee, the more subtle and potentially more serious constraints imposed by MCOs are directed at affiliated physicians. A duality of interests is present between MCO and enrollee and between physician and enrollee. The Hippocratic oath requires physicians to act in the patient's best interests. The AMA's Principles of Medical Ethics state, "A physician shall be dedicated to providing competent medical care, with compassion and respect for human dignity and rights," and "A physician shall . . . be honest in all professional interactions."[8] These guidelines suggest that patients' interests are primary as physicians connected to MCOs choose the level and content of care.

The physician is the fiduciary in the physician–patient relationship. It is perverse that a relationship necessitating such trust is influenced at all by financial incentives. Given that neutral financial incentives are likely to be impossible, it must be asked which type of payment best protects the interests of patients. Here, minimizing the interference of third parties must be the primary criterion, and the relationship that best achieves this result is fee-for-service practice. Because physicians are paid more for doing more, however, fee-for-service medicine has the incentive of overtreatment, with some increased risk to patients. On balance, however, the choices that patients make regarding third-party carriers, if any, and physicians continue the direct connection of traditional medicine and provide the best possibility of maintaining the trust so essential to this fiduciary relationship. It is unrealistic to expect physicians alone to resist the pressures of financial incentives—they need the help of their patients.

MCOs, however, determine the context that facilitates or inhibits physician responses. Initially, there is a self-selection bias when physicians choose in what setting and with whom they will contract. Physicians who cannot accept the rules imposed by an MCO will look elsewhere, although choices in this regard are becoming increasingly limited. Once a physician joins an MCO, management can use a range of actions to modify or direct behavior, including financial incentives and disincentives, treatment protocols, prior authorization of services, peer pressure (such as that achieved by disseminating practice profiles and comparisons with peers and best practices), nonrenewal, and dismissal. MCOs can limit referrals, especially outside the MCO; strictly control hospitalizations; establish quotas on the number of enrollees who must be seen per day, as in staff-model HMOs; and use a system of peer review. Peer pressure plays an important role in most constraints. Constraints are positive when they encourage judicious but appropriate use of resources. This may partly account for use of fewer ancillary services and hospital days by MCOs than fee-for-service providers.

Financial incentives and disincentives are high risk in terms of conflicts of interest; among these, physician-at-risk or capitated payments are among the most problematic. Bonuses may be based on use of ancillary services, referrals, and hospitalizations, and may be used as incentives or disincentives. The effect of a potential bonus is insidious in that clinical decision making may be affected subconsciously or in ways not fully appreciated, even by the physicians themselves. Patients are almost always ignorant of such incentives or relationships. A further problem with bonuses is that staff begin to view them as a usual and expected part of their compensation, and failing to pay them is likely to result in lower morale or other, even more negative consequences.

When do constraints become excessive and deny members needed services? When do constraints violate the principles of nonmaleficence and beneficence? Such questions are not easily answered because they are a function of the MCO's willingness, prompted by its (virtuous) managers acting as moral agents and the organization's conscience, to institute the safeguards that balance competitiveness and financial factors with furthering the interests of enrollees. Even when managers and clinical decision makers express the virtues of compassion and caring, media hyperbole and the political process may override clinical judgment, as when laws were passed to require 24-hour hospital stays for normal childbirth.

Other Constraints in MCOs

In addition to physician-oriented constraints, other types of constraints are found in the organization and management of MCOs. By employing a complicated process (e.g., significant committee involvement and several levels of review), the MCO may be slow to approve use of new procedures, techniques, or equipment that raise costs. Such complexities are found more often in not-for-profit than in investor-owned MCOs. The more complex processes in not-for-profit MCOs may result from a greater degree of democracy and not from deliberate efforts to diminish access. The effect may be the same, however. For-profit MCOs tend to use a narrower management pyramid that gives the CEO more authority and potentially greater efficiency.

MCOs may forgo purchasing high-technology equipment, or they may contract with physicians and hospitals that do not have such equipment. For example, the higher operating costs of teaching hospitals place them at a competitive disadvantage, which means they are less likely to have contracts with MCOs. Such strategies lower costs. If lower costs enhance financial integrity and guarantee the continued availability of services to enrollees, all parties have congruent interests. A conflict arises, however, between enrollees who might have benefited from access to the technology.

Controls on access, such as using primary care physicians as gatekeepers or case managers, limiting out-of-plan services, and specifying dollar limits on referrals and consultations, help MCOs curtail costs. Those in competitive environments, however, must show that enrollees who need services get them (or at least create a perception that this happens), lest they lose market share. In addition, indirect and retrospective controls on access occur through use of utilization review, which is conducted on resource consumption patterns of various types of services by physicians, with special focus on those that are high cost. Controls risk malpractice suits and negative publicity if limiting access and utilization are perceived as resulting in poor outcomes.

Dissatisfaction regarding access to treatment was reflected in a study of nonelderly, sick enrollees. Those in managed care were almost twice as likely (22% versus 13%) to state that they experienced major or minor problems obtaining treatment they or their physicians thought was necessary. The managed care group experienced greater difficulty (21% versus 15%) than the fee-for-service group in seeing a specialist in the past year when one was needed.[9] Data such as these support widespread anecdotal impressions that there is a cost–quality trade-off in managed care. In addition, the media regularly report horror stories describing alleged denials of (usually specialty) care to enrollees who suffer significant morbidity or death as a result. The issue of payment source and availability of services has not been lost on patients. Fee-for-service indemnity patients had higher levels of trust in their physicians than did patients whose physicians were in salaried, capitated, or fee-for-service managed care settings.[10] The ethical obligations of MCOs, whether for-profit or not-for-profit, are seen much differently by some commentators.[11]

Minimizing Conflicts of Interest and Other Conflicts

How do MCOs and their managers prevent or minimize conflicts of interest? An indispensable first step is a willingness to acknowledge that a duality of interests is inherent in the relationships between MCOs and enrollees, physicians and the MCO, and physicians and enrollees. Awareness permits avoidance or minimization. It is also obvious that third parties have legitimate interests in physician–patient encounters, but as third-party demands for information and control increase, "physicians must reassert their own moral authority and that of their patients."[12] Without the active cooperation of health services managers, such a task is likely to be impossible.

A system of checks and balances is also needed. One solution includes an ombudsman or customer relations specialist to assist enrollees. In addition, there should be due process procedures for persons who wish to have a decision reviewed. Federally qualified HMOs must have an effective grievance procedure for enrollees. This requirement provides some protection. For the requirement to be useful, however, enrollees must know that a problem has occurred; lack of knowledge is especially problematic when subtle quality of care issues arise. Enrollees are protected if they are able to participate effectively and if management is enlightened and the education and personal characteristics of staff involved are adequate.

MCOs may use the managing physician or gatekeeper concept to limit services provided to enrollees. Such roles are certain to cause conflicts between physicians' ethical obligations to foster the best interests of their patients and the economic expectations and constraints imposed on them by the MCO.[13] Internal audits of MCO utilization data or comparisons with external data from similar MCOs enable management to determine if utilization is in an acceptable range. Comparisons such as these alert managers to problems in the delivery of services that may result from a duality of interests. Awareness of the way in which conflicts of interest arise will help prevent them or minimize their effect. Such activities are essential if managers are to meet their ethical obligations to enrollees.

Mixing the employed medical staff of an MCO with voluntary, fee-for-service physicians raises several difficult questions.

Practice Pattern Problems Persist

Cedars-Sinai is a 400-bed community hospital located in a large East Coast metropolitan area. It has a reputation as a high-quality, low-cost provider. The medical staff at Cedars-Sinai comprise board-certified physicians who are overwhelmingly solo practitioners or members of two- or three-physician practices. No single- or multispecialty group practices are affiliated with Cedars-Sinai. Hospital governance and administration handle medical staff matters cautiously and conservatively.

In 1987, a large West Coast HMO established a presence and grew rapidly. Because of its fine reputation, Cedars-Sinai became a leading provider of services for the HMO, and many of the HMO's physician-employees have admitting privileges. Almost 20% of Cedars-Sinai's inpatient days are derived from HMO enrollees.

Following a review of the HMO's utilization patterns, a West Coast consultant noted the large difference in hospital days per 1,000 enrollees between the East and West Coast branches of the HMO. The HMO's clinical director was asked to assess how many days of care and, consequently, how many premium dollars could be saved by adopting the West Coast utilization level.

Word of this study came to the attention of Cedars-Sinai's CEO, who was immediately alarmed by the implications. She knew that reducing lengths of stay in any significant way by moving utilization patterns toward the West Coast experience would send shock waves through the majority of her medical staff—the voluntary, fee-for-service physicians who already believed that the HMO's physicians were underutilizing services. One consequence of such a disparity in patient-day utilization patterns could be a decision by her medical staff leadership not to reappoint the HMO's physician-employees to the medical staff because her voluntary medical staff would judge that the lengths of stay were inappropriately short and risked patient morbidity and mortality.

The CEO faces a true ethical dilemma: She has a duty of loyalty (fiduciary obligation) to the organization, but she also has a duty of beneficence to patients treated in the hospital and to potential patients in the community. Medical staff conflict will negatively affect the hospital's financial situation.

Yet, decreasing lengths of stay consistent with quality of care, patient safety, and patient satisfaction is desirable from the standpoint of patients and payers and meets the hospital's social responsibility as well. Evolutionary movement toward shorter lengths of stay may meet the needs of both groups, although neither is likely to consider it desirable.

Long-Term Cost Savings of Managed Care

As of this writing, the easy cost savings from managed care have been realized; the lower rate of health services inflation during the 1990s partly reflects this finding. The low-hanging fruit has been picked. Primarily, the savings resulted from lower payments to providers, with other payers subsidizing the deep discounts demanded and received by MCOs. Absent cross-subsidies, managed care could not have received the pricing it did and thus could not have shown the savings. For example, in the 1990s, U.S. Healthcare, a large HMO, doubled its profit margin in 2 years by cutting the fees paid to doctors and hospitals 12%–20%, not by enhancing productivity or quality.[14]

A 1995 Congressional Budget Office (CBO) report stated that "the most efficient health maintenance organizations cut patients' use of health services by 19.6% while maintaining levels of care roughly comparable to other types of health plans."[15] This statement is contradictory on its face; its accuracy hinges on how services and care were defined. The CBO identified two caveats. The first was that the finding applied only to staff- and group-model HMOs, which employ physicians; similar savings were not found in independent practice association–model HMOs, a type that is popular among enrollees. The second caveat was that even if all insured people enrolled in staff- and group-model HMOs, healthcare costs would not decrease 19.6%—administrative costs, pricing decisions, and doctor and hospital fees would also be factors. The study also questioned whether the successes of prepaid care among relatively younger, healthier individuals, who tend to choose HMOs, can be replicated among sicker patients, who tend to choose fee-for-service insurance. A major unknown is the amount that enrollees spent out-of-pocket for health services their plans did not cover, such as access to specialty referrals.

Managed competition was the cornerstone of the Clinton health plan in 1993. In that context, *managed* was a euphemism for government regulation and control. The accountable care organizations of the Obama healthcare plan passed in 2010 are similar in concept and effect. Given that basic benefits packages were mandated and that providers would have been highly regulated, savings might have occurred, but only in the short term. Significant economic costs would have been borne by providers, and there would have been large noneconomic costs to users, especially in the long term. In addition, the inevitable expenditure caps, as in the British National Health System or in Canada's global budgets, would have invariably led to less access for referrals and high-technology, high-cost procedures.

In the late 1990s and early in the third millennium, MCOs increased premiums significantly. In 2004, net income was projected to increase 16% to $6 billion on revenue of about $225 billion,[16] which produced a profit margin of less than 3%. In 2008, profits as a percent of revenues for healthcare insurance and managed care were just 2.2%.[17]

Short of capitation, the ability of MCOs to reduce or even control costs in the future will depend on how well they can begin "managing care." Financial incentives and disincentives to enrollees are likely to be important. Clinical practice guidelines, disease management, utilization control, and financial incentives and disincentives for physicians and health services organizations were interim steps in the evolution of managed care—itself a likely way station in the progression to direct contracting between employers or other groups and health services providers, thus eliminating the middle man.[18]

Ultimately, however, *managed care* must become *managed lives*. Healthcare costs are best controlled by reducing health risks, which inevitably means affecting lifestyles. Lifestyle initiatives may be economic, such as charging higher premiums for people with unhealthy habits; medical, such as early detection of disease or disenrolling noncompliant enrollees; or legal, such as providers or MCOs lobbying for passage of laws that promote healthful activities or limit those that are unhealthy.[19] In its latter stages, this evolution will bring us an Orwellian relationship with MCOs. Even then, delaying death from preventable diseases will only bring more people to slow, long-term deaths from chronic diseases, especially those of neurological etiology. Total costs to the health services system are likely to increase, not decrease.

CONCLUSION

The competitive environment in the field of health services brought with it the perception that marketing was essential. Almost universally during the 1980s, health services organizations engaged in marketing, at least at the level of building name recognition. For the not-for-profit organization especially, the question of whether to market raised a host of ethical issues that began with the basic question of the propriety of marketing itself and extended to issues such as creating demand and distinguishing among various types of demand.

Physicians are reacting to the constraints of third-party payers and managed care in one of two ways. More than a third admit to having deceived insurance companies to help patients by exaggerating an illness's severity so patients can be hospitalized longer, or billing for incorrect diagnoses and reporting nonexistent symptoms. More than half of physicians approve of such deceitful practices.[20] That physicians believe it is necessary to deceive third-party payers and risk civil and criminal penalties suggests major problems in that system of payment. The second reaction to third-party constraints is that physicians are refusing to participate. They are cutting their ties with insurers and asking patients to pay for their services directly and then seek reimbursement from the insurer. This has put patients in the middle and has forced payers to review their policies and relationships with physicians.[21] Some physicians simply decide to retire early or leave clinical practice entirely.[22] These problems cry out for solutions, especially since the trend appears to be accelerating.

Hospitals struggling with mountains of uncompensated care see offering better reimbursed services as a way to offset losses. "No margin, no mission" has become such an oft-repeated justification that it is almost cliché. More fiscally sound hospitals must ask themselves whether they are meeting a general duty under the principle of justice to offer unprofitable but necessary services that benefit the wider community.

As with all activities undertaken by the health services organization, philosophy and mission statements provide an ethical context for marketing. Managers should apply the virtues of honesty, candor, trustworthiness, and compassion in the organization's marketing. The principle of justice suggests that careful attention must be paid to the groups and medical conditions at which marketing is focused. Non–MCO health services organizations have the same ethical problems.

It behooves health services managers to read beyond the headlines and to be especially skeptical of claims that certain remedies are universal cures. Research findings must also be questioned, especially when studies from small samples or small universes are generalized to a wider population. Painting with a broad brush should alert everyone. As in life, when something sounds too good to be true, it probably is.

Institutional ethics committees (IECs) should assess prospectively and retrospectively the ethical issues raised in competition, marketing, and managed care. They should review the ethical implications of competition as it affects their patients, organization, and community. Marketing initiatives and their results should be understood from an ethical perspective, especially in terms of creating demand and the honesty and promise keeping involved. IECs can be valuable in monitoring care and outcomes to provide assurance that patients in managed care, as well as in other payment categories, receive the same, high-quality levels of care.

NOTES

1. Researchers: Risky heart attack therapy often unneeded. (1998, June 17). *CNN Interactive*. Retrieved January 12, 2004, from http://www.cnn.com/HEALTH/9806/17/mild.heart.attacks.
2. Anthony T. Corcoran, Pamela B. Peele, & Ronald M. Benoit. (2010). Cost comparison between watchful waiting with active surveillance and active treatment of clinically localized prostate cancer. *Urology 76*(3), pp. 703–707.
3. John J. Hanlon & George E. Pickett. (1990). *Public health: Administration and practice* (9th ed., p. 4). St. Louis: Times Mirror/Mosby College Publications.
4. American Hospital Association. (2010, September 11). *SHSMD advisory: Principles and practices for marketing and communication in hospitals and health systems*. Retrieved March 4, 2011, from http://www.shsmd.org/shsmd/resources/marketingcommunicationsadvisory.pdf.
5. Pam Belluck. (2009, May 25). Webcast your brain surgery? Hospitals see marketing tool. *New York Times*. Retrieved December 6, 2010, from http://www.nytimes.com/2009/05/25/health/25hospital.html?_r=1&scp=1&sq=webcast%20your%20brain%20surgery?&st=cse.
6. Gienna Shaw. (2010). Marketing: Are social media's rewards worth the risks? *HealthLeaders Media*. Retrieved March 4, 2011, from http://www.healthleadersmedia.com/content/235746/topic/WS_HLM2_MAG/Marketing-Are-Social-Medias-Rewards-Worth-the-Risks.html.
7. Peter Wehrwein. (1998, June). The big squeeze. *Managed Care Magazine*. Retrieved January 2, 2004, from http://www.managedcaremag.com/archives/9806/9806.squeeze.shtml.
8. American Medical Association. (2001, June). *AMA code of medical ethics*. Retrieved December 10, 2010, from http://www.ama-assn.org/ama/pub/physician-resources/medical-ethics/code-medical-ethics/principles-medical-ethics.shtml.
9. Sick patients not fond of managed care plans. (1995, October). *Medical Ethics Advisor*, p. 133, citing findings of a study conducted by the Harvard University School of Public Health.
10. Halina Brukner. (2001, February 15). Only human? The effect of financial productivity incentives on physicians' use of preventive care measures. *American Journal of Medicine 110*(3), pp. 226–228.
11. Allen Buchanan. (1998, August). Managed care: Rationing without justice, but not unjustly. *Journal of Health Politics, Policy and Law 23*(4), pp. 616–634.

12. Warren L. Holleman, David C. Edwards, & Christine C. Matson. (1994, Summer). Obligations of physicians to patients and third-party payers. *Journal of Clinical Ethics 5*(2), p. 120.
13. Edmund D. Pellegrino. (1994, Fall). Managed care and managed competition: Some ethical reflections. *Calyx 4*(4), p. 3.
14. Steven Findlay. (1994, October). The managed care dilemma. *Business and Health*, p. 66.
15. Spencer Rich. (1995, March 19). Study finds savings in some HMOs. *Washington Post*, p. A5.
16. Evan Pondel. (2003, October 22). HMO profits rising again; premium increases may fuel 16% gain. *Daily News of Los Angeles*. Retrieved March 5, 2011, from http://www.consumerwatchdog.org/story/hmo-profits-rising-again-premium-increases-may-fuel-16-gain.
17. Top industries: Most profitable. (2009, May 4). CNNMoney.com. Retrieved January 8, 2011, from http://money.cnn.com/magazines/fortune/fortune500/2009/performers/industries/profits/.
18. Wehrwein.
19. E. Haavi Morreim. (1995, November/December). Lifestyles of the risky and infamous: From managed care to managed lives. *Hastings Center Report 25*, pp. 5–6.
20. Doctors say they deceive insurers to help patients. (2000, April 12). *Washington Post*, p. A11; Ellen Goodman. (2000, April 15). Medical civil disobedience. *Washington Post*, p. A21. When third-party payers find physicians mischaracterizing services, they change the rules. In turn, physicians become more clever at finding ways to provide the services their patients need. This is a war of escalation between payers and physicians that leads from one deception to another.
21. Julie Appleby. (2000, July 20). Frustrated doctors rebel against insurers. *USA Today*, p. 1B.
22. Yuki Noguchi. (2003, December 23). No heart for the business: A cardiologist learns that fixing broken hearts is a tough way to make a living these days. *Washington Post*, p. F1.

CHAPTER 13

ETHICS IN RESOURCE ALLOCATION

E thical issues are integral to resource allocation decisions. Whether resource allocation affects populations or groups (macroallocation) or individuals (microallocation), it involves making choices. Decisions are based on explicit or implicit criteria. Some managers use subjective criteria such as social worth, usefulness to society, and need; others use more objective criteria such as selection through a lottery or queue or ability to pay once medical need has been determined. Values and philosophical statements about individuals and society underlie both, although these are usually implicit and may be only vaguely understood by decision makers.

Various methods and guidelines are used by decision makers in allocating resources. Often, decisions made by governments are based on economic or political motives. Like governments, health services organizations involve managers and clinicians in making macroallocation decisions. Microallocation in health services means making decisions about clinical treatment for individuals and involves nonclinician managers to a lesser extent. Important aspects of microallocation decision making are a physician's willingness to refer, a patient's geographic and economic access to services and technologies, and a patient's desire for treatment. Decisions at the micro level are often guided (in a sense, prejudged) by macroallocation decisions that the organization (or government) has made. Carefully husbanding resources is an important dimension of both macro- and microallocation decisions. Emphasis in the latter has led to efforts to minimize use of clinical resources when there is no reasonable hope of benefit.

As noted in Chapter 1, utilitarians judge the morality of an act by assessing the results produced and determining which course of action results in the greatest good for the greatest number. Economists and managers use this approach in cost–benefit analyses. Applying criteria of utility is only a partial answer, however. This narrow approach ignores considerations of human need, fairness, and justice, all of which health services managers find important.

MACROALLOCATION

Specific theories have been developed to suggest how macroallocation does or should occur. The concept of a right to healthcare is prominent in several theories. An extreme view is hyper-egalitarianism, which asserts that all treatments must be available to all persons needing them. Its corollary is that treatments not available to all should be available to none. This theory is an extreme expression of respect for persons and mandates that society recognize an inherent right to equal health services. Providing different levels of treatment implies that some persons are, in effect, given less respect than others are. Equal respect means receiving equal healthcare services, consistent with need. If this criterion cannot be met, the treatment should be available to none.

At the other end of the continuum are those who assert that health services are a privilege, not a right guaranteed by society. This hyper-individualistic position holds that health services providers, such as physicians, have no moral obligation to render services. In providing services, they act out of free will and humanitarian instinct. Hyper-individualists argue that if there were a right to healthcare, providers would be obliged to render services. An obligation (duty) to render services diminishes the freedom and dignity of providers and fails to recognize their inherent value and worth as human beings, thus violating the respect they are owed.

Between these extremes is the position that society has a duty to assist in developing, encouraging, and even providing health services. Fried argued that routine basic services ought to be available to all, a position known as the "decent minimum."[1] Beyond the decent minimum, this concept allows persons to purchase additional service as resources and interest permit. Contrast this approach with the Oregon Health Plan, which offers equal access to specified services for those covered by Medicaid. It prioritizes health services and pays for them to the extent that the legislature-approved budget allows. In effect, this rations services. Implicitly it uses hyper-egalitarianism, which, proponents argue, means sacrifice for some Medicaid recipients but equal, if limited, access for all.

Generally, exotic, high-technology services are limited because of location, cost, and referrals and are available on a different basis. Political decision making limits such services in publicly funded programs.

Governing bodies and managers of health services organizations face similar questions in macroallocation decisions. Typically, beneficence, fidelity (promise keeping), and justice are applied and supplemented by various of the virtues.

Ultimately, such values result in answers to questions of who gets what, when, where, and how. These questions are found in many issues, such as whether to build a new outpatient department, when to purchase a magnetic resonance imager, and how to allocate staff. Answering these questions requires careful attention to economic considerations. Financial well-being enables the organization to undertake its mission, a common aspect of which is serving the socially and economically disadvantaged.

The organization's mission and values provide the context for macroallocation decisions. General criteria that may be applied include 1) the needs of external (the service area), interface (physicians), and internal (staff and volunteers) stakeholders (but primarily the first) and 2) the goal of improving or providing high-quality services at a competitive price. Cost–benefit analyses are useful in measuring the desirability of projects, but these should be part of the general screening of projects. It is very likely that several proposals for macroallocation expenditures (e.g., programs, capital equipment, physical plant) will be allowed to proceed. It is from this list that organizational values and mission are applied for a final selection.

The Feasibility of Brain Electrical Activity Mapping

Brain electrical activity mapping (BEAM) is a relatively new technology used to image the brain. It significantly improves the ability to localize an abnormality. Responding to demands for the procedure from staff radiologists and local neurologists, and to reports in the literature on its usefulness, City Hospital decided to investigate the possibility of acquiring access to BEAM. Options included leasing, purchasing, and approaching nearby County Hospital about sharing its recently acquired BEAM machine.

A factor in the decision was uncertainty as to how changes in reimbursement would affect hospital revenues. These questions about reimbursement and a potential major expenditure of capital funds caused the chairman of the board to ask the chief executive officer to form a committee to evaluate options, including forgoing access to BEAM. This assessment would be used to make a final decision between BEAM and a proposed addition to the intensive care unit, a project that is strongly supported by the surgical staff and has already been delayed twice.

The board wanted to delay the decision on BEAM until the reimbursement implications were understood, but several attending physicians stated that

BEAM testing is critical to their practices. They said they prefer the nursing staff at City but felt that they will be forced to admit certain patients to County in order to use BEAM. A rumor surfaced among the medical staff that several prominent members were considering forming a consortium to purchase and operate BEAM and other diagnostic equipment in a professional office complex under construction.[2]

What are the important aspects of this case? First, the new technology will improve the quality of care. Second, its availability will affect the organization's financial situation—operating costs for BEAM are high, typically exceeding capital costs in a few years. Reimbursement issues complicate financial considerations. Third, the physicians are divided about the expenditure, and this adds to the complexity of medical staff politics. Fourth, BEAM is expensive technology, which makes the decision even more important and difficult.

The obvious starting point in solving this problem is to review the organizational philosophy and vision and mission statements. If City Hospital's mission is to serve special populations or needs, both BEAM and an ICU addition may use resources in a manner consistent with that mission. Are there even better uses for the resources? The various issues are not easily resolved, but internal decision processes, such as an ethics committee, can be of assistance. The expected context for decision making will be the organizational philosophy, as reflected in the strategic plan, which was described in Chapter 3. The technological imperative is present not only in delivering services to individual patients but also in macroallocation decisions.

In another example, senior management of a for-profit hospital system decided to spend $3.8 million for a piece of statuary while denying payment for heart transplants; this is a macroallocation decision with profound effects on service availability (microallocation). The statue was used to decorate the corporate offices.[3] No one expects the corporate offices of a multibillion-dollar organization to have Sheetrock walls and bare floors; it would seem, however, that the virtue of temperance ought to guide one's decisions in such situations.

MICROALLOCATION

One usually thinks of microallocation decisions in terms of exotic lifesaving treatment. All scarce resources require allocation, however, and that scarcity may be a function of time and circumstances.

Who Gets the Penicillin?

In 1943, penicillin was new and in short supply among U.S. armed forces in North Africa. Competitors for its use were two groups of soldiers suffering from infections that would respond to it: those with venereal disease and those with battle wounds. The chief surgical consultant advised that priority be given to the wounded; the theater medical commander directed that priority be given to soldiers with venereal disease, arguing that soldiers cured of venereal disease could be restored to fighting trim more rapidly, and that left untreated, such men represented a threat of spreading the infection. The decision to use the penicillin on soldiers with venereal disease was a pragmatic judgment consistent with the morality of utility in a situation where objectives—achieving maximum fighting power as rapidly as possible—were narrowly defined.[4]

Exclusively treating men infected with venereal disease is the morally correct choice only if the utilitarian criterion of returning the greatest number of troops to the line as quickly as possible is applied. This decision is made without judging either the relative worth of the soldiers in need of treatment or the way in which they came to require it.

A contemporary example of microallocation decisions involves non-American transplant recipients who obtain human organs from American donors. Often these patients come from countries in which technological impediments or religious and social customs prevent organ harvesting. They pay out-of-pocket rather than from private or public sources; the additional revenue makes them favored by transplant centers. In addition, they are generally willing to accept organs that may be "less fresh" or are not optimal tissue matches. Transplanting organs harvested in the United States into non-Americans raises legitimate concerns about priorities in a system in which American patients wait for organs while non-Americans receive them.

Theories of allocating exotic lifesaving treatment to individual patients have been developed by James Childress and Nicholas Rescher.[5] They address the problem of how decisions about who gets what should be made. Childress rejected the use of subjective criteria, such as worth to society, because such comparisons demean the potential recipient and run counter to a belief in the inherent dignity of each human being. His position is Kantian because it stresses respect for persons and its derivative, autonomy. He argued that a system that views all persons requiring treatment as equals recognizes inherent human worth. According to Childress, once medical criteria determine the need for and the appropriateness of therapy, opportunities for exotic lifesaving treatment should be available on a first-come, first-served basis or, alternatively, through some random selection process, such as a lottery.

A prominent ethicist, the late Paul Ramsey, agreed with Childress as to the desirability of a lottery or a policy of first-come, first-served that ignores the subjective judgments that one finds in other, criteria-oriented schemes. At the same time, Ramsey found nondiscriminatory, predetermined, and announced rules based on statistical medical probabilities to be acceptable. This view would, for example, permit groups such as the very young and the very old to be excluded from kidney dialysis programs.[6] This type of macroallocation criterion is used in the decision making of centralized European health systems.

Rescher's schema has two tiers. The first tier is devoted to basic screening and applies to groups of potential patients. It consists of factors such as constituency served, benefit to science, and likelihood of success by type of treatment or recipient. The second tier deals with individuals. It judges medical factors (e.g., relative likelihood of success, life expectancy) and social aspects, such as family role, potential future contributions, and past services rendered. Rescher stated that if all factors are equal, a random selection process should be used for the final choice. The social aspects caused Rescher the most difficulty because they rely heavily on value judgments. However, Rescher considered it irrational to make choices subject to chance alone once screening medical criteria are met.

Each of these microallocation theories has advantages and disadvantages, both moral and pragmatic. Each theory develops a formal or semiformal process that permits users to address issues and problems in an organized manner. Although the decision may not be satisfactory to all, the theories offer the advantage of an identified system that at least provides frameworks within which to make decisions. Given that medical criteria are met, a person's chances of being selected for exotic lifesaving treatment may be unpredictable (Childress), partially predictable (Ramsey), or almost totally predictable (Rescher). The basis for selection may hinge on largely subjective criteria (Rescher) or may be solely a matter of chance, and in that sense eminently fair to all who need the treatment (Childress) or all who meet the criteria for medical statistical probabilities (Ramsey).

Choices

Randy Glenn had just fallen asleep when the telephone rang. It was the night supervisor at the comprehensive care center and hospital at which Glenn was the chief executive officer. The supervisor was quite agitated and had trouble getting her words out. It took a few minutes for the message to become clear. One of Glenn's nightmares had come true: The four-bed ICU was full and an emergency case had just arrived.

The night supervisor explained that the new patient had been injured in a car accident. She had been stabilized in the emergency department but neither air medevac nor mobile ICU ambulance services were available. It was certain that she would not survive transfer by any other means. She needed to be admitted to the ICU within 2 hours.

The night supervisor then quickly described the patients currently occupying ICU beds:

- Patient A: 60-year-old woman, comatose, stroke victim who required respirator support, 27 days in the ICU; uncertain prognosis; retired; no family; city resident
- Patient B: 9-year-old boy with Down syndrome, acute respiratory infection; 4 days in ICU; family in adjacent city
- Patient C: 36-year-old man who had undergone an emergency appendectomy, developed severe wound infection and probable septicemia; source of infection unknown; requires ICU care for blood pressure instability secondary to sepsis; bachelor, mother lives in city
- Patient D: 12-year-old girl undergoing chemotherapy for leukemia with an experimental drug; has been in remission three times; monitoring of experimental protocol and potential reaction to drug requires ICU care; family in city
- New Patient: 24-year-old woman; college honor student in physics, scholarship winner; pregnant, engaged; no family known

The supervisor ended the telephone call by asking Glenn, "What should I do?" Indeed, what to do, thought Glenn, who suddenly wished the institutional ethics committee had been more active. Glenn pondered the alternatives as the garage door opened and the 10-minute ride to the center began.[7]

This is the classic "last bed in the ICU" ethical dilemma. Under Childress's and Ramsey's criteria, if all patients meet the medical criteria for ICU care, the new patient would be left to receive the best care she could get outside the ICU. Applying Rescher's criteria, the medical prognosis (likelihood of successful treatment) and the social aspects (potential future contributions) for one of the current patients are not as good as those for the new patient. Thus, one of the current patients should be removed from the ICU. None of the models allows the decision maker to abandon a patient unable to receive ICU care. All models would provide the best alternative care available.

General awareness of how choices are made may or may not enhance the public's view that health services organizations and the system act justly. Public scrutiny, however, will focus greater attention on decision criteria, the decision process, and the fairness of their application. Kantian principles of respect for persons and of not using persons as ends are reflected in Childress's approach, which stresses autonomy. Rescher's approach includes a mix of Kantian and utilitarian views and, most important, emphasizes justice, as described in Chapter 1. Some health services organizations make resource allocation decisions using formal ethical criteria—the preferred method. As with all macroallocation decisions, these criteria must be developed within the context of the organizational philosophy and the vision and mission statements.

Near-Futile Treatment

Some situations have all the elements of futility save one—the patient is not terminally ill. Sidney Miller's birth is such a case. Sidney was expected to die shortly after birth; aggressive intervention kept her alive, albeit with significant disabilities. In many respects, cases such as Sidney's are the most difficult of all. The literature has yet to use the concept of near-futile treatment, but it is appropriately distinguished from futile treatment. The Sidney Miller case should be borne in mind and distinguished from the discussion of futile treatment below.

Sidney Miller[8]

In 2003, Sidney Miller was 12 years of age. In 1991, she was a (23-week) premature infant delivered to Karla and Mark Miller at the Woman's Hospital of Texas in Houston. At birth, Karla's obstetrician told the Millers that the infant was unlikely to survive. The parents determined that Sidney should receive comfort care in the form of food, water, and warmth. She would survive or not on her own.

Other physicians recommended an experimental procedure that would likely result in brain damage or severe disability. Again, the parents chose comfort care. Hospital administrators overrode the Millers' decision and told them that an unwritten hospital policy and the "law" required that they resuscitate infants who weigh more than 500 grams (1.1 pounds).

The experimental treatment was undertaken. Sidney survived. At 12 years of age, her cognitive age is 3 months, she has cerebral palsy, and she cannot walk or talk. Sidney will require lifelong care.

The Millers sued. In 1998, a Texas jury awarded them $60.4 million against Columbia/HCA, the owners of the Woman's Hospital of Texas in Houston.

In 2000, a Texas court of appeals overturned the jury verdict, citing the state's advance medical directives law: "Parents are only allowed to withhold or withdraw life-sustaining medical treatment from a child where the child's condition has been certified in writing by a physician to be terminal." The appeals court did not address the countless other decisions to continue aggressive treatment of Sidney during 7 months of hospitalization.

In mid-2003, the Texas Supreme Court agreed with the appeals court. The Millers will receive nothing.

Ethical Issues in the Miller Case   The ethical issues of Sidney Miller's case are clouded by questions of applicable law. The federal Child Abuse Prevention and Treatment Act Amendments of 1984 (PL 98-457) allow physicians to decline to treat a newborn when the infant is chronically and irreversibly comatose, when treating would only prolong dying or not correct all life-threatening conditions, or when treatment would be virtually futile and inhumane. The Texas court of appeals did not refer to the federal law, citing instead state law requiring that a physician certify in writing that the infant's condition is terminal. Apparently, such a determination had not been made.

Ethicists are in broad agreement that withholding and withdrawing life-sustaining treatment are morally indistinguishable. The psychology of these two actions is very different, however. Withdrawing life-sustaining treatment seems to cause death, and family and caregivers may find it difficult to recognize that the underlying medical condition or the disease process causes death, not the act of withdrawing life-sustaining treatment. When it is certain that continuing to treat is futile (no hope of benefit), caregivers and decision makers will have less difficulty discontinuing treatment. Paradoxically, Karla Miller could have had a legal abortion, even while in labor, had she chosen to do so.

It is unclear if the hospital actually had a written policy (or policies) regarding the role of parents in cases like this. The principle of justice (fairness) requires that the hospital's policy regarding aggressive resuscitation and a trial period on a ventilator be communicated to the Millers before the start of labor. This information would have allowed an informed choice; they might have chosen to abort the fetus, or seek medical care elsewhere.

Sidney was hospitalized for 7 months; the costs of care totaled millions of dollars. Regardless of payment source, one must question whether these resources were used wisely. It may be time to reconsider expenditures with such limited positive results. In the case of premature infants, however, this debate must factor in the high levels of uncertainty in making accurate prognoses.

FUTILITY THEORY

Modern technology allows clinicians to support life far into the dying process. Applying technology when there is a probability or even hope of benefit raises few ethical issues. Treatment continued beyond hope of benefit suggests futility. Applying the futility concept has been described as a unilateral do-not-resuscitate (DNR) order, a decision made by physicians using a physiologic definition.[9] At its root, futility theory focuses on the absence of benefit from continued treatment. Quality of life is not expressly considered, even though it cannot be ignored as a psychological factor that the physician may implicitly consider. Futility guidelines address the issue of demands for treatment that clinicians judge to offer no hope of benefit. Rare, almost miraculous recoveries haunt decision makers and cloud futility theory and its application. Such patients improve months or even years after reasonable hope of benefit from life-sustaining treatment should have ended. Sometimes, the improvement is dramatic.[10,11]

Futile treatment invariably raises questions of resource consumption and economics. A skeptic might ask whether economics are really the driving force. Similar questions have been raised about advance medical directives (AMDs), which are touted as giving patients control but almost always only limit services. Some futile treatment policies specifically address resource consumption and the moral obligation of the health services organization to use its resources judiciously.

Background

In many ways, futility theory is old wine in new bottles. Its origins lie in the distinction between ordinary and extraordinary care, which is restated here. *Ordinary care* is all medicines, treatments, and operations that offer reasonable hope of benefit and that can be obtained without excessive expense, pain, or other inconvenience. *Extraordinary care* is all medicines, treatments, and operations that cannot be obtained or used without excessive expense, pain, or inconvenience, or that, if used, would not offer a reasonable hope of benefit. This definition makes it ethical to withhold any medicine, treatment, or operation that offers no reasonable hope of benefit or that cannot be obtained or used without excessive expense, pain, or inconvenience. A common mistake is to define ordinary as usual or customary treatment; this results in statements such as "Ill persons must always be given food and water because this is ordinary (i.e., usual and customary) care."

Futility theory has quantitative and qualitative aspects. The *quantitative* aspect is concerned with the probability of success if a treatment were attempted or continued. Probability of success means that the treatment can be successfully performed and achieve its intended purpose. So, for example, tube feeding will sustain the life of a patient in a persistent vegetative state (PVS), but it will not restore cognition. This highlights the importance of viewing care as a continuum, not an isolated event. More than two-thirds of states allow patients (through AMDs), and their proxies and surrogates, to make decisions about withdrawing or withholding artificial hydration and nutrition in cases of PVS without judicial intervention or assistance.[12]

Qualitative assumes a successful treatment that achieves its intended purpose, but it asks whether the result is such that the treatment ought to be undertaken. The quantitative determination is made by clinical experts. The qualitative determination (judgment) can be made only by the patient or, as necessary, the patient's surrogate. The concept of futility limits the qualitative decision.

Three basic variations of circumstances raise questions of futile treatment. The first is that patients demand services that offer no reasonable hope of benefit. Lacking data, this situation may be an urban myth or a largely incorrect perception. AMDs generally limit medical intervention, although they may demand services that clinicians later deem futile.

A second type of futile treatment occurs when organizations insist on providing treatment that surrogates have determined offers no reasonable hope of benefit and should end. The cases of Karen Ann Quinlan and Nancy Beth Cruzan illustrate such policies (especially Cruzan, whose continued treatment was required by state law). Quinlan and Cruzan suggest that futility policies are better directed toward legislators, organizations, and staff than patients and families.

The third type occurs when treatment is continued because surrogate decision makers demand it. An example is the case of Helga Wanglie, a Minneapolis woman in PVS whose husband demanded all efforts to keep her alive, despite a prognosis that doing so offered no reasonable hope of benefit.[13] Another example is Baby K, an anencephalic infant whose mother would not authorize a DNR order, but rather insisted that all treatment continue.

Baby K

The legal case captioned *In the Matter of Baby K** began in 1992, when a baby girl with anencephaly was born at Fairfax Hospital in northern

*The identities of the mother and child were sealed by the court and were not revealed until after the U.S. Supreme Court refused to review the federal appeals court decision.

Virginia. This case raises several ethical issues; the focus here is on resource allocation and the organization's obligations when futile treatment
is demanded.

This case is distinguished from others involving infants with anencephaly in that the mother demanded that everything be done for Baby K.
In the realm of ethics, decisions about infants with anencephaly raise questions of futile treatment. In politics, such emotionally charged situations
are almost beyond public debate, and politicians will undoubtedly flee any
discussion of them.

Anencephaly is a rare congenital anomaly in which the cerebral cortex
of the brain has not developed and the top of the skull and scalp are absent.
It is estimated that 1,000–2,000 infants with anencephaly are born annu-
ally in the United States. Most die within hours or days of birth, with or
without intervention. Some are born with better-developed brain stems
and live for weeks or months. Rarely do infants with anencephaly live longer. Baby K was an exception and lived 2 years, with the need for intermit-
tent aggressive intervention.

Clinical Aspects   Baby K's anencephaly had been diagnosed prena-
tally. The mother, Ms. H, continued the pregnancy despite the recommendations of her obstetrician and a neonatologist that termination would
be best. Baby K's father was not married to her mother and was not involved in her care or the decision making about it. He did, however, support efforts to have a DNR order written.

Baby K was delivered by cesarean section. She was born permanently
unconscious and could not see, hear, or otherwise interact with her environment. Brain stem functions were limited to feeding and respiratory
reflexes, and she reflexively responded to sound or touch. Mechanical ventilation was begun at birth, but it served no therapeutic or palliative purpose because the underlying anencephaly was untreatable.

Ethical and Legal Aspects   The physicians urged the mother to authorize a DNR order, but she refused and would not authorize discontinuation of the ventilator. Ms. H and Baby K's physicians met with a
specially appointed three-person panel of the hospital ethics committee,
two of whom were physicians (a family practitioner and a psychiatrist).
The third member was a minister. The panel "concluded that Baby K's
ventilator treatment should end because 'such care was futile' and decided
to 'wait a reasonable time for the family to help the caregiver terminate
aggressive therapy.'"[14] If the mother refused to follow the advice, the panel

recommended that the hospital seek a legal solution. Ms. H rejected the ethics panel's recommendation.

Baby K was successfully weaned from the ventilator. After disagreement about treatment, Fairfax Hospital sought to move her to another hospital, but other hospitals with pediatric ICUs declined. Six weeks after the birth, Ms. H allowed Baby K to be transferred to a nursing facility on the condition that Baby K could be readmitted to the hospital if respiratory problems recurred. Indeed, Baby K was brought to the hospital in respiratory distress several times after the transfer. Between acute episodes, Baby K remained at the nursing facility and did not require life-sustaining treatment except for occasional use of a ventilator.

Trial Court   To protect itself legally, Fairfax Hospital sought a declaratory judgment in federal district court that it would not violate the Emergency Medical Treatment and Active Labor Act (EMTALA) of 1986 (PL 99-272), the Rehabilitation Act of 1973 (PL 93-112), or the Americans with Disabilities Act (ADA) of 1990 (PL 101-336) by refusing to administer life-sustaining treatment to an infant with anencephaly. The EMTALA requires that emergency departments (ED) in hospitals that receive Medicare funds must treat all who arrive at the ED with emergency medical conditions and continue treatment until the person can be transferred safely. The Rehabilitation Act and the ADA prohibit discrimination because of handicap or disability, respectively.

The hospital conceded that respiratory distress is an emergency condition but argued that the EMTALA should be interpreted to include an exception for treatment deemed "futile" or "inhumane" by hospital physicians. The trial judge found no such exception in the EMTALA; regardless, he reasoned, the exception would not apply to Baby K because her breathing could be restored and therefore mechanical ventilation could not be considered futile or inhumane. The trial court also found that Baby K's condition was a handicap and a disability, and therefore that the hospital could not legally refuse treatment (per the Rehabilitation Act and the ADA, respectively). Denying care to Baby K would constitute discrimination. The trial court ruled further that as a general matter of law, absent a finding of neglect or abuse, parents have a constitutionally protected right under the 14th Amendment's due process clause to raise children as they see fit and to make decisions about their medical treatment. The judge concluded that when parents disagree, the courts should support the parent who decides in favor of life. The attorney appointed by the court as guardian *ad litem* (guardian for the purposes of a legal proceeding) for

Baby K agreed with the hospital. Fairfax Hospital appealed the trial court decision.

Appeals Court   In a 2 to 1 decision, the 4th U.S. Circuit Court of Appeals affirmed the trial court decision. It ruled that the EMTALA requires hospitals receiving Medicare funds to provide care in life-threatening situations, regardless of the patient's condition. The appeals court determined that because the hospital had a duty to render medically stabilizing treatment under the EMTALA, there was no need to determine the hospital's obligations under other federal statutes or the laws of Virginia.

The majority agreed with the hospital that the standard of care for infants with anencephaly is to provide only warmth, hydration, and nutrition. Nevertheless, it held that the statutory language was unambiguous and included no such limitation. The majority declined to legislate from the bench:

> It is beyond the limits of our judicial function to address the moral or ethical propriety of providing emergency stabilizing medical treatment to anencephalic infants. We are bound to interpret federal statutes in accordance with their language and any expressed congressional intent.[15]

The dissenting judge argued that the EMTALA was enacted to prevent patients from being "dumped" for economic reasons, that dumping was not an issue for Baby K, and that therefore the statute should not apply. Baby K's respiratory failures related to anencephaly; her necessary care should be viewed as a continuum in which no medical treatment can improve her condition of permanent unconsciousness.

Aftermath   Before the appeals court decision in 1993, Fairfax Hospital issued a statement:

> We believe that continuing to provide extraordinary measures to prolong the dying process is medically and ethically inappropriate, and not in the best interests of this infant. . . . The hospital and its physicians remain ready to provide appropriate medical care, which in this case includes nutrition, hydration, and warmth.[16]

In 1994, the U.S. Supreme Court refused to hear an appeal from the appeals court decision.

Baby K had a grim prognosis but lived far longer than other infants with her condition. She died in April 1995, 2 years after her birth. Private insurance and Medicaid covered her medical bills of almost $500,000, approximately half of which was the cost of hospital services. Hospital officials' denial that economics motivated their legal action is supported by the fact that all hospital services had been paid.[17]

Analysis   Anencephaly had been diagnosed months before Baby K's birth. If the physicians believed mechanical ventilation was medically inappropriate, this should have been made clear to Ms. H at that time. She should have been encouraged to find alternative sources of physician and hospital care, which may have been impossible through her health plan. It is certain, however, that had Ms. H refused to follow the physicians' recommendation or had she been unable to find a physician and a hospital to provide the care she wanted, Fairfax Hospital and its physicians would have had no choice but to continue treating Baby K.

If mechanical ventilation were to be used, the goal of the intervention (e.g., confirmation of the diagnosis) should have been specified and respiratory support should have continued only until that goal was reached or found to be unattainable. Ms. H might have reneged on an agreement to discontinue respiratory support, however, which would have put the physicians and hospital back where they started.

Hospital administration and legal counsel seem to have overreacted. They should have supported the physicians in their application of existing medical standards and encouraged further discussions with Ms. H through the ethics committee and its special panel. Such efforts could have continued even after Baby K was discharged to the nursing facility. By going to court, they turned an issue of medical practice and medical ethics into a legal issue. Having once undertaken legal proceedings, the hospital effectively lost control of the situation—highly undesirable by any measure. Court proceedings are always difficult, expensive, unpredictable, and intensive in terms of energy and emotion. The publicity surrounding such cases is often a public relations nightmare, regardless of the result.

The appeals court decision rejected the argument that the medical standard of care should be used implicitly to guide interpretation of the EMTALA. This substantially limits the discretion of providers in terms of the circumstances that justify withholding or withdrawing care where patients have not or cannot express their wishes regarding life-sustaining treatment. Meeting the standard of care may protect physicians and hospitals from malpractice actions, which are governed by state law, but it does not protect them from liability under federal law.

The extent to which the ethics committee or its special panel sought to solve the problem from an ethical standpoint is unclear. Rarely do ethics committees make decisions, but their evaluative, educative, and consultative roles are well-known. In terms of the educative and consultative roles, all efforts should have been made to continue a dialogue with Ms. H until a resolution acceptable to both sides was reached. Here, however, they advised only on the question of futility and how clinical decisions should be addressed. Such a role is too passive.

In addition, one must question whether it was wise to focus on the medical dimensions of the case by appointing physicians as two of the three members of the special panel. Ms. H must have been knowledgeable about the clinical (scientific) aspects of anencephaly, but she chose to ignore them. This decision suggests the need to focus on the psychosocial dimensions, a task likely best undertaken by nonphysicians. The role of the member of the clergy and whether Ms. H was of his faith are unknown.

Because the ethics subcommittee and Baby K's mother were at loggerheads, mediation could have been attempted as a way to resolve the dispute. A mediator is a neutral person who works with the parties to develop an acceptable solution, which may be a compromise. In such situations, keeping the parties talking is essential to success.

Summary   The U.S. Supreme Court may consider a similar case in the future and reverse the decision in Baby K. Meanwhile, Congress can amend the EMTALA and other federal law to allow treatment to be withheld or withdrawn when caregivers judge it to be futile or inhumane. Such exceptions are found in the Child Abuse Amendments of 1984 (PL 98-457), which were enacted to prevent denial of treatment to infants with disabilities. The problem for Congress is that the political context will make it virtually impossible to deny parents the right to demand treatment even when it is deemed futile or inhumane by caregivers.

The challenge for health services organizations in cases such as Baby K will be to meld the concerns of family, caregivers, and organization in a way that eliminates or minimizes futile and inhumane treatment while meeting federal and state laws, organizational values, and the personal ethics of those involved.

Futile Treatment Guidelines

Increasingly, health services organizations, especially acute care hospitals, have futile treatment guidelines or policies. Developing and adopting them have been stimulated by the perception that patients and their surrogates demand treatment that clinicians have determined has little, if any, likelihood of benefiting the patient. Consent and autonomy drive initial phases of decision making for patients able to participate. Patients should be given the information to make an informed choice about options for treatment (or nontreatment). Especially to be tempered are unattainable goals of treatment or unrealistic expectations of medical science. Patients bear the brunt of continued treatment; this makes them more willing than surrogate decision makers to limit what is done. When patients' decisions (or demands) will not result in efficacious medical treatment or will only prolong suffering and the dying process, clinicians have a moral obligation to withhold or withdraw treatment. Typically, guidelines regarding withholding or withdrawing life-sustaining treatment require agreement of both attending and consulting physicians that the treatment is futile.

Decisions about appropriateness of continued medical treatment are made within the context of the purposes of medical care:

> There is . . . general agreement that the goals of standard medical treatment are to cure, restore, improve or maintain some level of a person's ability to think, feel, and interact with others and the environment. Medical interventions that have little likelihood of achieving any of these treatment goals can be considered futile.[18]

The futility guidelines for Trinity Health, a nationwide, faith-based health-care system, begin by positing the religious context for the guidelines, describing the role of the patient in decision making and the importance of professional integrity of caregivers, as well as the need for stewardship of resources. The guidelines continue by defining medically futile treatment and providing examples.[19] Trinity Health defines medically futile treatment as any treatment that, within a reasonable degree of medical probability, has little likelihood of

- Having any positive physiological effect on the patient's condition; or
- Reversing the patient's imminent dying; or
- Restoring the patient's ability to function as a person, i.e., his/her cognitive, affective and interactive functions.[20]

Several aspects of these futility guidelines are notable: 1) the criteria are stated in the alternative (e.g., if reversing imminent dying is likely by applying a treatment, that treatment is not futile); 2) there is no consideration of "quality of life," either as judged by the patient or someone else; and 3) there is no specific attention to the economic dimensions of the treatment being rendered.

Examples of futile treatment given by the Trinity Health guidelines include continued ventilator support for a patient who meets brain death criteria, cardiopulmonary resuscitation (CPR) for a patient with end-stage cancer that has metastasized or a patient with multiple organ failure, and aggressive therapies for a PVS or permanently comatose patient. The guidelines also outline a process for making decisions about medical futility. Steps include the following:[21]

1. Judgment that a treatment is futile is made by agreement of the attending physician, medical consultants, and caregiving team.
2. The attending physician informs the competent patient or surrogate, as appropriate, that the treatment judged medically futile will not be started or will be stopped, if already under way. Assurance will be given that comfort care will be provided.
3. If the competent patient or surrogate (as appropriate) agrees, appropriate orders will be written in the chart.
4. Lacking agreement, the ethics committee is consulted. The ethics committee determines that the guidelines' criteria have been met and assists with communication and negotiation between the parties involved.
5. Judgments about futile treatment involving incompetent patients without a surrogate will be reviewed by the ethics committee. If it concurs the attending physician will document the process in the chart and write appropriate orders.
6. If, after the ethics committee concurs with the attending physician that a treatment is medically futile, a competent patient or surrogate, as appropriate, refuses to agree, a mediator will be used to try to resolve the dispute.
7. If the patient or surrogate chooses to remain in the facility or if they remain because no alternative facility can be found the medically futile treatment will: a. not be started, b. (be) started or continued for a goal-specific or time-limited trial as the result of mediation, or, c. if started, will be discontinued.

The guidelines end by providing direction for situations in which physicians and caregivers disagree regarding potentially futile treatments. Here, the ethics committee is a significant part of the process. Emphasis is also placed on the need for ongoing dialogue with patients or surrogates. Using a mediator, who is a neutral third party, is useful to resolve disagreements as to the course of treatment, or its discontinuation. Since both parties must agree to the solution, 7b in the preceding guidelines offers the best possibility for resolving the dispute.

Futile treatment guidelines or policies should emphasize that physicians have no moral (or legal) obligation to provide treatment that they judge to be inappropriate. Physicians' professional integrity is compromised and they fail to meet their duty to their patients if they provide treatment that is of no benefit or offers no hope of benefit. Physicians fail, too, in their ethical obligation to make effective use of resources if they are used by patients for whom they offer neither benefit nor hope of benefit.

In all but five states, providers may refuse to deliver medical treatment the patient has requested. A majority of states do not require providers to act contrary to generally accepted standards of care. Eleven states permit physicians to decline to comply with healthcare decisions for reasons of conscience or personal belief. Fourteen permit providers to withhold or withdraw medical treatment based on moral convictions or religious beliefs. Oregon permits healthcare institutions or staff members to decline to act contrary to philosophical beliefs.[22] California's noncompliance provision for physicians and hospitals applies if a requested treatment "requires medically ineffective healthcare or healthcare contrary to generally accepted healthcare standards applicable to the healthcare provider or institution."[23] Similarly, the Texas Advance Directives Act (1999, known as the Texas Futile Care Law) allows a healthcare facility to discontinue life-sustaining treatment ten days after giving written notice, so long as the treating physicians judge the treatment to be medically inappropriate.[24] Despite such laws, it is doubtful that either physicians or hospitals will refuse to provide treatment that they deem futile, except after a considerable period of life-sustaining treatment and when the prognosis is unequivocal. The potential is too great for accusations from the public and media that passive, involuntary euthanasia is occurring or that patients are being treated inhumanely. Reaction to highly publicized futile treatment cases show significant levels of ignorance among the public. In this milieu, enforcing futile treatment guidelines could cause a public relations fiasco. Health services organizations should have guidelines or a policy on futile treatment, nonetheless.

The presence of guidelines will encourage physicians to take steps to withhold or withdraw futile treatment, if doing so is appropriate. Thus encouraged, their frank discussions with patients or surrogates may yield results consistent with futile treatment guidelines. By informing patients or surrogates of their moral objection to continuing treatment because it is medically inappropriate and harmful, physicians may gain assent without invoking the organization's guidelines. The "transfer out" option is probably not viable: patients will likely be too ill to transfer, or no facility will take them. However, a discussion of transfer out is useful to convince patients or surrogates how serious the problem is. Transferring out becomes even more difficult if all hospitals in a region agree to a common set of futile treatment guidelines. City-wide guidelines have been developed in Knoxville, Tennessee, and Houston, Texas. Thus, after a reasonable time without an alternative source of care, the organization must act to withhold or withdraw futile treatment.

The concept of futile treatment is not without its critics, however, as shown in the following case.[25]

Knowing Whether or When to Stop

An 18-year-old woman suffered severe brain injuries in a car accident in 1987. After a few weeks in a coma, she opened her eyes but was totally nonresponsive for 15 months. Then nurses noticed a hopeful sign when she twice seemed to obey their orders to move her leg or to close her eyes. These responses were rare, but 2 months later her physicians administered drugs to improve alertness and her condition slowly improved. Over time, she learned to answer multiple-choice questions and calculate simple math problems using eye blinks. At one point, she communicated, "Mom, I love you."

Three years after the accident, she was communicating regularly with eye blinks and could move her arms somewhat. After 5 years, she could mouth words and short phrases. Although her attention span was limited to 15 minutes, she liked to be pampered and took pleasure in teasing her nurses. Her favorite joke was pretending not to know their identities.

Her mother was overjoyed; she reveled in each small bit of progress. The young woman was sent home 5 years and 2 months after the injury, completely dependent on others. Her rehabilitation had cost well over $1 million.[26]

This tragic case suggests some of the difficulties of applying futile treatment guidelines. By emerging from PVS, this patient had a rare, almost miraculous outcome. Treatment had been continued at her family's insistence. Had the futile treatment guidelines been applied, she would have died.

Implications

Futility theory goes well beyond the contemporary concept of autonomy. Patient autonomy is a negative right, the right to be free from unwanted treatment—to be able to say no. Futility theory limits what is asserted as a positive right, the right to demand treatment—even when there is no medical benefit to receiving it. From an ethical standpoint, it is generally agreed that no positive rights exist.

Futility theory seeks to deal with the issues of extraordinary, disproportionate, and burdensome care. The decision maker is the physician. The preceding sample guidelines stated that there is a need to educate and inform the patient. The patient and/or family need not concur with the decision, however. Futility theory is very different from shared decision making in what is considered the ideal, nonpaternalistic physician–patient relationship. In fact, the problem that futility theory purports to address may be only partly attributable to patient demands. Research documents many shortcomings in the care of patients who are seriously ill and dying, especially the effectiveness of patient–physician communication.

The findings of the Study to Understand Prognoses and Preferences for Outcomes and Risks of Treatments (SUPPORT) research are compelling:

> [The] Study to Understand Prognoses and Preferences for Outcomes and Risks of Treatments patients were seriously ill, and their dying proved to be predictable, yet discussion and decisions substantially in advance of death were uncommon. Nearly half of all DNR orders were written in the last 2 days of life. The final hospitalization for half of patients included more than 8 days in generally undesirable states: in an ICU, receiving mechanical ventilation, or comatose. Families reported that half of the patients who were able to communicate in their last few days spent most of the time in moderate or severe pain.[27]

These results occurred in the intervention phase of the SUPPORT study, despite the presence of nurses whose task was to improve communication and encourage the patient and family to engage in an informed and collaborative decision-making process with a well-informed physician. The authors concluded that additional proactive and forceful measures may be needed. It was estimated that patients meeting SUPPORT criteria account for approximately 400,000 hospital admissions per year in the United States. Such findings seem to confirm the seemingly harsh approach in the previously listed futile treatment guidelines, but there is reason for caution.

In a corollary to the first phase of SUPPORT, investigators examined the impact of prognosis-based futility guidelines on survival and hospital length of stay on a cohort of adults with serious illness. They calculated the hospital days that would not be used if, on the third day, life-sustaining treatment had been stopped or not initiated for patients with an estimated 2-month survival chance of 1% or less. They found that only 10.8% of hospital days would have been saved and concluded that only modest savings would have resulted.[28]

If a large number of patients demand futile treatment, futile treatment guidelines will have several important effects: voluntary passive euthanasia (i.e., patient and/or surrogates have consented) will exist in theory but will be rarely necessary. Involuntary passive euthanasia (i.e., patient and/or surrogates have not consented) will increase dramatically. Futile treatment guidelines may cause physicians to feel less obligated to talk to their patients and surrogates.

An apparent contradiction exists between science and the quality of life suggested in the previously noted definition of futile treatment. This contradiction raises the question of whether a paternalistic quality of life decision is masquerading as scientific, objective decision making. If so, futile treatment guidelines are a large step back for patient autonomy—a return to the physician paternalism of the Hippocratic tradition.

Another possible result is that the right to die may become a duty to die. Do futile treatment policies put health services organizations and providers on a slippery slope? Will the policies become broader and increasingly focused on the quality of life that clinicians determine would be acceptable to the patient? These questions can be answered only in retrospect, in itself not a cheery prospect.

Summary

Absent data showing that patients and surrogates commonly demand treatment that caregivers consider futile, it is possible that futility guidelines are solving a nonproblem. In addition, the SUPPORT investigators' findings as to economic impact should be explored further.

If the problem exists, however, the first alternative solution is the status quo—patients and/or surrogates must agree to discontinue treatment after physicians determine it is futile. An adjunct to this alternative is to enhance the communication skills of physicians and other caregivers. It may be that patients and surrogates inadequately understand the prognosis. Health professionals such as nurses and social services staff may be used more effectively, for example. The task should not be left only to physicians and ethics committees since both are likely to be much more daunting to patients and surrogates.

COMPLEMENTS TO FUTILE TREATMENT GUIDELINES

Allow Natural Death

Allow natural death (AND) is ordered when a terminally ill patient (or surrogate) decides to forgo interventions such as CPR to sustain life. Essentially, AND is a DNR order. The meaning of DNR and its effects are difficult to communicate to patients and families. Further, DNR may suggest that the patient will receive insufficient care because there is no CPR or similar efforts. These two aspects of DNR argue against continuing to use it when AND has the same results. Patients who are AND receive comfort care, including hydration, nutrition, and pain control. Providing water and food artificially is a separate decision, but denying it is within the parameters of AND. Avoided are significant treatments that intervene to slow the dying process for someone who is terminally ill.

Palliative Care

The World Health Organization defines palliative care as

> an approach that improves the quality of life of patients and their families facing the problem associated with life-threatening illness, through the prevention and relief of suffering by means of early identification and impeccable assessment and treatment of pain and other problems, physical, psychosocial and spiritual.[29]

In addition to pain relief, palliative care regards dying as a normal part of life; it neither hastens nor postpones death. Important in its application is a team-based support system for patients and families. Palliative care intends to enhance the quality of life and positively influence the course of illness. It may be used in conjunction with therapies that are intended to prolong life, such as chemotherapy. It may include other interventions to understand and manage clinical complications.[30]

A corollary to palliative care is palliative sedation to unconsciousness (PSU). PSU is limited to terminally patients. Even here, however, it is reserved for "cases in which severe symptoms persist despite intensive interdisciplinary efforts to find a tolerable palliative treatment that does not affect the patient's level of consciousness."[31] The consensus in medicine is that PSU is a medical treatment; thus, it is not active euthanasia.[32] PSU is similar to terminal sedation, which was discussed in Chapter 11. PSU or terminal sedation have the indirect effect of shortening life, even though that was not intended. The patient's intense pain necessitates palliation to an extent that death is hastened. The rule of double effect applies to PSU and terminal sedation. The act of reducing or eliminating pain is good; the agent intends only the good effect. The death that is hastened was not intended. Both PSU and terminal sedation border on voluntary (or involuntary) active euthanasia. This line is crossed if palliation is excessive relative to the patient's pain.

Quantitative Assessment

Increasingly, there are objective means of predicting patient survival or the probability of a good clinical outcome. One such system is the Acute Physiological and Chronic Health Evaluation (APACHE) system. It can be used to assist decision makers (patients and/or surrogates) in understanding the best course of action. APACHE was developed at the George Washington University Hospital in 1981. APACHE II, introduced in 1985, was a simplified approach that used 12 acute physiological variables, age, and chronic health status to predict the probable outcomes of treatment. Further refinements produced APACHE III in 1990[33] and APPACHE IV in 2006.[34] Systems such as APACHE promote the efficient use of critical care resources, especially ICUs. Patients too well or too sick should not be admitted to ICU; the former have no need for its technology, the latter die despite it.[35] Scoring systems that quantify the probability of survival give patients, surrogates, and physicians an important supplement to their decision making.

Societal Changes

The quantitative assessment described above provides an objective assessment of probability of success of treatment. Other approaches require changes in thinking about end-of-life care. A solution that is more long range is to change the presumption about treatment. At present, it is presumed that all interventions are to be provided absent directives to the contrary. This presumption, reflecting Baconian theory about science conquering nature, has been reinforced in the law. Recognizing the limits of medicine requires a return to the Hippocratic tradition.[36] The new presumption could be that after diagnosis of a terminal illness or PVS, treatment will be provided only if it is probable that the patient will benefit from it.

Another alternative is to develop and apply a community standard. Implementation would not be easy, but all health services organizations can participate in its operational aspects. Here, the idea is to protect society's resources. Its contemporary manifestation is communitarianism, a concept championed by Amitai Etzioni. Communitarianism involves recognizing that there are resource limits and cooperatively working within them. Services are provided within the framework of limits—an approach similar to the Oregon Health plan (which is Oregon Medicaid).[37]

CONCLUSION

Questions of resource allocation are common to all health services organizations. Both macro- and microallocation issues are becoming more important as economic constraints increase, and it is crucial that the organizational philosophy and the vision and mission statements guide these decisions. This guidance requires a level of precision and specificity lacking in many organizations. This deficit must be overcome.

Hospitals with significant uncompensated care may offer services reimbursed at a higher rate to offset losses. Fiscally sound health services organizations must ask whether they are meeting their obligations under the principle of justice to offer unprofitable but needed services that benefit the wider community. They also must ask if they are meeting a duty of general beneficence to use surpluses to assist persons who might require services.

Futile treatment guidelines are becoming common. Before developing them, the extent of the problem should be determined. Other remedies, such as more effective education on AMDs and improving the processes of getting AMDs on the medical record, may be more effective. The most important use for futile treatment guidelines may be to provide moral and administrative support for physicians, whose clinical practice will benefit from defining and understanding futile treatment. In turn, the guidelines may be used to convince patients or surrogates that treatment without reasonable hope of benefit should be withheld or withdrawn.

NOTES

1. Charles Fried. (1976, February). Equality and rights in medical care. *Hastings Center Report 6*, pp. 29–34.
2. From Beaufort B. Longest, Jr., & Kurt Darr. (2008). Healthcare technology. In *Managing health services organizations and systems* (5th. ed., pp. 156–157). Baltimore: Health Professions Press; adapted by permission.
3. Milt Freudenheim. (2003, May 23). Art, commerce and a heart transplant denied. *New York Times*, p. C1.
4. From Jonathon S. Rakich, Beaufort B. Longest, Jr., & Kurt Darr. (1985). *Managing health services organizations* (2nd ed., pp. 139–140). Philadelphia: W.B. Saunders; adapted by permission.
5. James E Childress. (1970, Winter). Who shall live when not all can live? *Soundings: An Interdisciplinary Journal 53*(4), pp. 339–355; Nicholas Rescher. (1969, April). The allocation of exotic medical lifesaving therapy. *Ethics 79*(3), pp. 173–186.
6. Paul Ramsey. (1970). *The patient as person* (p. 252). New Haven, CT: Yale University Press.
7. From Beaufort B. Longest, Jr., Jonathon S. Rakich, & Kurt Darr. (2000). Ethics. In *Managing health services organizations and systems* (4th. ed., pp. 676–677). Baltimore: Health Professions Press; adapted by permission.
8. Sources for the Sidney Miller case: Kris Axtman. (2003, March 27). Baby case tests rights of parents. *Christian Science Monitor*. Retrieved March 28, 2011, from http://www.csmonitor.com/2003/0327/p01s01-usju.html; Vida Foubister.

(2001, February 5). Texas court overturns ruling on resuscitation of premature baby. *American Medical News*. Retrieved May 6, 2004, from http://www .ama-assn.org/amednews/2001/02/05/prsb0205.htm; Traci Neal. (2002). Who has the right to decide when to save the sickest babies? *Hartford Advocate*. Retrieved May 6, 2004, from http://old.hartfordadvocate.com/articles/pulling theplug.html; Anthony J. Sebok. (2002, December 2). When a hospital ignores parents' request to let their newborn die, is it a tort? *FindLaw*. Retrieved March 28, 2011, from http://writ.news.findlaw.com/sebok/20021202.html.

9. David B. Waisel & Robert D. Truog. (1995, February 15). The cardiopulmonary resuscitation-not-indicated order: Futility revisited. *Annals of Internal Medicine 122*(4), pp. 304–308.

10. Man in coma awakes, believes Reagan is still president. (2003, July 10). *Washington Times*, p. A10.

11. Wesley J. Smith. (2001, July 23)."Futile care" and its friends. *Weekly Standard*. Retrieved May 3, 2004, from http://www.weeklystandard.com/Utilities/ printer_preview.asp?idArticle=230&R=9E37234FA; Wesley J. Smith. (2002, December). Futile care theory and medical fascism: The duty to die. *FrontPage Magazine*. Retrieved March 28, 2011, from http://www.indiadivine.org/ audarya/ayurveda-health-wellbeing/969400-futile-care-theory-medical-fas cism.html.

12. Dan Larriviere & Richard J. Bonnie. (2006, June). Terminating artificial nutrition and hydration in persistent vegetative state patients: Current and proposed state laws. *Neurology 66*, pp. 1624–1628.

13. In re Wanglie, No. PX-91-283 (Minn. Prob. Ct. Hennepin County June 28, 1991), reprinted in A. Capron. (1991, September). In re Helga Wanglie. *Hastings Center Report 21*(5), p. 26.

14. *In the matter of Baby "K."* 832 F. Supp. 1022 (E.D. Va. July 1, 1993).

15. *In the matter of Baby "K."* 16 F. 3d 590 (4th Cir., February 10, 1994).

16. Bill Miller & Marylou Tousignant. (1993, September 25). Mother fights hospital to keep infant alive. *Washington Post*, p. A14.

17. Marylou Tousignant & Bill Miller. (1995, April 7). Death of "Baby K" leaves a legacy of legal precedents. *Washington Post*, p. B3.

18. Trinity Health. (2001, December). *Q&A: Guidelines on medically futile treatment*. Novi, MI: Author.

19. Trinity Health. (2001, December). *Trinity Health guidelines on medically futile treatment*. Novi, MI: Author.

20. *Ibid.*

21. *Ibid.*

22. Monica Sethi. (2007, December). A patient's right to direct own health care vs. a physician's right to decline to provide treatment. *Bifocal 29*(2), pp. 27–28.

23. Veda Foubister. (2000, August 14). California law facilitates advance directives for end-of-life medical care. *American Medical News*. Retrieved November 14, 2003, from http://www.ama-assn.org/amednews/2000/08/14/prsb0814.htm.

24. The Texas Advance Directives Act, § 166.046. (1999). Retrieved December 29, 2010, from http://www.statutes.legis.state.tx.us/docs/Hs/htm/HS.166.htm.

25. Nancy Valko. (2003). Futility policies and the duty to die. *Voices 18*(1). Retrieved March 24, 2004, from http://www.wf-f.org/03-1-Futility.html.

26. Nancy L. Childs & Walt N. Mercer. (1996). Brief report: Late improvement in consciousness after post-traumatic vegetative state. *New England Journal of Medicine 334*(1), pp. 24–25; "Permanent" coma can be misnomer, Texas case shows. (1996, January 4). *Washington Post*, p. A16.

27. The SUPPORT Principal Investigators. (1995, November 22/29). A controlled trial to improve care for seriously ill hospitalized patients: The Study to Understand Prognoses and Preferences for Outcomes and Risks of Treatments (SUPPORT). *Journal of the American Medical Association 274*(20), p. 1595.

28. Joan M. Teno, Donald Murphy, Joanne Lynn, Anna Tosteson, Norman Desbiens, Alfred E. Connors, Jr., Mary Beth Hamel, Albert Wu, Russell Phillips, Neil Wenger, Frank Harrell, Jr., & William A. Knaus for the SUPPORT Investigators. (1994, November). Prognosis-based guidelines: Does anyone win? *Journal of the American Gerontological Society 42*, pp. 1202–1207.

29. World Health Organization. (2011). *WHO definition of palliative care*. Retrieved March 6, 2011, from http://www.who.int/cancer/palliative/definition/en/#.

30. *Ibid.*

31. Jeffrey T. Berger. (2010, May/June). Rethinking guidelines for the use of palliative sedation. *Hastings Center Report 40*(3), p. 33.

32. *Ibid.*

33. SATELLIFE. (2002, December 28). *Critical care medicine: Introduction*. Retrieved January 9, 2004, from http://www.healthnet.org.np/resource/thesis/anes/Introduction.PDF.

34. K. Strand & H. Flaatten. (2008). Severity scoring in the ICU: A review. *Acta Anaesthesiologica Scandinavica 53*, p. 470.

35. SATELLIFE. (2002, December 28). *Critical care medicine: Literature review*. Retrieved January 9, 2004, from http://www.healthnet.org.np/resource/thesis/anes/Introduction.PDF.

36. Nancy S. Jecker. (1991, May/June). Knowing when to stop: The limits of medicine. *Hastings Center Report 21*(3), pp. 5–8.

37. Amitai Etzioni. (2003). Organ donation: A communitarian approach. *Kennedy Institute of Ethics Journal 13*(1), pp. 1–18.

Chapter 14

Social Responsibility

Three dimensions of the social responsibility of health services organizations are examined in this chapter; generally, they are framed as contrasting service with financial performance. One dimension is protecting and enhancing organization assets while maximizing community benefit. A second is the moral obligation of health services organizations to provide services appropriate to a patient's needs, with no hint of decision making based on nonrelevant factors such as age, payment status, race, or sex. The third dimension of social responsibility considered is the organization's obligation to protect the commonweal—in terms of both private resources and public sources such as Medicare and Medicaid.

COMMUNITY BENEFIT

Controlling costs and improving efficiency should be of concern to administrative staff. They ultimately benefit the community and should be a focus for clinicians.

Different Settings, Different Costs

In late 1991, Metropolitan Hospital undertook successful negotiations for a 50–50 joint venture with a six-physician group of gastroenterologists to establish a freestanding endoscopy center. This agreement was a natural outgrowth of a long-term affiliation with the same single-specialty group whose members had been on the active staff at Metropolitan for more than 10 years. These six physicians performed two-thirds of the endoscopies at Metropolitan.

Alice Macalin, a member of Metropolitan's staff, manages the center as well as inpatient endoscopy services at Metropolitan. Cost data showed that supply costs at the center were almost 35% lower than for endoscopies performed in the hospital. Initially, it was thought that the higher acuity level of patients undergoing endoscopy at the hospital increased costs significantly, but investigation showed this had only a marginal effect.

Macalin noted significant differences in attitudes among the physicians, depending on where they were working. As center director, Macalin is often approached by the physicians with cost-savings ideas, such as switching to reusables for certain supplies. The physicians took it upon themselves to ask technologists to remind them of the cost of expensive disposables before they opened the package. In addition, they tracked one another to determine who might be overusing supplies or using expensive supplies when less expensive alternatives were suitable. On their own, the physicians discussed ways to increase operational efficiency at the center, and they devised a scheduling change to better fill down time.

Little of this interest in cost reduction transferred to the hospital. When practicing at Metropolitan, the physicians are not deliberately wasteful, but they are noticeably less interested in developing or initiating cost savings. Macalin had hoped that the patterns from the center would transfer automatically to the hospital, but after almost a year this had occurred only marginally and cost differences continued to be significant. She knew something should be done, but what?

Waste is an ethical issue. Obviously, the financial implications of even shared ownership make the physicians much more interested in improving efficiency at the center. Changing physicians' attitudes about the use of resources is a major challenge for managers and is reflected in efforts to tie physicians into the economic health of the organization through such arrangements as physician–hospital organizations. Macalin could attempt to force changes, but doing so would risk both physician antipathy and apathy. Applying expectations and patterns from the center to the hospital would be interpreted by physicians as interfering with professional judgment and decision making; after all, the patients are hospitalized when endoscopies are performed in Metropolitan. Education and working patiently with the physicians to gain their understanding of the applicability and transferability of efficiency from the center to the hospital are essential activities for Macalin as she exhibits the virtue of thrift. Improving efficiency (general duty of beneficence) benefits the community by reducing costs, thus making health services more affordable and accessible.

In addition to reducing waste, health services organizations have a moral obligation to collect debts owed to them. Not-for-profit organizations are expected to provide uncompensated care—services that provide community benefit—to retain their special tax status. Yet, they should, and arguably must, take reasonable steps to collect monies legally owed to them. Part of a health services organization's fiduciary obligation to its service area is to maintain its financial status. Aggressive debt collection raises ethical issues, however, even if the law allows the actions taken by the organization.

Pursuit[1]

Memorial Hospital is a 250-bed, not-for-profit organization. It is financially successful but has chronic problems with accounts receivable (AR) and writes off more bad debt each year than comparable-size not-for-profit hospitals. Memorial hired a financial consultant who told them to become much more aggressive in collecting patient debts. The consultant recommended filing lawsuits against debtors, garnishing patients' wages, and seizing their income tax refunds. When the new tactics were explained, some senior managers demurred. Ultimately, however, the chief executive officer (CEO) and chief financial officer (CFO) decided to use the legal but extreme methods that had been recommended.

As an ultimate expression of collection efforts, debtors who missed court appearances were arrested pursuant to an order issued by the presiding judge. These orders resulted from a court's authority to punish those who fail to appear as directed.* Some debtors were jailed briefly, until bail was posted. The collection efforts caused bankruptcy for others.

When the media became aware of Memorial's debt collection policy, critical stories were published. One astute reporter noted that the uninsured were being asked to pay charges rather than the discounted rates paid by payers who had contracts with the hospital. Charges are typically much higher than discounted rates.

Memorial's CEO and CFO were very pleased with the reduction in the amount and aging of AR, but governing body members began asking questions about the collections practice of one another and of the CEO.

The case describes an ethical dilemma for health services organizations. The oft-repeated mantra "no margin, no mission" fits here. One must ask whether hospitals are meeting their duty of fidelity to their service area, patients, and staff if they fail to make significant efforts to collect what is owed them. In addition, organizations have vendors to whom timely payment must be made lest essential goods and services become unavailable. Hospitals further defend such practices by noting that they must collect

---

*Various jurisdictions call them *body attachments, civil arrest warrants, bench warrants,* or *writs of capias.* Technically, they are not punishment for the debt but for flouting the court's authority.

the debts they are owed because costs are increasing even as reimbursement from third-party payers declines. It must be asked whether practices such as body attachments treat the debtor (and former patient) with dignity and respect. The patient owes respect to the organization and its needs, as well, however, and the organization may have been unable to get the debtor's attention any other way. Certainly, the bad press diminishes the organization's reputation and community standing. Positive for the organization, however, is that public knowledge about extreme collection practices will cause self-selection—patients unwilling or unable to pay for services will go elsewhere. Thus, the hospital's financial situation is improved, even as access may be lessened.

Hospitals' financial problems are exacerbated by the millions of uninsured. Those without health insurance vary significantly by region and state. Estimates of the uninsured range from 45 to 50 million. Knowing the composition of those estimates is essential to understanding the implications of being "uninsured." About 25% of the uninsured are eligible for Medicaid or the State Children's Health Insurance Program but have not enrolled. Another 20% of the "uninsured" are technically not Americans—they are illegal aliens. A significant percentage—estimated at three-quarters—of the uninsured have the financial means to purchase insurance but choose not to do so. Further, most of the uninsured are young and, generally, in good health. They have little incentive to pay the higher insurance premiums that community rating requires, which subsidize those in older age brackets. Finally, because most Americans obtain health insurance through employment, most uninsured are actually uninsured for only a short period as they move between jobs.[2] At its core, however, discussion of the uninsured should center on the effect that insurance status has on mortality. Lack of a discernible difference in morality rates between the insured and uninsured provides crucial information about both the importance of insurance status and the value of access to healthcare.[3]

We've Earned It, We'll Keep It!

Freeland Hospital is a not-for-profit, general acute care hospital located in an affluent suburban neighborhood. Its Medicare census is less than 20%, and it receives less than 1% of its revenues from Medicaid. Uncollectibles are less than 3%. Freeland Hospital's current financial situation is sound.

Sherwood Shurman had been the CEO of Freeland for almost 20 years and is justifiably proud of the changes and improvements that he has achieved during his tenure. One improvement has been to establish the Freeland Hospital Foundation, Inc., which receives charitable donations as well as excess of income over expense from the operations of Freeland Hospital. In only 10 years, the Foundation has accumulated $12 million; $2 million were used to acquire equipment.

Occasionally, board members question whether the hospital is sufficiently socially conscious. The most common suggestion is that Freeland ought to establish an outpatient clinic in the inner city, where access to primary care is limited. Shurman has assiduously avoided acting on these informal recommendations.

Shurman hired a marketing director, Maureen O'Riley, and asked her to identify new initiatives for Freeland. O'Riley's market research resulted in a plan that included programs for respite care, addiction treatment, and rehabilitation medicine. O'Riley noted that there are no competing programs in their service area and that expected demand will be covered by private-pay patients or nongovernmental third-party payers, at least the former of whom are likely to pay charges. Shurman was enthusiastic about the suggestions and asked the board to review the proposal.

Shurman was shocked when the plan met significant resistance. No member of the board disputed the well-documented need and the potential demand for the proposed programs. Instead, they were troubled by the prospect of generating additional revenues and adding them to the endowment. Several members indicated that they would support the new programs only if a large part of any surplus were used to assist the city's underserved areas. Others mentioned social consciousness; one even used the word guilt to describe her feelings about having so much while others had so little. The proposal was tabled.

Shurman was angry as he left the board meeting but took care not to allow others to see his state of mind. After a few minutes' reflection on the meeting, he asked to meet with his chief operating officer, Maria Sanchez. Shurman told Sanchez what had happened and asked her to solicit any equipment requests submitted by the medical staff and to ensure that they were in his office by week's end. He told Sanchez to dust off the plans that had been developed several years earlier to build a staff education wing and the more recent request from the oncology department for an expanded unit. As Sanchez left, Shurman thought to himself that he would be damned if he would see his hard work and fiscal success wasted on a harebrained scheme to provide primary care to a population that was the city's responsibility.

Freeland Hospital is financially sound. Some board members recognize a broader social responsibility for the hospital, whereas Shurman has a narrow view of Freeland's role. The questions raised by the board should have been addressed in the hospital's philosophy and vision and mission statements, and these documents should be reviewed for guidance—or amended. If no attention has been given to Freeland's broader social responsibility, this fundamental issue must be addressed before decisions are made about the marketing plan and the recommended programs. It is folly to proceed without a clear direction and a consensus to pursue this responsibility.

The service area concept is Shurman's strongest reason for opposing the board's interest in aiding the city's underserved. The inner city appears to be out of Freeland's service area. Is it just (fair) to take resources from Freeland's service area and redirect them to individuals elsewhere, regardless of how compelling the reason is? This view suggests that Freeland should reduce its surpluses and simultaneously benefit its service area by reducing charges. This action would directly benefit those whom it serves. Alternatively, Freeland could identify health needs that are not adequately insured or are not likely to be highly sought by private payers but are important nonetheless. Examples include mental health programs and various counseling services.

Shurman's attitude seems extraordinarily parochial, while the board's attitude may be too altruistic. A wide middle ground exists to accommodate both. It is reasonable to study what role Freeland could play in meeting the health needs of the wider community, whether or not it is in Freeland's service area. Additional information may make the answer apparent.

Historical attitudes about competition, lack of profit motive, and not-for-profit status have both helped and hindered the health services system. The absence of economic incentives has contributed to health services organizations feeling good about themselves, since they were doing good rather than concentrating on performing well and efficiently.

A health services organization loses public confidence if it appears not to be working in the community's best health services interests. The conflict is between protecting its financial integrity—an ethical obligation of the organization linked to its role of providing services to the community—and serving patients.

Not-for-profit health services organizations, especially hospitals, commonly name units, wings, lobbies, and programs for persons and organizations that have made substantial contributions to them. Sometimes these donations bring with them "baggage" that causes a negative reaction from members of the public. Without these donations, however, many health services providers could not survive financially and likely could not offer costly specialized services and the high levels of medical technology that allow them to be of maximum benefit to their patients.

Please, What's that Name Again?[4]

A $10 million donation prompted Columbus Children's Hospital in Ohio to name its emergency department and trauma center for the retailer Abercrombie &

Fitch (A&F). The result was an unexpected storm of protest from a coalition of 15 children's organizations and 80 individuals who contended that naming the new center for A&F sends the wrong message to children and parents. At issue are the provocative advertising and revealing clothing that A&F directs at teens and pre-teens in its marketing program. The coalition claims that this makes A&F "among the worst corporate predators" for "sexualizing and objectifying children."

The hospital defended its decision by stating that it had chosen to name the center for A&F because of its significant philanthropy. It was a way to honor the gift and recognize the tremendous support that A&F had given the hospital. The spokesman took issue with allegations that the hospital had sold naming rights to A&F. He noted that a nonprofit hospital accepts gifts as a way to support its mission.

This case is emblematic of the types of problems that can arise from corporate giving; there are strong elements of a quid pro quo. As noted previously, there may be elements of managerial self-aggrandizement and differing interests when vendors make donations. The above case suggests the negative reaction when moral criteria are applied to donors. Some constituencies assert that the source of the wealth must be considered when accepting a charitable gift.

Is wealth value-free? If it carries a stigma, how long does that stigma last? Should an alcohol rehabilitation center be named for a distiller of spirits after its parent corporation makes a large contribution? Is a pornographer's (ill-gotten) wealth forever tainted and unacceptable, even though he now wishes to do good works with it? These examples show what many may consider unacceptable sources of charitable giving. If the motive is doing good works, perhaps the organization should accept the gift to allow donors to expiate their guilt, as well as to benefit from the resources. Forgiveness should be instinctive to human beings. Would its gifts be acceptable were A&F to pledge to discontinue its sexualized advertising to teens and preteens?

SIMILAR NEED, DISSIMILAR TREATMENT

It is likely fruitless to set a goal to provide the same services for all persons with the same medical need. The numbers and types of variables involved are staggering. For example, access is limited by geography, availability and capability of providers, individual desire to receive services, a subculture's attitudes about health, physicians' ability or willingness to treat or refer, insurance status, financial circumstances, mental state, and dozens of other attributes of individuals and the health services system. The problems of equity (fairness) are legion and probably unresolvable, regardless of how health services are organized, provided, or financed. Even systems with universal access have disparities in use or access because of system expenditures for services and technology, socioeconomic class, geography, and physicians' willingness to refer patients. Given the number of factors and the certainty that variability in service access and use are inevitable, it is nonetheless important that providers seek to identify these types of problems and make reasonable efforts to eliminate them or minimize their effects. Disparities begin far upstream. In the past, the National Cancer Institute (part of the National Institutes of Health) has spent less than 1% of its budget on end-of-life research and training.[5]

Ageism appears to be present in parts of the health services system. For example, although older adults are at greater risk of dying from heart disorders, cancer, and influenza/pneumonia, there is evidence that they do not get the most aggressive forms of treatment and diagnostic and preventive care, which is standard for younger patients. The disparity may result from a notion that older adults cannot tolerate more aggressive treatment or do not want it, neither of which is necessarily true. There is also evidence that physicians are less likely to suggest that these individuals participate in screening for various cancers or receive influenza vaccinations.[6] Other disparities are present at the end of life. African Americans constitute 14% of the U.S. population but only 8.7% of hospice patients—despite a higher incidence of cancer and higher mortality rates than Caucasians. In 2009, 80.5% of hospice patients were white/Caucasian.[7] This research did not account for these disparities. In addition to variation in hospice use by ethnicity, there is wide geographic variation in use of the Medicare hospice benefit by older individuals.[8]

Research at five teaching hospitals found disparities in using cardiopulmonary resuscitation (CPR). CPR was more likely to be used for men, younger patients, African Americans, patients whose reported preferences were for CPR, and those who had higher physician estimates for 2-month survival. Rates also vary significantly by geographic location and diagnosis.[9]

A sample of 1.56 million nursing facility residents found that African Americans are approximately one-third as likely as Caucasians to have living wills and one-fifth as likely to have do-not-resuscitate (DNR) orders. Hispanics are approximately one-third as likely as Caucasians to have DNR orders but just as likely to have living wills. The researchers concluded that the presence of advance care plans is related to race, even after controlling for health and other demographic factors.[10]

Another dimension of DNR orders is whether they are written equitably for patients with different diseases but similar prognoses. A 1995 study reported that DNR orders are written more often for older patients, women, and patients with dementia or incontinence and less often for patients who are African American, have Medicaid insurance, or are in rural hospitals.[11] Similar disparities were found in an earlier study in which DNR orders were much more likely to be written for patients with AIDS or inoperable lung cancer than for patients with other diseases with equally poor prognoses, such as cirrhosis or heart failure.[12]

General concerns have been raised regarding the unequal treatment of individuals who are dying:

> Ample evidence exists that the process of dying is less than optimal. Too many dying patients suffer unnecessary physical symptoms such as pain, dyspnoea, nausea, and vomiting; too many suffer untreated depression, anxiety, and hopelessness; and too many feel they have lost their dignity. It is the perception that dying is a painful process filled with unnecessary suffering and indignity that fuels campaigns— and public support—for legalizing euthanasia and physician-assisted suicide.[13]

Reforms suggested include training physicians, nurses, and other providers to communicate better with dying patients; improving management of pain, anorexia, insomnia, fatigue, and other physical symptoms; improving diagnosis and treatment of depression; referring dying patients to hospice care earlier; improving palliation; and facilitating dying at home.[14] Patients who have DNR orders apparently receive no less contact from staff and visitors than those who do not have DNR orders, however.[15]

Variation in types and amounts of care also occurs by region of the country. It is well-known that the rates at which various surgical and medical treatments are used vary widely by state, region, and even county. Apparently, these variations are a function of how physicians practice medicine. Not unexpected, then, is wide variation in the use (prevalence) of tube feeding by state. A study of patients 65 years of age and older who had severe cognitive impairment, including total dependence in eating, and who resided in nursing facilities in nine states showed wide variation in use of tube feeding. Prevalence ranged from a low of 7.5% in Maine to a high of 40.1% in Mississippi. The other seven states studied ranked between. Differences in state law may have contributed to some variation, but the authors concluded that after adjusting for clinical and demographic variables, there are true differences in the prevalence of tube feedings in the nine states studied. In addition, there are differences in use of tube feeding by race, with Caucasian residents being less than half as likely as other ethnic groups to receive this treatment.[16] Sometimes, the availability of services results from a payment system that makes it impossible for providers to survive financially. One example is the attribution of hospital closures to inadequate payment from managed care and other contracting practices, thus reducing access to both emergency department (ED) and general hospital services. Between 1991 and 2001, nearly one in five hospitals with EDs closed.[17] Between 1993 and 2003, the number of EDs decreased by 425.[18]

Between the extremes of hyper-egalitarianism and hyper-individualism is the position that society has a duty to assist in developing, encouraging, and even providing health services. Fried argued that routine basic services ought to be available to all, a view known as *the decent minimum*.[19] More exotic high-technology services are limited by factors such as location, cost, and referrals and must be available on a different basis. Drawing this line is a political decision and depends on society's willingness to provide the resources needed. The Oregon Medicaid plan was referenced earlier. It allocates the budget against a priority list of services available to all who are eligible for the program.

Hospital EDs go on ambulance diversion (i.e., the EDs close) when they are at capacity and cannot safely accept more patients. The need for diversion is communicated to the centers that dispatch ambulances, and the ambulances are directed elsewhere. It is common for busy EDs to go on diversion, as shown in the following case.

The Emergency Department

University Hospital, a private, partially investor-owned academic health center hospital, is located in a major East Coast metropolitan area. Its ED is the city's busiest. Two years ago, closure of the city-owned hospital eliminated the major source of services for persons who are uninsured or medically indigent. The city established a fund to pay private providers such as University Hospital for the uncompensated care it provided to city residents.

The city-owned ambulance service has a policy to take patients to the closest available ED that can provide the services the patient needs. Ambulance dispatchers are informed when an ED is at capacity, and ambulances are rerouted to other EDs. The decision to close an ED is made by the ED director.

University's ED director determined that her ED was at capacity and told a staff member to call the dispatch center to request temporary reroute of patients being moved by ambulance. The call was made, but communication failed at the dispatch center. When an emergency medical technician (EMT) radioed to tell University's ED that they were bringing in a patient, the ED director asked what the patient's medical problem was and from where she was being brought. The EMT told her the patient was from the inner city. The ED director then told the EMT that University's ED was on reroute. The EMT decided that the reason he was told that University's ED was on reroute was because the patient was coming from the inner city, was likely a minority, and was probably uninsured. This belief caused several EMTs to file a complaint with the city health department. An investigation followed.

The investigation found that the ED was on diversion when the EMT called and that the decision was consistent with city guidelines. This case suggests problems of general perception, allegations of bias, and miscommunication. The EMTs' conclusion that the decision was made on nonmedical grounds suggests a preexisting poor relationship with University Hospital. Improving that relationship should receive early attention from the hospital and EMTs. The EMTs' perception of biased decision making can be improved over time by the hospital's determining its source; and, if there is substance behind the perception, by the hospital's making the necessary changes to prevent that perception from continuing. Even if substance is lacking, the hospital does not want perception to drive reality. Regardless, it will take a long-term effort on University Hospital's part to improve relations with the EMTs.

It is argued that rationing is the only way to bring fairness (justice) to the healthcare system. This position is supported by identifying the extraordinarily high cost of early "last-chance therapies," such as totally implantable artificial hearts, left ventricular assist devices, and Herceptin, a drug to treat metastatic breast cancer.[20] More ultra-expensive therapies are likely to follow. Any system that guarantees a decent minimum of primary care and specialty services is unlikely to be able to afford to pay for ultra-expensive services that might be available and demanded by all. The concept of meritocracy—the idea that those with greater, lawfully acquired wealth may choose to buy more services—is usually accepted by all but the most hard-core hyper-egalitarians.

The microallocation decisions that health services providers make constantly result in rationing. The last bed in the ICU case study in Chapter 13 is a classic example. Yet, there are many others, most of which are more subtle and less easily identified—for example, allocation of donor organs, blood products in short supply, and even general medical-surgical beds. Macroallocation decisions that have the effect of rationing occur as well.[21]

THE COMMONWEAL

Macroallocation

It is at the macro level that healthcare costs and their effect on the commonweal are most dramatic. Despite claims of a scientific basis, very little of what physicians do has been proved effective using the scientific gold standard of a random, double-blind study. Modern medical practice is based on tradition, pragmatism, inertia, logic, and long-held assumptions that remain scientifically unverified. The estimates of wasteful, ineffective treatments in the $2.5 trillion spent on U.S. healthcare in 2009 are as high as $650 billion, or approximately 25%. Other estimates are that 20% or more of all costs could be eliminated without harm to anyone, and that 40% of specialist visits and 25% of hospital stays are unnecessary. Areas in which healthcare costs might be reduced include excessive high-tech imaging, overuse of psychotropic drugs, unnecessary investigations of fainting spells, overtreating for back and neck pain, inappropriate use of cardiovascular stents and angioplasty, and overuse of knee arthroscopy in arthritis. Several factors contribute to the lack of interest in knowing the efficacy of generally accepted medical treatments: political cowardice, the many sectors in the system that benefit from overuse and waste, and the view of the public that good medicine requires numerous interventions, especially those that use high tech.[22] There is some hope that the issues of waste, overuse, and inappropriate use of medical resources and technology will be addressed as financial constraints in the public and private sectors stimulate a greater search for savings.

American Hospital Association (AHA) data show that in 2009, hospitals provided $39.1 billion in uncompensated care.[23] This was a large increase from the $22.3 billion provided in 2002,[24] which, in turn, was a large increase from the $16 billion spent in 1995.[25] The AHA defines *uncompensated care* as the sum of charity care and bad debt valued at the cost to the hospital of the services provided. It excludes other unfunded costs of care, such as underpayment from Medicaid and Medicare.[26] Other health services organizations define *uncompensated care* to include costs in excess of payments received for Medicare and Medicaid services.[27] In 2009, the 5,008 hospitals registered with the AHA had average uncompensated care costs of 6%.[28] Major publicly owned teaching hospitals and urban government hospitals have an uncompensated care rate that is typically two to three times higher.[29] The concern during the 1990s that hospitals would reduce uncompensated care to counter payment shortfalls from Medicare and Medicaid, as well as price discounts negotiated by managed care plans, did not materialize.[30] Hospitals' commitment to treat those unable to pay continues largely unabated.

During the 1990s, a number of not-for-profit hospitals were converted to investor-owned (for-profit) status, a development that seems related to declining economic performance of the not-for-profits. From 1991 to 1997, there were 431 conversions. The uncompensated care provided by the converted entities decreased from 5.3% to 4.7%, approximately equal to a $400,000 reduction in per hospital spending. The decline was more substantial in public facilities that became investor-owned, which had reductions from 5.2% to 2.5% of total expenses, or about $800,000 less per hospital per year. Overall, changing from not-for-profit to investor-owned status resulted in a reduction of about 13% in the amount of uncompensated care that was provided.[31] The concern is that numerous conversions of hospitals to investor-owned will diminish sources of care for the uninsured or those unable to pay.

Comparisons of not-for-profit and investor-owned hospitals offer insights into uncompensated care. Analyzing 1993 data, a study of 116 Tennessee hospitals, approximately one-third of which were investor-owned, showed that as a percentage of expenses, not-for-profit hospitals provided more uncompensated care than did investor-owned hospitals. Average differences were not large, however. The median for all Tennessee hospitals was 8.4%; the median for not-for-profit and investor-owned hospitals was 8.9% and 8.1%, respectively. Notably, the value of taxes paid by investor-owned hospitals was not included in calculating direct and indirect contributions to programs such as Medicare and Medicaid. Taxes include federal and state income taxes and sales, property, and local business taxes.[32] Findings in Tennessee were similar to those reported by the Medicare Payment Advisory Commission: investor-owned and not-for-profit hospitals provided substantially the same amount of uncompensated care in 1999 as a percentage of costs, 4.2% and 4.6%, respectively.[33]

The tax variable was considered in a study undertaken by the Virginia Health Services Cost Review Council, an independent state data commission. Using 1993 data, it ranked 88 acute care hospitals in Virginia via 18 productivity and efficiency variables. A variable used to measure community benefits provided by each hospital proved controversial. *Community support* was defined as the percentage of a hospital's total expenses for charity care, bad debt, and all taxes. Including taxes placed for-profit hospitals ahead of most not-for-profit hospitals. A Virginia Hospital Association analysis, which excluded two state-supported university hospitals, found that 13 for-profit hospitals used 14% of their operating expenses for community support as compared with the 73 not-for-profit hospitals that spent 7.7%. Commenting on the data, members of the investor-owned sector argued that taxes should be included because they support local communities, as should Medicaid and Medicare. Conversely, members of the not-for-profit sector asserted that including taxes is misleading because most taxes are state and federal income taxes, which may or may not be used for local healthcare programs.[34]

Data from California hospitals, who provided uncompensated care totaling $1.5 billion in 2000, provides another perspective on the problem. When using the expanded definition of uncompensated care (i.e., including the costs in excess of payments for Medicare and Medicaid services), however, the total jumps to $5.3 billion. Not-for-profit hospitals provided 61% of uncompensated care. Government-owned hospitals provided twice as much uncompensated care per bed as not-for-profit hospitals, and thrice as much as investor-owned hospitals.[35]

In 2006, the Congressional Budget Office of the U.S. Congress reported relatively little difference in the two types of hospitals. As a share of hospitals' operating expenses, not-for-profit hospitals provided 4.7% uncompensated care compared with 4.2% at for-profits. For-profit hospitals, however, provide fewer specialized services, such as emergency services and labor and delivery.[36] Such specialized services tend to generate more costs than revenue.

Such studies are often marred by methodological problems; the definitive study may never be done. It is clear, however, that caution must be used in attributing motives and results solely to ownership. Since 1983, the AHA has not provided data on uncompensated care that distinguish not-for-profit and investor-owned hospitals.

Microallocation

Macroallocation decisions affect microallocation. Failure to fund a program, clinic, or center means, for example, that there are too few or no resources available for services to individual patients. Within these limits are dynamics that can cause what appears to be a lack of humanitarian motives or a failure to be interested in the well-being of those with healthcare needs.

Free Clinic Woes[37]

As the director of Franklin Creek District Health Department, Jane Porterfield was proud of herself. She had gotten a small grant from a local corporation for a part-time receptionist and had received free use of an old store in one of her counties—the county that was most rural. She also had gotten two big-city physicians who were willing to travel to that store twice a week. She had all she needed to start a free clinic.

The primary care clinic would be available for those in the rural county who were working but unable to afford health insurance. In other words, they were too poor to afford an individual health plan but probably too rich to be eligible for Medicaid. Because all services were to be free, the state would furnish special help, such as free malpractice insurance coverage for the doctors.

Furthermore, the state health department had given Jane's health department approval to hold a childhood vaccine program in the same rural building twice a month. This would make it possible to increase the number of rural children who got immunized according to the state timetables.

Jane was at her desk preparing an agenda for the next board of health meeting, with all this good news on it. She felt that she was really making a difference in her region.

Suddenly, there was knock on her office door.

Jane looked up to see a member of the board of health Dr. Karen Matthewsen. Jane felt Karen was the best board member that they had. Karen was a country doctor who worked in the rural county where Jane's concerns were the strongest, and Karen was a champion of the medically indigent throughout the whole region.

"Come in, Karen," Jane said with enthusiasm. "You can perhaps give me some help drawing up the agenda item about the wonderful new free clinic and vaccine program."

"Well, that is why I wanted to come see you, Jane—I am worried about those new developments." Karen said these words as she sat down in the guest chair by Jane's desk. Karen was clearly upset.

"But you were the biggest champion for the dispossessed on our board. I thought you would be tickled pink to see more services opening where the need is so great." Jane was also getting a little upset. This reaction from her old friend was not expected.

"As you know, Jane, I see more poor patients than any other doctor in the area, and I must say that it is tough enough to make a living in a rural county without having neighboring doctors come in and give free care. I know they are not supposed to take my Medicaid patients, but I operate on a close margin—closer than you might expect—and the loss of even underpaying self-pay patients and maybe some Medicaid ones, too, is problematic. Some patients might even prefer your services to going on Medicaid, while I work to get my uninsured patients covered by Medicaid and never turn a Medicaid patient down.

"Furthermore, lots of residents in our rural county could use the new childhood vaccine programs you are offering, and these vaccines represent 20% of my practice net income every summer in the month before school opens."

Jane countered by noting that the free clinic would be encouraging eligible individuals to sign up for Medicaid and to see local doctors, but Karen noted that the free clinic would not be operating but two half days a week, and with volunteer labor, it would be unlikely to do a lot of follow-up and paperwork.

"No," Karen said, looking Jane straight in the eye. "I must say that, for the first time, I am against a new health department program aimed at the indigent. I believe country doctors like me need to be free of well-meaning government initiatives that are redundant, with private enterprises already struggling financially. I plan to vote against the clinic."

This case presents several ethical issues. Most prominent is the conflict of interest that arises as Dr. Matthewsen tries to meet her duties as a board member of the health department and her appropriate duty of self-interest to keep her medical practice solvent. This case, however, is included to highlight the concerns raised by private practice physicians when a publically funded clinic is being established. Clearly, Ms. Porterfield did not understand the interests of all the stakeholders that might be affected by the health department's otherwise-desirable initiative. Although it is hard to believe that anyone could oppose a "free" clinic, this case illustrates such a situation.

The tragic case of Jesica Santillan riveted the public's attention in early 2003. It has elements of both resource allocation and social responsibility, but the case is discussed here because it highlights important issues of social responsibility and the obligation of U.S. health services providers to treat illegal aliens.

Jesica Santillan[38]

Jesica Santillan was 17 years old when she died. She had been born near Guadalajara, Mexico, with congenital cardiac insufficiency. Her family smuggled her into the U.S. to obtain the heart/lung transplant she needed to stay alive. Jesica was placed on the transplant list at Duke University Hospital. North Carolinian Mack Mahony, who had become a family friend, helped raise the $500,000 needed to pay for the transplant.

The United Network of Organ Sharing (UNOS) manages a nationwide organ matching system under contract with the federal government. Its criteria allow 5% of organs transplanted at any hospital to be used for illegal aliens or foreign nationals.

Although Jesica was on the transplant list, she was not on the list of potential recipients for the heart and lungs that were available—she was not a match. Nonetheless, the transplant coordinator and Jesica's doctor discussed giving the available organs to her. Neither realized that she was not on the list as being a match.

Jesica received the mismatched heart-lung transplant on February 7, 2003. It was soon apparent that her body was rejecting the organs. A correctly matched heart and lungs were transplanted, but her condition worsened. Jesica was declared brain dead at 1:25 P.M. on February 23. Life support was stopped at 5:00 P.M.

North Carolina law defines someone who is brain dead as no longer having life to support. Thus, life support may be ended without obtaining consent.

The Santillan family objected to the decision to discontinue life support. Mack Mahony asked for time to obtain a second opinion as to Jesica's condition. No extension of time was given, however.

This is an emotionally wrenching story of a young woman fighting for life. Despite her critical medical condition, there was every reason to believe she could have been saved. The following elements of the situation involve ethical issues: medical errors, the microallocation decision by Duke University Hospital in the first transplant, the microallocation by Duke University Hospital in the second transplant (preferential treatment, low probability of success), a non–U.S. citizen receiving scarce organs, and the macroallocation criteria developed by UNOS.

Crossing the ethical-legal boundary are the medical errors committed by staff at Duke University Hospital. The medical errors here did not involve the surgeons' technique or other treatment. Rather, they resulted from the failure of the processes that supported the transplant activity—processes developed and maintained by management. The hospital and its staff failed to meet their ethical duties of nonmaleficence and beneficence in the care provided to Jesica.

The ethical principle of justice is found in two microallocation decisions made at Duke University Hospital. The first has to do with the decision to allow an illegal alien to receive the transplant, regardless of the availability of funds and organs. Perhaps fresh in the minds of Duke's clinicians and administrators was the experience involving the Cleveland Clinic, which, in similar circumstances, initially refused to provide a liver transplant to an illegal alien. It bowed to political pressure from a Hispanic city councilman, however, and provided the treatment. The principle of justice also arises in the microallocation decision Duke University Hospital made when it transplanted a second (correctly matched) set of heart and lungs. Questions about preferential treatment abound in that one patient received a second set of organs, which were transplanted despite a very low probability of success.

Finally, there is the issue of macroallocation of organs to non–U.S. citizens, which is even more questionable for illegal aliens. Given the scarcity of transplantable organs, it seems morally unjust that non–U.S. citizens receive any at all. After all, non–U.S. citizens contribute no organs to the pool of organs available for transplantation. Indeed, anecdotal evidence suggests that many noncitizens come from cultures where organ donation is religiously or socially unacceptable. It is noteworthy that the Santillans declined to donate any of Jesica's organs.[39] The Santillan case strongly suggests that UNOS reconsider its position on allocation of organs to non–U.S. citizens—especially illegal aliens, who bring with them the double problem of a greatly enlarged service area and, typically, no resources to pay the costs of care.

How Can We Afford This?

A 63-year-old woman slipped into an irreversible coma after having two heart attacks. Three years later she was still a patient in an acute care hospital. Her aggregate unpaid bill totaled $750,000 after private insurance coverage lapsed. The insurer argued that the patient was receiving only custodial care, and therefore it would not pay for acute care. According to state law, the patient could be transferred to another facility only if she were declared mentally incompetent. Hospital efforts to achieve this through court action caused much adverse publicity in the community. Ultimately, the hospital failed to achieve its goal of discharging the woman from the hospital, and she died there.

The organization and its managers faced an ethical dilemma—their ongoing relationship with a patient who no longer needed acute care. The principles of beneficence and nonmaleficence and the virtues of caring and compassion prevented them from abandoning the patient, but the uncompensated costs of her care increasingly conflicted with the hospital's obligation to maintain its financial integrity, which was necessary to serving the community. Thus, managers failed to meet the virtues of loyalty and thrift. This large, financially healthy hospital could absorb the losses attributable to this patient, but the issue of resource allocation remains, nonetheless. The cost of a microallocation decision—continued treatment for someone unable to benefit from hospital care—would have overwhelmed the ability of many other hospitals to provide services to the community (macroallocation).

It is trite to characterize this case as a public relations failure, but the hospital might have gained community understanding had it been more forthright and communicative in describing the problem and the dilemma it faced in moving the woman to a more suitable alternative facility. Changing legal requirements so that mental status is but one criterion for making such decisions is important and should be championed by the hospital's trade association.

Noncompliant patients pose a special problem in microallocation decisions. Typically, they have chronic health problems that need continuing, periodic treatment, such as the dialysis that treats end-stage renal disease. These patients may be noncompliant in following a dietary and medication regimen, submitting to scheduled treatment, or they may behave such that staff cannot treat them. The organization is morally obligated to facilitate treatment for all patients needing its services. However, those with significant behavioral problems or who do not comply with their treatment regimen should be discharged from the program, with proper attention to legal requirements.

A new dimension to the policy issue of uncompensated care is raised when non–U.S. citizens are taken to U.S. hospitals for treatment. It has been reported that ambulances from Mexico are using unguarded border crossings to bring illegal aliens to U.S. hospitals after the patients were denied care in Mexican hospitals because they could not pay. U.S. hospitals must provide services because of the Emergency Medical Treatment and Active Labor Act (EMTALA) of 1986 (42 USC § 1395dd.), which makes no distinction between citizens and illegal aliens. Some federal monies have been made available to offset the burden of meeting EMTALA service demands from illegals. Adding significantly to costs is providing helicopter transport from border hospitals to inland medical centers when more sophisticated treatment is needed. It has been estimated that hospitals along the Mexican border have lost more than $200 million in unreimbursed costs for treating illegal aliens, and the losses show no signs of abating. Some verge on bankruptcy; others have been forced to close their EDs. The result is compromised access for legal immigrants and U.S. citizens. A study found that 77 U.S. hospitals along the Mexican border face a medical emergency. Numerous reports describe the financial plight of hospitals on the Mexican border that are providing large amounts of uncompensated care to non-American patients.

The federal government is responsible for the integrity of the nation's borders; yet, it has been unwilling to effectively address illegal immigration, so the financial burden has fallen on the hospitals.[40] The injustice of this situation and its negative effect on legal immigrants and U.S. citizens served by these hospitals are patent. Absent effective action, hospitals will fall further into financial decline and may close—to the detriment of all whom they were meant to serve.

CONCLUSION

This chapter examined some of the issues attendant to the social responsibility of health services organizations, primarily hospitals. Although organizations have an ethical obligation to husband resources, there are ethical limits, for instance, to how aggressively they should collect monies owed them. Also, sharp business practices should be avoided because they are inconsistent with various virtues and the principle of respect for persons. The virtues are fully consistent with the organization's efforts to protect and enhance its assets while maximizing patient and community benefit.

Through their managers, health services organizations are morally obliged to provide services that meet the patient's needs without considering nonrelevant factors such as age, payment status, race, or sex. Persistent variations in provisions of medical services appear to be more a function of how physicians practice medicine than deliberate expressions of bias. What is identified as ageism may be as much an expression of the culture's emphasis on youth as it is a bias against older adults. Ethically unacceptable, however, are implicit judgments about poor quality of life. Health services managers must identify and eliminate any hint of systemic or personal bias in medical decision making and delivery of services.

Protecting the commonweal—the sum of private and public resources—is a more ethereal responsibility. Much of what can or should be done is beyond the control of health services managers. Nonetheless, wasteful programs, regardless of funding source, and those of lesser clinical quality or that unnecessarily put the public at risk, must be eliminated. Husbanding resources is an ethical obligation for managers, because all resources, regardless of ownership, are part of the commonweal.

NOTES

1. Lucette Lagnado. (2003, October 30). Hospitals try extreme measures to collect their overdue debts. *Wall Street Journal*, p. A1.
2. Tanner, Michael D. (2009, August 17). Who are the uninsured? *Philadelphia Inquirer*. Retrieved March 26, 2011, from http://www.cato.org/pub_display.php?pub_id=10449.
3. June E. O'Neill & Dave M. O'Neill. (2010). *Who are the uninsured? An analysis of America's uninsured population, their characteristics and their health (p. 4)*. Washington, DC: Employment Policies Institute.

4. Adapted from Stuart Elliott. (2008, March 12). When a corporate donate raises protests. *New York Times*. Retrieved March 8, 2011, from http://www.nytimes.com/2008/03/12/business/media/12adco.html?sq=.

5. Susan Okie. (2001, June 20). Better cancer care urged: Focus on cure hurts treatment of symptoms, study finds. *Washington Post*, p. A14.

6. Joyce Howard Price. (2003, December 1). Seniors medical care poses bias question. *Washington Times*, p. A1.

7. National Hospice and Palliative Care Organization. (2010). *NHPCO facts and figures: Hospice care in America (p. 7)*. Alexandria, VA: Author.

8. Beth A. Virnig, Sara Kind, Marshall McBean, & Elliott Fisher. (2000, September). Geographic variation in hospice use prior to death. *Journal of the American Geriatrics Society 48*(9), pp. 1117–1125.

9. Sarah J. Goodlin, Zhenshao Zhong, Joanne Lynn, Joan M. Teno, Julie P. Fago, Normal Desbiens, Alfred F. Connors, Jr., Neil S. Wenger, & Russell S. Phillips. (1999, December 22). Factors associated with use of cardiopulmonary resuscitation in seriously ill hospitalized adults. *Journal of the American Medical Association 282*(24), 2333–2339.

10. Howard B. Degenholtz, Robert A. Arnold, Alan Meisel, & Judith R. Lave. (2002, February). Persistence of racial disparities in advance care plan documents among nursing home residents. *Journal of the American Geriatrics Society 50*(2), pp. 378–381.

11. Neil S. Wenger, Marjorie L. Pearson, Katherine A. Desmond, Ellen R. Harrison, Lisa V. Rubenstein, William H. Rogers, & Katherine L. Kahn. (1995, October 23). Epidemiology of do-not-resuscitate orders: Disparity by age, diagnosis, gender, race, and functional impairment. *Archives of Internal Medicine 155*, pp. 2056–2062.

12. Robert M. Wachter, John M. Luce, Norman Hearst, & Bernard Lo. (1989, September). Decisions about resuscitation: Inequities among patients with different diseases but similar prognoses. *Annals of Internal Medicine 3*(6), pp. 525–532.

13. Ezekiel J. Emanuel. (2001, June 9). Euthanasia: Where the Netherlands leads will the world follow? No. Legalisation is a diversion from improving care for the dying. *British Medical Journal 322*(7299), pp. 1376–1377.

14. *Ibid.*

15. Very sick patients left all alone, Georgetown study finds. (2001, December 3). *American Medical News*. Retrieved November 14, 2003, from http://www.ama-assn.org/amednews/2001/12/03/prbf1203.htm.

16. Judith C. Ahronheim, Michael Mulvihill, Carol Sieger, Pil Park, & Brant E. Fries. (2001, February). State practice variations in the use of tube feedings for nursing home residents with severe cognitive impairment. *Journal of the American Geriatrics Society 49*(2), pp. 148–152.

17. Maureen Glabman. (2003, June). Managed care makes it tough for some hospitals to stay afloat. *Managed Care Magazine*. Retrieved January 2, 2004, from http://www.managedcaremag.com/archives/0306/0306.er.html.

18. Institute of Medicine Report Brief. (2006, June). *The future of emergency care in the United States health system*. Retrieved December 18, 2010, from http://www.iom.edu/~/media/Files/Report%20Files/2006/Hospital-Based-Emergency-Care-At-the-Breaking-Point/EmergencyCare.ashx.

19. Charles Fried. (1976, February). Equality and rights in medical care. *Hastings Center Report 6(2)*, pp. 29–34.
20. Leonard M. Fleck. (2002, March/April). Rationing: Don't give up. *Hastings Center Report 32*(2), pp. 35–36.
21. Greta Anand. (2003, September 12). The big secret in health care: Rationing is here. *Wall Street Journal*, p. A1.
22. Robert Langreth. (2009, November 30). Useless medicine. *Forbes 184*(10), pp. 64, 66, 68, 70, 72.
23. American Hospital Association. (2010, December). *Uncompensated hospital care cost fact sheet (p. 1)*. Chicago. Author.
24. Mary Ann Costello. (2004, February 18). Nation's hospitals provided $22.3 billion in uncompensated care in 2002. *AHA News Now*, p. 1.
25. David Burda. (1995, May 8). Hospitals' care for poor rises slowly. *Modern Healthcare 25*(19), p. 30.
26. American Hospital Association, p. 1.
27. Health First. (2003). *What are not-for-profit/community-minded hospitals? What it means to your community.* Retrieved March 26, 2011, from http://www.health -first.org/about_us/not_for_profit.cfm.
28. American Hospital Association, p. 4.
29. National Association of Public Hospitals and Health Systems. (2011). *2009 annual survey: Safety net hospitals and health systems fulfill mission in uncertain times.* Retrieved March 26, 2011, from http://www.naph.org/Main-Menu-Category/ Publications/Safety-Net-Financing/2009-Characteristics-Survey-Research -Brief.aspx?FT=.pdf.
30. Burda, p. 30.
31. K.E. Thorpe, C.S. Florence, & E.E. Seiber. (2000). Hospital conversion, margins and the provision of uncompensated care. *Health Affairs 19*(6), pp. 187–199.
32. David Burda. (1995, April 24). Tennessee for-profits lag in care for poor. *Modern Healthcare 25*(17), pp. 70, 72, 74.
33. *Statement of the Federation of American Hospitals: Hospitals' non-profit status: Federal Trade Commission and Department of Justice hearings on health care and competition law and policy* (2003, April 10) (testimony of Eugene Anthony Fay). Retrieved March 29, 2011, from http://www.ftc.gov/ogc/healthcarehearings/ docs/030410fay.pdf.
34. David Burda. (1995, May 8). For-profits, not-for-profits reignite battle. *Modern Healthcare 25*(19), pp. 28, 30.
35. Sarah Yang. (2003, October 27). New briefs find relatively few hospitals providing bulk of charity care in the state. *UC Berkeley News*. Retrieved January 6, 2004, from http://www.berkeley.edu/news/media/releases/2003/10/27_char ity.shtml.
36. Congress of the United States, Congressional Budget Office. (2006, December). *Nonprofit hospitals and the provision of community benefits.* Retrieved March 8, 2011, from http://www.cbo.gov/ftpdocs/76xx/doc7695/12-06-Nonprofit .pdf.
37. Written by Gary E. Crum, Ph.D., MPH, Executive Director, Graduate Medical Education Consortium, University of Virginia at Wise. Used with permission.

38. Sources for the Jesica Santillan case: Angela Heywood Bible & Sarah Avery. (2003, February 24). *At odds over Jesica's last hours.* Retrieved May 4, 2004, from http://organtx.org/ethics/mismatch.htm; Donna Gregory. (2003, February 23). Santillan family planning lawsuit. *MSNBC News*; A. Comarow. (2003, July 28). Jesica's Story. *U.S. News & World Report 135*(3), p. 51; Michelle Malkin. (2003, March 18). Illegal alien health care has crippling effects on citizens. *Insight on the News.* Retrieved May 4, 2004, from http://www.findarticles.com/cf_0/m1571/7_19/98923512/p1/article.jhtml.
39. Thomas H. Maugh. (2003, February). Mexican teen dies after her 2nd transplant. *Orlando Sentinel.* Retrieved March 25, 2011, from http://articles.orlandosentinel.com/2003-02-23/news/0302230324_1_blood-life-support-transplant.
40. Jerry Seper. (2002, December 12). Mexican medics take sick to U.S.: Americans left to pick up tab. *Washington Times*, p. A1.

ORGANIZATIONAL PHILOSOPHIES AND MISSION STATEMENTS

COMMITMENT, MISSION, VISION, AND VALUES STATEMENT OF SUTTER HEALTH

Our Commitment

We go to those in need.

> "Charity care isn't just a slogan at Sutter Health; it's a deep felt commitment. Everyone gets the same high-quality care and treatment at our facilities from our care providers regardless of their ability to pay."
> —Jim Gray, Sutter Health Board of Directors

Sutter Health's mission focuses beyond the walls of our care facilities and out into the community. School based clinics, mobile clinics, transportation services, language assistance and prevention and wellness strategies are among the ways Sutter Health seeks to put its "mission into action."

Our Mission Statement

Vision and Values We enhance the well-being of people in the communities we serve through a not-for-profit commitment to compassion and excellence in health care services.

Vision Sutter Health leads the transformation of health care to achieve the highest levels of quality, access and affordability.

Values

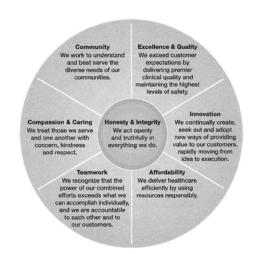

Retrieved April 4, 2011, from http://www.sutterhealth.org/about/comben/commitment/index.html

MISSION, CORE VALUES, AND
VISION STATEMENT OF TRINITY HEALTH

Mission

> We serve together in Trinity Health,
> in the spirit of the Gospel,
> to heal body, mind and spirit,
> to improve the health of our communities
> and to steward the resources entrusted to us.

Core Values

Respect   We value and esteem every human person because each and every one is created by God, in the image of God. Everyone, regardless of title or position, income, education or status, race, religion or ethnicity has a dignity that is sacred. We treasure and hold human life sacred from its simplest beginnings until its end. (Gen. 1:26; Luke 9:47-48; John 10:10)

Social Justice   In this age of globalization and instant communication, we more quickly recognize our common humanity. We recognize as well the great gaps in economy, health, education and development among the peoples of this earth. Social justice commits us to the common good so that all may have their basic needs met. We recognize health and access to healthcare as a basic human right and seek to provide and advocate for it. (Wisdom 9:2f; Isaiah 32:16-18.)

Compassion   People come to us when they are in need and in distress. In the spirit of Jesus, we recognize their need and seek to respond to it. We reach out to them in their pain and suffering and care for them in body, mind and spirit. The ability to feel and to respond to the suffering of others is an essential value in our ministry of healthcare, no matter where we serve. We recognize also that those we cannot cure we can still love, care for and be with in their suffering. (Mark 1:40f; Mark 10:51; Luke 4:40 Luke 10:30-37; Romans 12:15; I Cor. 13:4-7)

Care of the Poor and Underserved   God hears the cry of the poor and so, with respect and compassion, we seek out the poor and underserved as a special focus of our healthcare ministry. It is those without resources of their own who need us most. We seek to care not only for their immediate needs but also to change the structures that keep them in unhealthy environments and inhumane conditions. Through our ministry of health care and our persistent advocacy, we seek to serve the poor and underserved of our communities. We too hear the cry of the poor and underserved. (Acts 4:32-35; James 2:15)

Excellence　The scriptures look to the day when there will be a new heaven and a new earth, when creation will be made perfect. Our vision is no less. In all we do, we reach for more-greater respect, fuller justice, deeper compassion, better care, less poverty. We are impatient to do better and hold ourselves accountable for continuous improvement in the services we offer. (Matthew 25:14-23; II Corinthians. 9:6; Revelations 21:1)

Vision

Inspired by our Catholic faith tradition, Trinity Health will be distinguished by an unrelenting focus on clinical and service outcomes as we seek to create excellence in the care experience. Trinity Health will become the most trusted health partner for life.

The Vision focuses on a "trinity" of themes:

- A commitment to our founding purpose to strengthen Catholic health care

- An emphasis on providing a personal care experience in our Ministry Organizations

- The importance of building trusting relationships with all of our constituencies: patients, associates, physicians and communities

Retrieved April 4, 2011, from http://www.trinity-health.org/body.cfm?id=19

MISSION AND VISION STATEMENT OF
THE GEORGE WASHINGTON UNIVERSITY MEDICAL CENTER

Mission

- Teaching with creativity and dedication

- Healing with quality and compassion

- Discovering with imagination and innovation

Working together in our nation's capital, with integrity and resolve, The George Washington University Medical Center is committed to improving the health and well-being of our local, national and global communities.

Vision

The George Washington University Medical Center will improve the health and well-being of our local, national and global communities by:

- Developing tomorrow's leaders

- Delivering high-quality health care

- Advancing scientific discovery and translating discoveries into action

- Harnessing new technology

- Establishing community partnerships

- Fostering multidisciplinary collaboration

- Pursuing alliances unique to our location.

Retrieved April 4, 2011, from http://www.gwumc.edu/about/ourmission

MISSION, VALUES, AND SUPPORTING
STATEMENTS OF MOUNTAINVIEW REGIONAL MEDICAL CENTER

Mission

Create and maintain a caring environment where our healthcare team exemplifies clinical and service excellence within our regional community.

Values and Supporting Statements

Safety   We will create a safe environment, which promotes confidence and emphasizes high ethical standards.

Compassion   We will foster a compassionate and caring atmosphere for our patients, their families and guests.

Teamwork   We will support a positive working environment, which encourages collaboration, communication and pride among our employees, medical staff, administration, volunteers and the community.

Efficiency   We will, individually and collectively, be known for clinical and service excellence by providing high-quality, efficient healthcare.

Retrieved April 4, 2011, from http://www.mountainviewregional.com/About/Pages/Mission%20and%20Vision.aspx

MISSION, PRIMARY VALUE, AND VALUE STATEMENTS OF MAYO CLINIC

Mission

To inspire hope and contribute to health and well-being by providing the best care to every patient through integrated clinical practice, education and research.

Primary value

The needs of the patient come first.

Value statements

These values, which guide Mayo Clinic's mission to this day, are an expression of the vision and intent of our founders, the original Mayo physicians and the Sisters of Saint Francis.

Respect Treat everyone in our diverse community, including patients, their families and colleagues, with dignity.

Compassion Provide the best care, treating patients and family members with sensitivity and empathy.

Integrity Adhere to the highest standards of professionalism, ethics and personal responsibility, worthy of the trust our patients place in us.

Healing Inspire hope and nurture the well-being of the whole person, respecting physical, emotional and spiritual needs.

Teamwork Value the contributions of all, blending the skills of individual staff members in unsurpassed collaboration.

Excellence Deliver the best outcomes and highest quality service through the dedicated effort of every team member.

Innovation Infuse and energize the organization, enhancing the lives of those we serve, through the creative ideas and unique talents of each employee.

Stewardship Sustain and reinvest in our mission and extended communities by wisely managing our human, natural and material resources.

Retrieved April 4, 2011, from http://www.mayoclinic.org/about/missionvalues.html
Reprinted with permission.

MISSION, PRINCIPLES OF SERVICE, AND CORE VALUES STATEMENT OF SUNRISE SENIOR LIVING

Each team member at every Sunrise community is trained to understand the value of our mission, Principles of Service and Core Values, and are encouraged to be guided by them in all they do for our residents every day. These are the hallmarks of Sunrise.

Our Mission

Right from the beginning, Sunrise's mission has been to champion quality of life for all seniors. Sunrise's Founders, Paul and Terry Klaassen, developed their resident-centered philosophy of care based on deep convictions about how to achieve the best quality of life for each individual. Those beliefs are now the foundation of the Principles of Service and Core Values that guide and focus our team members at all of our senior living communities.

Our Principles of Service

Everyone who works at Sunrise is guided by these six Principles of Service.

Preserving Dignity

We value the life experiences of every senior and give each the respect they deserve. For example, in our Reminiscence Neighborhoods, residents living with Alzheimer's disease and other forms of memory loss are guided to engage in meaningful activities that give them a sense of purpose and create pleasant days.

Nurturing the Spirit

We care for the whole person—mind, body and spirit. Our team members care not only for the physical needs of our residents, but are committed to providing opportunities for social interaction, mental exercise and spiritual fulfilment that suit the tastes and preferences of each resident.

Celebrating Individuality

We recognize that every one of our residents is unique. Each one has a life story we want to hear and understand, with personal tastes and preferences that will be respected.

Enabling Freedom of Choice

We empower seniors to live as they wish by offering choices. Options are a way of life at Sunrise, whether it's in the dining room where there's always a special menu of daily options along with à la carte favorites, or in a resident's suite, where they can wake up as late or as early as they want—just like they've always done.

Encouraging Independence

We encourage our residents' right to self-reliance in whatever ways possible. Our communities are specially designed to encourage mobility in a safe environment, and care managers are trained to support our residents' choices whenever possible.

Involving Family and Friends

We welcome family and friends to participate in all community activities and events. There are no "visiting hours" at Sunrise, and we encourage visitors to spend time with residents at any time of day or night. Our care managers and community leaders regularly communicate with family members to ensure we are providing the very best service for our residents.

Our Core Values

Sunrise works to ensure these core values are instilled in all of our team members:

Passion

Joy in Service

Stewardship

Respect

Trust

Retrieved April 4, 2011, from http://www.sunriseseniorliving.com/the-sunrise-difference/principles-and-values.aspx

ETHICAL CODES

THE HIPPOCRATIC OATH: CLASSICAL VERSION

I swear by Apollo Physician and Asclepius and Hygieia and Panaceia and all the gods and goddesses, making them my witnesses, that I will fulfill according to my ability and judgment this oath and this covenant:

To hold him who has taught me this art as equal to my parents and to live my life in partnership with him, and if he is in need of money to give him a share of mine, and to regard his offspring as equal to my brothers in male lineage and to teach them this art—if they desire to learn it—without fee and covenant; to give a share of precepts and oral instruction and all the other learning to my sons and to the sons of him who has instructed me and to pupils who have signed the covenant and have taken an oath according to the medical law, but no one else.

I will apply dietetic measures for the benefit of the sick according to my ability and judgment; I will keep them from harm and injustice.

I will neither give a deadly drug to anybody who asked for it, nor will I make a suggestion to this effect. Similarly I will not give to a woman an abortive remedy. In purity and holiness I will guard my life and my art.

I will not use the knife, not even on sufferers from stone, but will withdraw in favor of such men as are engaged in this work.

Whatever houses I may visit, I will come for the benefit of the sick, remaining free of all intentional injustice, of all mischief and in particular of sexual relations with both female and male persons, be they free or slaves.

What I may see or hear in the course of the treatment or even outside of the treatment in regard to the life of men, which on no account one must spread abroad, I will keep to myself, holding such things shameful to be spoken about.

If I fulfill this oath and do not violate it, may it be granted to me to enjoy life and art, being honored with fame among all men for all time to come; if I transgress it and swear falsely, may the opposite of all this be my lot.

Retrieved April 4, 2011, from http://www.pbs.org/wgbh/nova/doctors/oath_classical. html. Translation from the Greek by Ludwig Edelstein. From *The Hippocratic Oath: Text, Translation, and Interpretation*, by Ludwig Edelstein. Baltimore: Johns Hopkins Press, 1943.

AMERICAN COLLEGE OF HEALTHCARE EXECUTIVES (ACHE) CODE OF ETHICS

Preamble

The purpose of the Code of Ethics of the American College of Healthcare Executives is to serve as a standard of conduct for affiliates. It contains standards of ethical behavior for healthcare executives in their professional relationships. These relationships include colleagues, patients or others served; members of the healthcare executive's organization and other organizations, the community, and society as a whole.

The Code of Ethics also incorporates standards of ethical behavior governing individual behavior, particularly when that conduct directly relates to the role and identity of the healthcare executive.

The fundamental objectives of the healthcare management profession are to maintain or enhance the overall quality of life, dignity and well-being of every individual needing healthcare service and to create a more equitable, accessible, effective and efficient healthcare system.

Healthcare executives have an obligation to act in ways that will merit the trust, confidence, and respect of healthcare professionals and the general public. Therefore, healthcare executives should lead lives that embody an exemplary system of values and ethics.

In fulfilling their commitments and obligations to patients or others served, healthcare executives function as moral advocates and models. Since every management decision affects the health and well-being of both individuals and communities, healthcare executives must carefully evaluate the possible outcomes of their decisions. In organizations that deliver healthcare services, they must work to safeguard and foster the rights, interests and prerogatives of patients or others served.

The role of moral advocate requires that healthcare executives take actions necessary to promote such rights, interests and prerogatives.

Being a model means that decisions and actions will reflect personal integrity and ethical leadership that others will seek to emulate.

I. The Healthcare Executive's Responsibilities to the Profession of Healthcare Management

The healthcare executive shall:

A. Uphold the Code of Ethics and mission of the American College of Healthcare Executives;

B. Conduct professional activities with honesty, integrity, respect, fairness and good faith in a manner that will reflect well upon the profession;

C. Comply with all laws and regulations pertaining to healthcare management in the jurisdictions in which the healthcare executive is located or conducts professional activities;

D. Maintain competence and proficiency in healthcare management by implementing a personal program of assessment and continuing professional education;

E. Avoid the improper exploitation of professional relationships for personal gain;

F. Disclose financial and other conflicts of interest;

G. Use this Code to further the interests of the profession and not for selfish reasons;

H. Respect professional confidences;

I. Enhance the dignity and image of the healthcare management profession through positive public information programs; and

J. Refrain from participating in any activity that demeans the credibility and dignity of the healthcare management profession.

II. The Healthcare Executive's Responsibilities to Patients or Others Served

The healthcare executive shall, within the scope of his or her authority:

A. Work to ensure the existence of a process to evaluate the quality of care or service rendered;

B. Avoid practicing or facilitating discrimination and institute safeguards to prevent discriminatory organizational practices;

C. Work to ensure the existence of a process that will advise patients or others served of the rights, opportunities, responsibilities and risks regarding available healthcare services;

D. Work to ensure that there is a process in place to facilitate the resolution of conflicts that may arise when values of patients and their families differ from those of employees and physicians;

E. Demonstrate zero tolerance for any abuse of power that compromises patients or others served;

F. Work to provide a process that ensures the autonomy and self-determination of patients or others served; and

G. Work to ensure the existence of procedures that will safeguard the confidentiality and privacy of patients or others served.

III. The Healthcare Executive's Responsibilities to the Organization

The healthcare executive shall, within the scope of his or her authority:

A. Provide healthcare services consistent with available resources, and when there are limited resources, work to ensure the existence of a resource allocation process that considers ethical ramifications;

B. Conduct both competitive and cooperative activities in ways that improve community healthcare services;

C. Lead the organization in the use and improvement of standards of management and sound business practices;

D. Respect the customs and practices of patients or others served, consistent with the organization's philosophy;

E. Be truthful in all forms of professional and organizational communication, and avoid disseminating information that is false, misleading or deceptive;

F. Report negative financial and other information promptly and accurately, and initiate appropriate action;

G. Prevent fraud and abuse and aggressive accounting practices that may result in disputable financial reports;

H. Create an organizational environment in which both clinical and management mistakes are minimized and, when they do occur, are disclosed and addressed effectively;

I. Implement an organizational code of ethics and monitor compliance; and

J. Provide ethics resources to staff to address organizational and clinical issues.

IV. The Healthcare Executive's Responsibilities to Employees

Healthcare executives have ethical and professional obligations to the employees they manage that encompass but are not limited to:

A. Creating a work environment that promotes ethical conduct by employees;

B. Providing a work environment that encourages a free expression of ethical concerns and provides mechanisms for discussing and addressing such concerns;

C. Providing a work environment that discourages harassment, sexual and other; coercion of any kind, especially to perform illegal or unethical acts; and discrimination on the basis of race, ethnicity, creed, gender, sexual orientation, age, or disability;

D. Providing a work environment that promotes the proper use of employees' knowledge and skills;

E. Providing a safe work environment; and

F. Establishing appropriate grievance and appeals mechanisms.

V. The Healthcare Executive's Responsibilities to Community and Society

The healthcare executive shall:

A. Work to identify and meet the healthcare needs of the community;

B. Work to support access to healthcare services for all people;

C. Encourage and participate in public dialogue on healthcare policy issues, and advocate solutions that will improve health status and promote quality healthcare;

D. Apply short-and long-term assessments to management decisions affecting both community and society; and

E. Provide prospective patients and others with adequate and accurate information, enabling them to make enlightened decisions regarding services.

VI. The Healthcare Executive's Responsibility to Report Violations of the Code

An affiliate of ACHE who has reasonable grounds to believe that another affiliate has violated this Code has a duty to communicate such facts to the Ethics Committee.

Retrieved April 4, 2011, from http://www.ache.org/abt_ache/ACHECodeofEthics-2007 .pdf.

AMERICAN COLLEGE OF HEALTH CARE ADMINISTRATORS (ACHCA) CODE OF ETHICS

Preamble

The preservation of the highest standards of integrity and ethical principles is vital to the successful discharge of the professional responsibilities of all long-term health care administrators. This Code of Ethics has been promulgated by the American College of Health Care Administrators (ACHCA) in an effort to stress the fundamental rules considered essential to this basic purpose. It shall be the obligation of members to seek to avoid not only conduct specifically proscribed by the code, but also conduct that is inconsistent with its spirit and purpose. Failure to specify any particular responsibility or practice in this Code of Ethics should not be construed as denial of the existence of other responsibilities or practices. Recognizing that the ultimate responsibility for applying standards and ethics falls upon the individual, the ACHCA establishes the following Code of Ethics to make clear its expectation of the membership.

Expectation I

Individuals shall hold paramount the welfare of persons for whom care is provided.

Prescriptions: The Health Care Administrator shall:

- Strive to provide to all those entrusted to his or her care the highest quality of appropriate services possible in light of resources or other constraints.

- Operate the facility consistent with laws, regulations, and standards of practice recognized in the field of health care administration.

- Consistent with law and professional standards, protect the confidentiality of information regarding individual recipients of care.

- Perform administrative duties with the personal integrity that will earn the confidence, trust, and respect of the general public.

Take appropriate steps to avoid discrimination on basis of race, color, sex, religion, age, national origin, handicap, marital status, ancestry, or any other factor that is illegally discriminatory or not related to bona fide requirements of quality care.

Proscription: The Health Care Administrator shall not:

- Disclose professional or personal information regarding recipients of service to unauthorized personnel unless required by law or to protect the public welfare.

Expectation II

Individuals shall maintain high standards of professional competence.

Prescriptions: The Health Care Administrator shall:

- Possess and maintain the competencies necessary to effectively perform his or her responsibilities.
- Practice administration in accordance with capabilities and proficiencies and, when appropriate, seek counsel from qualified others.
- Actively strive to enhance knowledge of and expertise in long-term care administration through continuing education and professional development.

Proscriptions: The Health Care Administrator shall not:

- Misrepresent qualifications, education, experience, or affiliations.
- Provide services other than those for which he or she is prepared and qualified to perform.

Expectation III

Individuals shall strive, in all matters relating to their professional functions, to maintain a professional posture that places paramount the interests of the facility and its residents.

Prescriptions: The Health Care Administrator shall:

- Avoid partisanship and provide a forum for the fair resolution of any disputes which may arise in service delivery or facility management.
- Disclose to the governing body or other authority as may be appropriate, any actual or potential circumstance concerning him or her that might reasonably be thought to create a conflict of interest or have a substantial adverse impact on the facility or its residents.

Proscription: The Health Care Administrator shall not:

- Participate in activities that reasonably may be thought to create a conflict of interest or have the potential to have a substantial adverse impact on the facility or its residents.

Expectation IV

Individuals shall honor their responsibilities to the public, their profession, and their relationships with colleagues and members of related professions.

Prescriptions: The Health Care Administrator shall:

- Foster increased knowledge within the profession of health care administration and support research efforts toward this end.

- Participate with others in the community to plan for and provide a full range of health care services.

- Share areas of expertise with colleagues, students, and the general public to increase awareness and promote understanding of health care in general and the profession in particular.

- Inform the ACHCA Standards and Ethics Committee of actual or potential violations of this Code of Ethics, and fully cooperate with ACHCA's sanctioned inquiries into matters of professional conduct related to this Code of Ethics.

Proscription: The Health Care Administrator shall not:

- Defend, support, or ignore unethical conduct perpetrated by colleagues, peers or students.

From American College of Health Care Administrators (ACHCA). Retrieved April 4, 2011, from http://www.achca.org/index.php/about-achca. Reprinted by permission.

AMERICAN MEDICAL ASSOCIATION
PRINCIPLES OF MEDICAL ETHICS

Preamble

The medical profession has long subscribed to a body of ethical statements developed primarily for the benefit of the patient. As a member of this profession, a physician must recognize responsibility to patients first and foremost, as well as to society, to other health professionals, and to self. The following Principles adopted by the American Medical Association are not laws, but standards of conduct which define the essentials of honorable behavior for the physician.

Principles of Medical Ethics

I.   A physician shall be dedicated to providing competent medical care, with compassion and respect for human dignity and rights.

II. A physician shall uphold the standards of professionalism, be honest in all professional interactions, and strive to report physicians deficient in character or competence, or engaging in fraud or deception, to appropriate entities.

III. A physician shall respect the law and also recognize a responsibility to seek changes in those requirements which are contrary to the best interests of the patient.

IV. A physician shall respect the rights of patients, colleagues, and other health professionals, and shall safeguard patient confidences and privacy within the constraints of the law.

V.   A physician shall continue to study, apply, and advance scientific knowledge, maintain a commitment to medical education, make relevant information available to patients, colleagues, and the public, obtain consultation, and use the talents of other health professionals when indicated.

VI. A physician shall, in the provision of appropriate patient care, except in emergencies, be free to choose whom to serve, with whom to associate, and the environment in which to provide medical care.

VII. A physician shall recognize a responsibility to participate in activities contributing to the improvement of the community and the betterment of public health.

VIII. A physician shall, while caring for a patient, regard responsibility to the patient as paramount.

IX. A physician shall support access to medical care for all people.

Retrieved April 4, 2011, from http://www.ama-assn.org/ama/pub/physician-resources/medical-ethics/code-medical-ethics/principles-medical-ethics.page. Adopted June 1957; revised June 1980; revised June 2001.

AMERICAN MEDICAL ASSOCIATION
COUNCIL ON ETHICAL AND JUDICIAL AFFAIRS

Fundamental Elements of the Patient–Physician Relationship

From ancient times, physicians have recognized that the health and well-being of patients depends upon a collaborative effort between physician and patient. Patients share with physicians the responsibility for their own health care. The patient-physician relationship is of greatest benefit to patients when they bring medical problems to the attention of their physicians in a timely fashion, provide information about their medical condition to the best of their ability, and work with their physicians in a mutually respectful alliance. Physicians can best contribute to this alliance by serving as their patients' advocate and by fostering these rights:

1. The patient has the right to receive information from physicians and to discuss the benefits, risks, and costs of appropriate treatment alternatives. Patients should receive guidance from their physicians as to the optimal course of action. Patients are also entitled to obtain copies or summaries of their medical records, to have their questions answered, to be advised of potential conflicts of interest that their physicians might have, and to receive independent professional opinions.

2. The patient has the right to make decisions regarding the health care that is recommended by his or her physician. Accordingly, patients may accept or refuse any recommended medical treatment.

3. The patient has the right to courtesy, respect, dignity, responsiveness, and timely attention to his or her needs.

4. The patient has the right to confidentiality. The physician should not reveal confidential communications or information without the consent of the patient, unless provided for by law or by the need to protect the welfare of the individual or the public interest.

5. The patient has the right to continuity of health care. The physician has an obligation to cooperate in the coordination of medically indicated care with other health care providers treating the patient. The physician may not discontinue treatment of a patient as long as further treatment is medically indicated, without giving the patient reasonable assistance and sufficient opportunity to make alternative arrangements for care.

6. The patient has a basic right to have available adequate health care. Physicians, along with the rest of society, should continue to work toward this goal. Fulfillment of this right is dependent on society providing resources so that no patient is deprived of necessary care because of an inability to pay for the care. Physicians should continue their traditional assumption of a part of the responsibility for the medical care of those who cannot afford essential health care. Physicians should advocate for patients in dealing with third parties when appropriate.
(I, IV, V, VIII, IX)

From Council on Ethical and Judicial Affairs of the American Medical Association. Issued June 1992 based on the report "Fundamental Elements of the Patient–Physician Relationship," adopted June 1990 (JAMA, 1990; 262: 3/33); Updated 1993. Retrieved April 4, 2011, from https://ssl3.ama-assn.org/apps/ecomm/PolicyFinderForm.pl?site=www.ama-assn.org&uri=%2fama1%2fpub%2fupload%2fmm%2fPolicyFinder%2fpolicyfiles%2fHnE%2fE-10.01.HTM

CODE OF ETHICS FOR NURSES
FROM THE AMERICAN NURSES ASSOCIATION (ANA)

1. The nurse, in all professional relationships, practices with compassion and respect for the inherent dignity, worth, and uniqueness of every individual, unrestricted by considerations of social or economic status, personal attributes, or the nature of health problems.

2. The nurse's primary commitment is to the patient, whether an individual, family, group, or community.

3. The nurse promotes, advocates for, and strives to protect the health, safety, and rights of the patient.

4. The nurse is responsible and accountable for individual nursing practice and determines the appropriate delegation of tasks consistent with the nurse's obligation to provide optimum patient care.

5. The nurse owes the same duties to self as to others, including the responsibility to preserve integrity and safety, to maintain competence, and to continue personal and professional growth.

6. The nurse participates in establishing, maintaining, and improving health care environments and conditions of employment conducive to the provision of quality health care and consistent with the values of the profession through individual and collective action.

7. The nurse participates in the advancement of the profession through contributions to practice, education, administration, and knowledge development.

8. The nurse collaborates with other health professionals and the public in promoting community, national, and international efforts to meet health needs.

9. The profession of nursing, as represented by associations and their members, is responsible for articulating nursing values, for maintaining the integrity of the profession and its practice, and for shaping social policy.

From American Nurses Association. (2001). *Code of Ethics for Nurses.* Washington, DC: Author. Reprinted by permission.

SELECT BIBLIOGRAPHY

Ackoff, R.L. (1999). *Re-creating the corporation: A design of organizations for the 21st century.* New York: Oxford University Press.

Adler, M.J. (1978). *Aristotle for everybody: Difficult thought made easy.* New York: Macmillan.

Armstrong, A. (2006). Towards a strong virtue ethics for nursing practice. *Nursing Philosophy* 7,110–124.

Association of American Medical Colleges (2010). In the interest of patients: Recommendations for physician financial relationships and clinical decision making. *Report of the Task Force on Financial Conflicts of Interests.*

Baily, M.A. (2003, January/February). Managed care organizations and the rationing problem. *The Hastings Center Report, 33*(1), 34–42.

Barie, P., Hughes, D., & Ullery, B. (2008). The contemporary approach to the care of Jehovah's Witnesses. *The Journal of Trauma, Injury, Infection, and Critical Care, 65*:1, 237–247.

Battin, M.P. (1995). *Ethical issues in suicide.* Upper Saddle River, NJ: Prentice Hall.

Battin, M.P. "Terminal sedation: Pulling the sheet over our eyes." *The Hastings Center Report* 38:5 (Sep–Oct 2008): 27–30.

Beauchamp, T.L., & Childress, J.F. (2001). *Principles of biomedical ethics I* (5th ed.). New York: Oxford University Press.

Beauchamp, T.L., & Walters, L. (Eds.). (1999). *Contemporary issues in bioethics* (5th ed.). Belmont, CA: Wadsworth Group.

Beauchamp, T.L., Walters, L., Kahn, J.P. & Mastroianni, A.C. (eds.). (2007). *Contemporary issues in bioethics* (7th ed.). Belmont, CA: Wadsworth Group.

Begley, A. M. (2005). Practising virtue: A challenge to the view that a virtue centered approach to ethics lacks practical content. *Nursing Ethics 12*:6, 622–637.

Begley, A. M. (2008). Truth-telling, honesty and compassion: A virtue-based exploration of a dilemma in practice. *International Journal of Nursing Practice,1,* 336–341.

Bell, J. & Breslin, J. M. (2008). Healthcare provider moral distress as a leadership challenge. *JONA's Healthcare Law, Ethics, and Regulation, 10*:4, 94–97.

Blacksher, E. "Carrots and sticks to promote healthy behaviors: A policy update." *The Hastings Center Report* 38:3 (May–Jun 2008): 13–18.

Boatright, J.R. (2003). *Ethics and the conduct of business* (4th ed). Upper Saddle River, NJ: Prentice Hall.

Brock, D.W. (2008). Conscientious objection by physicians and pharmacists: Who is obligated to do what and why? *Theories of Medical Bioethics, 2,* 187–200.

Buchanan, A. (1998, August). Managed care: Rationing without justice, but not unjustly. *Journal of Health Politics, Policy and Law, 23*(4), 616–634.

Callahan, D. (2003, March/April). Too much of a good thing: How splendid technologies can go wrong. *The Hastings Center Report, 33*(2), 19–22.

Chervenak, F.A., & McCullough, L.B. (2001, April). The moral foundation of medical leadership: The professional virtues of the physician as fiduciary of the patient. *American Journal of Obstetrics and Gynecology, 184*(5), 875–880.

Deal, T.E., & Kennedy, A.A. (1982, reissued 2000). *Corporate cultures: The rites and rituals of corporate life.* New York: Perseus Books Group.

DeGeorge, R.T. (2009). *Business ethics* (7th ed.). Upper Saddle River, NJ: Prentice Hall.

Doukas, D.J. (2003). Where is the virtue in professionalism? *Cambridge Quarterly of Healthcare Ethics, 12,* 147–154.

Emanuel, E.J. (2000, May/June). Justice and managed care: Four principles for the just allocation of health care resources. *The Hastings Center Report, 30*(3), 8–16.

Frankena, W.K. (1988). *Ethics* (2nd ed.). Upper Saddle River, NJ: Prentice Hall.

Gallagher, E., Alcock, D., Diem, E., Angus, D., & Medves, J. (2002, March/April). Ethical dilemmas in home care case management. *The Journal of Healthcare Management,* 85–97.

Gallagher, J.A., & Goodstein, J. (2002). Fulfilling institutional responsibilities in health care: Organizational ethics and the role of mission discernment. *Business Ethics Quarterly, 12*(4), 433–450.

Gallagher, T.H., Waterman, A.D., Ebers, A.G., Fraser, V.J., & Levinson, W. (2003, February 26). Patients' and physicians' attitudes regarding the disclosure of medical errors. *Journal of the American Medical Association, 289*(8), 1001–1007.

Gert, H.J. (2002, September/October). Avoiding surprises: A model for informing patients. *The Hastings Center Report 32*(5), 23–32.

Gold, A. (2010). Physicians' right of conscience, beyond politics. *Journal of Law, Medicine, and Ethics,* Spring, 2010, 134–142.

Hall, R.T. (2000). *An introduction to healthcare organizational ethics.* New York: Oxford University Press.

Hodkinson, K. (2008). How should a nurse approach truth-telling? A virtue ethics perspective. *Nursing Philosophy 9,* 248–256.

Jansen, L.A., & Sulmasy, D.P. (2003, July/August). Bioethics, conflicts of interest, the limits of transparency. *The Hastings Center Report, 33*(4), 40–43.

Jennings, B., Gray, B.H., Sharpe, V.A., Weiss, L., & Fleischman, A.R. (2002, July/August). Ethics and trusteeship for health care: Hospital board service in turbulent times. *The Hastings Center Report, 32*(Suppl.), S1–S27.

Jonsen, A.R., & Toulmin, S. (1988). *The abuse of casuistry: A history of moral reasoning.* Berkeley: University of California Press.

Keown, J. (2002). *Euthanasia, ethics and public policy: An argument against legalization.* New York: Cambridge University Press.

Kollas, C. & Boyer-Kollas, B. (2006). Closing the Schiavo case: An analysis of legal reasoning. *Journal of Palliative Medicine, 9*:5, 1145–1163.

LeBar, M. (2009). Virtue ethics and deontic constraints. *Ethics 119* (July, 2009), 642–671.

Lee, D.E. (2003, January/February). Physician-assisted suicide: A conservative critique of intervention. *The Hastings Center Report, 33*(1), 17–19.

Loewy, E.H. (2001, February 12). Terminal sedation, self-starvation, and orchestrating the end of life. *Archives of Internal Medicine, 161*(3), 329–332.

Monagle, J.F., & Thomasma, D.C. (1994). *Health care ethics: Critical issues.* Sudbury, MA: Jones and Bartlett.

Morreim, E.H. (1995, November/December). Lifestyles of the risky and infamous. *The Hastings Center Report, 25,* 5–12.

Nelkin, D., & Andrews, L. (1998, September/October). *Homo economicus:* Commercialization of body tissues in the age of biotechnology. *The Hastings Center Report, 28*(5), 30–39.

Nelson, W.A. and Donnellan, J. "An executive-driven ethical culture." *Healthcare Executive* 24:6 (Nov–Dec 2009): 44–46.

Nuland, S.B. (1995). *How we die: Reflections on life's final chapter.* New York: Vintage Books.

Oakley, J., & Cocking, D. (2001). *Virtue ethics and professional roles.* New York: Oxford University Press.

Office of Inspector General of the U.S. Department of Health and Human Services and the American Health Lawyers Association. (2003, April 2). *Corporate responsibility and corporate compliance: A resource for health care boards of directors.* Retrieved March 9, 2004, from http://oig.hhs.gov/fraud/docs/complianceguid ance/ 040203CorpRespRsceGuide.pdf

Onwuteaka-Philipsen, B.D., Pasman, H. R., van der Heide, A. (2010). The last phase of life: Who requests and who receives euthanasia or physician-assisted suicide? *Medical Care, 48*:7, 596–603.

Pellegrino, E.D. (1994, Fall). Managed care and managed competition: Some ethical reflections. *Calyx, 4*(4), 1–5.

Pellegrino, E.D., & Thomasma, D.C. (1988). *For the patient's good: The restoration of beneficence in health care.* New York: Oxford University Press.

President's Commission for the Study of Ethical Problems in Medicine and Biomedical and Behavioral Research. (1981). *Defining death: A report on the medical, legal and ethical issues in the determination of death.* Washington, DC: U.S. Government Printing Office.

President's Commission for the Study of Ethical Problems in Medicine and Biomedical and Behavioral Research. (1981). *Protecting human subjects: The adequacy and uniformity of federal rules and their implementation.* Washington, DC: U.S. Government Printing Office.

President's Commission for the Study of Ethical Problems in Medicine and Biomedical and Behavioral Research. (1981). *Whistleblowing in biomedical research: Policies and procedures for responding to reports of misconduct.* Washington, DC: U.S. Government Printing Office.

President's Commission for the Study of Ethical Problems in Medicine and Biomedical and Behavioral Research. (1982). *Compensating for research injuries: A report on the ethical and legal implications for programs to redress injured subjects. Volume 2.* Washington, DC: U.S. Government Printing Office.

President's Commission for the Study of Ethical Problems in Medicine and Biomedical and Behavioral Research. (1982). *Making health care decisions: A report on the ethical and legal implications of informed consent in the patient–practitioner relationship. Volume 1: Report.* Washington, DC: U.S. Government Printing Office.

President's Commission for the Study of Ethical Problems in Medicine and Biomedical and Behavioral Research. (1982). *Making health care decisions: A report on the ethical and legal implications of informed consent in the patient–practitioner relationship. Volume 2: Appendices, Empirical studies of informed consent.* Washington, DC: U.S. Government Printing Office.

President's Commission for the Study of Ethical Problems in Medicine and Biomedical and Behavioral Research. (1982). *Splicing life: A report on the social and ethical issues of genetic engineering with human beings.* Washington, DC: U.S. Government Printing Office.

President's Commission for the Study of Ethical Problems in Medicine and Biomedical and Behavioral Research. (1983). *Deciding to forego life-sustaining treatment: A report on the ethical, medical, and legal issues in treatment decisions.* Washington, DC: U.S. Government Printing Office.

President's Commission for the Study of Ethical Problems in Medicine and Biomedical and Behavioral Research. (1983). *Implementing human research regulations: Second biennial report on the adequacy and uniformity of federal rules and policies, and of their implementation, for the protection of human subjects.* Washington, DC: U.S. Government Printing Office.

President's Commission for the Study of Ethical Problems in Medicine and Biomedical and Behavioral Research. (1983). *Screening and counseling for genetic conditions: The ethical, social, and legal implications of genetic screening, counseling, and education programs.* Washington, DC: U.S. Government Printing Office.

President's Commission for the Study of Ethical Problems in Medicine and Biomedical and Behavioral Research. (1983). *Securing access to health care: A report on the ethical implications of differences in the availability of health services. Volume 1: Report.* Washington, DC: U.S. Government Printing Office.

President's Commission for the Study of Ethical Problems in Medicine and Biomedical and Behavioral Research. (1983). *Securing access to health care: A report on the ethical implications of differences in the availability of health services. Volume 2: Appendices, Sociocultural and philosophical studies.* Washington, DC: U.S. Government Printing Office.

President's Commission for the Study of Ethical Problems in Medicine and Biomedical and Behavioral Research. (1983). *Securing access to health care: A report on the ethical implications of differences in the availability of health services. Volume 3: Appendices, Empirical, legal, and conceptual studies.* Washington, DC: U.S. Government Printing Office.

President's Commission for the Study of Ethical Problems in Medicine and Biomedical and Behavioral Research. (1983). *Summing up: Final report on studies of the ethical and legal problems in medicine and biomedical and behavioral research.* Washington, DC: U.S. Government Printing Office.

Prinz, J. (2009). The normativity challenge: cultural psychology provides the real threat to virtue ethics. *Ethics, 13*, 117–144.

Reiser, S.J. (1994, November/December). The ethical life of health care organizations. *The Hastings Center Report, 24*, 29–35.

Repenshek, M. & Slosar, J. P. (2004). Medically assisted nutrition and hydration: A contribution to the dialogue. *Hastings Center Report 34*:6, 3–16.

Schneiderman, L.J., Fein, J.E., & Dubler, N. (2001, November/December). The limits of dispute resolution. *The Hastings Center Report, 31*(6), 10–12.

Schneiderman, L. J.; Gilmer, T.; & Teetzel, H. (2003). Effect of ethics consultations on nonbeneficial life-sustaining treatments in the intensive care setting: A randomized controlled trial. *Journal of the American Medical Association, 290*:9, 1166–1172.

Segal, S., Gelfand, B., Hurwitz, S., Berkowitz, L., Ashley, S., Nadel, E., & Katz, J. (2010). Plagiarism in residency application essays. *Annals of Internal Medicine, 153*,112–120.

Spencer, E.M., Mills, A.E., Rorty, M.V., & Werhane, P.H. (2000). *Organization ethics in health care.* New York: Oxford University Press.

Sullivan, W.M. (1999, March/April). What is left of professionalism after managed care? *The Hastings Center Report, 29*:2, 7–13.

Swanton, C. (2003). *Virtue ethics: A pluralistic view.* New York: Oxford University Press.

Teisberg, E.O., Porter, M.E., & Brown, G.B. (1994, July/August). Making competition in health care work. *Harvard Business Review* 72:4, 131–141.

Van Z.L. (2009). Agent-based virtue ethics and the problem of action guidance. *Journal of Moral Philosophy 6*, 50–69.

Vinten, G. (1994). *Whistleblowing: Subversion or corporate citizenship?* New York: St. Martin's Press.

Weber, L.J. (2001). *Business ethics in healthcare: Beyond compliance.* Bloomington: Indiana University Press.

Winkler, E.C. and Gruen, R.L. "First principles: Substantive ethics for healthcare organizations." *Journal of Healthcare Management 50*:2 (Mar–Apr 2005): 109–120.

Wocial, L. (2008). An urgent call for ethics education. *The American Journal of Bioethics, 8*:4, 21–23.

Wright, S. and Ziegelstein, R. (2004). Writing more informative letters of reference. *Journal of General Internal Medicine, 19*, 588–593.

INDEX

Page numbers followed by f, t, or n indicate
figures, tables, or notes, respectively.

Morphine, 249, 250–251
Morrow, Henrietta, 249, 250–251, 252
MountainView Regional Medical Center, 61, 367

Naming rights, 342–343
National Health Service, 279–280
Natural law, 15, 19, 30, 33
Near-futile treatment, 316–317
Need
    demand vs., 289–295
    dissimilar treatment and, 343–347
Negligence, consent and, 215
Nepotism, 128–129
Netherlands, physician-assisted suicide and, 270, 271–274, 279, 280
Nightengale, Dr., 298–299
Nightingale Pledge, 85
Nihilism, defined, 1
Noncompliant patients, 355
Nonmaleficence
    application of, 31–33
    consent and, 215–216
    double effect and, 251
    ordinary vs. extraordinary care and, 249
    overview of principle, 29
Nonprogrammed decisions, 43
Normative ethics, defined, 1
Not-for-profit, conversion to for-profit, 349
Nuremberg Code, 107
Nurses. *See also* American Nurses Association
    code of ethics for, 85–86, 87
    organizational ethical issues and, 163–165
Nursing facility managers, 81–82
Nutrition. *See* Artificial hydration and nutrition

Obama healthcare plan, 304–305
Obitoria, 276–277
Occupational Safety and Health Act of 1970 (OSHA), HIV/AIDS and, 166–167
Office of Government Ethics (OGE), 77
Ombudsman programs, 195, 225, 302
Oral consent, 216
Ordinances, as formal sources of law, 6
Ordinary care
    extraordinary care vs., 249–250
    formerly competent patients and, 254
    futility theory and, 318
    nonmaleficence and, 29, 32
    persistent vegetative state and, 257

Oregon, physician-assisted suicide and, 266–267, 268–270, 277, 280
Oregon Health Plan (Oregon Medicaid Plan), 310, 332, 346
Organizational culture, 90–91, 197
Organizational ethical issues
    in appraisal of managerial performance, 171–173
    consent and, 224–228
    infant care review committees and, 118–120
    institutional ethics committees and, 98–107, 105t
    institutional review boards and, 107–118
    in new relationships with medical staff, 170–171
    organizational context of relationships and, 149–152
    organizational information and, 152–156
    overview of, 176–177
    overview of responses to, 97, 121
    professional credentials and, 173–176
    in relations with nonphysician staff, 163–170
    in relationships with governing body, 156–159, 157f
    in relationships with medical staff, 159–163
    specialized assistance for response to, 120–121
Organizational information, 152–156
Organizational philosophies
    achieving congruence of, 72–73
    artificial hydration and nutrition and, 253
    codes of ethics and, 90–91
    consent and, 224–225
    culture as pheromone and, 59–60
    development of, 54–59, 57f
    examples of, 362–370
    mission statement development and, 66–67
    overview of, 2, 53–54, 72–73
    personal ethic and, 38–39, 49–50
    philosophy statement content and, 60–66
    reconsideration of, 67–70
    resource allocation and, 312
    strategic management and, 72
    understanding patient bills of rights and, 70–72
    whistle-blowing and, 197
Organizational responses to ethical issues
    consent and, 224–225